LIFELONG
NUTRITION

LIFELONG NUTRITION

MARGARET McWILLIAMS

Ph.D.,R.D.
Professor Emeritus of Food and Nutrition
California State University, Los Angeles

PLYCON PRESS

Cover Photos (front and back) by:
  Alexei Prohoroff Photography
  prohoroffphoto.homestead.com

Plycon Press
2555 Duraznitos Pl.
Ramona, CA 92065
(760)788-9455; FAX: (760)788-4627
plyconpress.com

ISBN 0-916434-17-6

Printed in the United States of America

DEDICATION

To my children and their families,
All of whom have added great joy and
Enlightenment to me for many years!

PREFACE

Nutrition is a subject that assumes a variety of subtle meanings as you proceed through life, meanings which probably vary quite a bit from person to person. However, the importance of applying good nutrition from the very start of life and all the way into the senior years cannot be ignored by anybody. The way you look and feel at any age is shaped significantly by the nutrients you provide your body from the foods you choose and the amounts you eat.

Ideally, good nutrition begins at birth and continues on through childhood and then the adult and senior years. At first, parents are responsible for feeding infants a healthy diet in appropriate amounts; to this role is added that of role model on eating for good health as children begin to assert their own food preferences in childhood and on through the teens. The transition to assuming personal responsibility for good nutrition is a gradual process as children progress through school and finally live independently. In the adult years, the habits that have been established previously tend to dominate eating patterns and even to determine the food patterns that young parents may begin to establish in their children. Thus, dietary consequences, either good or bad, tend to be perpetuated. The important issue is that the patterns being perpetuated are consistent with achieving and maintaining optimal health.

This book focuses on the roles of the nutrients in the body and the consequences of deficiencies and excesses at various times throughout life. Emphasis is given to the early years because of their importance in developing and maintaining a healthy body through good nutrition. Attention is given to ways of integrating lifestyles and food choices to meet individual preferences and nutritional needs. The discussions about nutrition in the adult years recognize the many challenges that today's adults face and suggest ways that good nutrition and a healthy lifestyle can be achieved realistically.

This is a particularly challenging time for the study of nutrition because there is a great deal of emphasis on nutrition on all fronts, with the media often heading the chorus to bring nutrition "facts" to the public. The result is that awareness and appreciation of the importance of nutrition have increased, but so also has the confusion on just how a person needs to eat. The abundance of misinformation (emphatically presented as the gospel) breeds insecurity in some people and a disillusioned attitude in others. Never has there been a greater stampede to buy unnecessary food and nutrition supplements. The amount of money being wasted on various supplements is far more than enough to put a totally adequate diet of wholesome foods on the table. Not only does that food taste better, but it also is far more effective and safer nutritionally than are many of the high dose supplements that fearful and particularly concerned people tend to buy and consume.

This book presents a reasoned and in-depth look at nutritional needs and practical, healthful applications for people throughout the life cycle. The varying levels of need for nutrients at different stages of life are examined in detail so that healthful eating approaches are presented for all ages. Students of dietetics and nutrition and other individuals will find this book helpful, not only in professional practice, but also in their own lives. Here's to healthy eating!

Margaret McWilliams
Redondo Beach, California

CONTENTS

SECTION ONE

The Foundation

CHAPTER ONE

Nutrition Basics

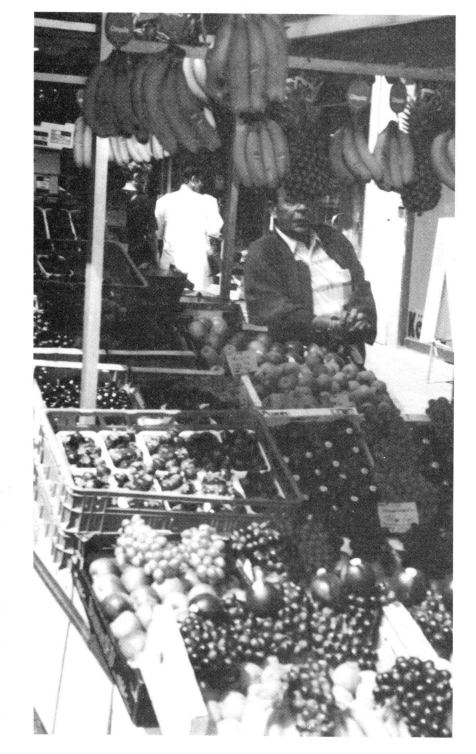

OVERVIEW

Vital to every individual, whether an infant or an adult, is a sound, healthy body. Key to achieving this goal is good nutrition. How simple this sounds! However, in real life you will find a wide range of ideas and suggestions about how you and others should eat; some of these may be excellent, while others may actually be contrary to achieving good nutrition. This chapter serves as a road map to the general subject of nutrition and to eating for good health.

The other chapters provide an understanding of how nutrition interrelates to the development of mind and body from

1

*conception through the adolescent years. You will explore
ways of promoting good dietary patterns in children at various ages. Doubtless, you will find that helping children of
all ages eat to achieve optimal health presents intellectual
and also very practical challenges. Not surprisingly, children usually have their own ideas on what they want to eat!
After all, why should we expect them to be different from
ourselves?*

*Each person, whether a child or a mature adult, determines
how much of which foods he or she will actually eat. Even
babies signal loudly when they need more food or when
their feeding is over. As children leave infancy behind and
move toward independence, potential food choices
become rather complex, yet decisions are made primarily
on an individual basis. It is because of this independence
in making food decisions that an understanding of nutrition
is so vital to us all.*

INTRODUCING THE NUTRIENTS

At first glance, the approximately 50 nutrients people
need for growth and maintenance of health may seem overwhelming, but they can be studied when they are divided into
groups of related substances. The nutrients present in the
largest quantities in the food we eat happen to be the nutrients
we need in the greatest amounts. These are the energy nutrients.
Specifically, the energy nutrients (carbohydrates, lipids, and
proteins) are the sources which give your body the energy needed
for moving and doing work, as well as for such vital activities as
breathing and pumping blood. Minerals (a category of more than
20 nutrients) perform a variety of functions, although they are
not sources of energy. Vitamins are regulatory substances
needed in even smaller amounts than minerals. At present,
thirteen vitamins are recognized as essential nutrients. The list
of nutrients ends with water, the fluid so vital to life.

THE ENERGY NUTRIENTS

CARBOHYDRATES

*CARBOHYDRATES
Hydrates of carbon;
compounds important
as sources of energy
for the body.*

Carbohydrates are organic compounds composed of
carbon, hydrogen, and oxygen. Because the ratio of hydrogen to

MONOSACCHARIDE
Smallest unit classified as a carbohydrate; includes glucose, fructose, and galactose.

DISACCHARIDE
Carbohydrates called sugars; composed of two monosaccharide units joined together.

SUCROSE
Often called sugar; composed of one unit of glucose and one of fructose.

MALTOSE
Disaccharide composed of two units of glucose.

oxygen is essentially the same as in water, these substances are classified chemically as hydrates of carbon. Among the best known carbohydrates are sugar, starch, and cellulose.

TYPES   The simplest of the carbohydrates are called the monosaccharides (Table 1.1). Even the most abundant of the monosaccharides (glucose, fructose, and galactose) are not found in foods in very large amounts. Nevertheless, these monosaccharides are familiar because they can be joined with a second monosaccharide unit to make a slightly more complex carbohydrate. The resulting carbohydrates are called disaccharides, and they are commonly found in foods. Sucrose, the carbohydrate often simply called sugar, is actually made up of one unit of glucose and one of fructose. Other fairly common disaccharides are maltose (made up of two units of glucose) and lactose (one unit of glucose and one of galactose).

The complex carbohydrates are called polysaccharides (the prefix "poly" means "many"). Starch is a familiar polysaccharide and is made up entirely of units of glucose. Cellulose is also made up of glucose units. However, these units are fastened together in a unique linkage, which explains the very different

TABLE 1.1   Summary of the Classification, Food Sources, and Functions of Carbohydrates

Classification	Food Sources	Functions
Monosaccharides (glucose, fructose, and galactose)	Candy, honey, syrups, fruits, jellies, jams, brown sugar, maple sugar, granulated sugar	Source of energy (4 kcal/gm) for all body functions, including glucose for grain.
Disaccharides (sucrose, lactose, and maltose)		Spare protein for its special functions.
Polysaccharides Digestible: Starch (amylose and amylopectin)	Cereals, legumes (peas, beans, etc.), bread, potatoes	Metabolism of fats.
Indigestible: Cellulose, Pectin, Gums	Bran of cereals (whole-grain cereals), fruits, vegetables, seaweeds, seeds, plant exudates	Roughage to promote motility of food mass in gastrointestinal tract (aid in preventing constipation and inhibiting colon cancer and diverticulosis).

role this polysaccharide performs in nutrition. Pectin is yet another example of a polysaccharide, being a combination of galactose derivatives. Gums are composed of a variety of simpler carbohydrate units.

SOURCES   The simple carbohydrates — the sugars — are found in plant foods, with sugar beets and sugarcane the primary sources for the production of granulated sugar (Table 1.1). Maple syrup, corn syrup, and fruits are other excellent sources of the various sugars. Honey produced by bees is one of the few examples of sugars from the animal kingdom.

Starch is abundant in legumes and cereals. Flour milled from wheat, as used in a vast array of bread, cakes, and other baked products, is a good source of starch. Some vegetables are also high in starch. Fruits and vegetables are valuable sources of cellulose, and some are also used as sources of pectin.

FUNCTIONS   Carbohydrates are generally valued as excellent sources of energy. For each gram of pure carbohydrate digested by humans, four kilocalories of energy will become available (Table 1.1). When the diet contains adequate amounts of carbohydrates, they help to spare protein to carry out its unique functions in the body. The body also needs glucose to provide the energy for the brain. Another reason carbohydates are important is their role in deriving energy from fats. When fats are broken down in the body, the small fragments released combine with a carbohydrate derivative to complete utilization of the fat. Unless carbohydrates are present in sufficient quantities, these fragments will accumulate as ketone bodies, creating a health hazard.

Cellulose, pectin, and a few other complex carbohydrates cannot be digested by people. Although they do not function in the ways described in the preceding paragraph, they play an extremely important role as roughage in stimulating the gastrointestinal tract. Vigorous contractions promote the movement of food residues through the tract for elimination, thus avoiding constipation. Undigested carbohydrates are referred to collectively as fiber.

Carbohydrates can have a few negative effects. For example, sugars have been shown to be cariogenic (promoting the development of dental caries), making it important to practice good dental hygiene by brushing the teeth after eating sweets.

LACTOSE
Disaccharide composed of one unit of glucose and one of galactose.

POLYSACCHARIDE
Carbohydrates consisting of many saccharide units; starch, cellulose, and pectin are examples.

KILOCALORIE
Unit used to express the amount of energy required to raise 1 kg of water 1°C (from 15°C to 16°C).

FIBER
Cellulose, pectin, and a few other carbohydrates, such as gums, that are important in preventing constipation.

CARIOGENIC
Fostering the development of dental caries; sticky candies are examples of sugar-containing products that can be harmful to dental health.

DIGESTION
Breakdown of
compounds in food
into components
capable of being
absorbed into the body
to help meet nutri-
tional demands.

SALIVARY AMYLASE
Starch-splitting
enzyme secreted in the
saliva to initiate the
digestion of starch in
the mouth.

ENZYME
Protein capable of
altering the rate of a
chemical reaction
without being
changed itself; an
organic catalyst.

DEXTRINS
Carbohydrates
composed of numerous
glucose units linked
together, but in
somewhat shorter
chains than those of
starch.

PANCREATIC AMYLASE
Enzyme formed in the
pancreas and trans-
ported to the small
intestine where it acts
on starch and starch
fragments to digest
these complex
molecules to maltose.

MALTASE
Enzyme in the
microvilli of the small
intestine that breaks
maltose into its two
component units of
glucose.

Many people seem to be constantly coping with the problem of excess weight. People with a "sweet tooth" like candies and sweet desserts and may find that they are gaining weight simply because they are eating too many high-energy foods. This excess weight problem is not solely due to eating too many carbohydrate-rich foods; it results from eating foods that provide more energy than is needed for maintenance and activity. The appeal of carbohydrate-rich foods may cause some people to eat more than they really require, and this continuing excessive consumption leads to problems in weight control. It is not, however, a normal feature of carbohydrates to cause obesity; they are essential components of any diet.

DIGESTION AND ABSORPTION Foods must undergo chemical changes (digestion) in preparation for individual components to be absorbed through the lining of the small intestine and other regions in the gastrointestinal tract. The first site of carbohydrate digestion is the mouth (Fig. 1.1), where the teeth mechanically break food into smaller pieces and saliva is mixed with the food for easier transport through the tract. Saliva contains salivary amylase (also called ptyalin), a digestive enzyme which initiates the splitting of the large molecules of starch into ever-shortening chains of glucose units.

From the mouth, the food mass moves through the esophagus and into the stomach. The salivary amylase, which has been mixed with the starch in the mouth, is carried to the stomach and continues to break down the starch until the stomach acid halts the action. The starch fragments (called dextrins) eventually leave the stomach and move into the small intestine. There the action of pancreatic amylase, followed by the action of maltase, results in the release of free molecules of glucose. Glucose is absorbed through the wall of the small intestine.

Sugar digestion is somewhat different from the action on starches. Sucrose (table sugar) is unchanged until it is held in the stomach. Hydrochloric acid in the stomach effects some digestion into the two monosaccharides (glucose and fructose) comprising sucrose. Most of the sucrose and other sugars which may be present proceed into the small intestine without having been digested. In the microvilli of the small intestine, the enzymes that split the disaccharides into the component monosaccharides needed for absorption are found: maltase is available to split maltose into two units of glucose, sucrose to

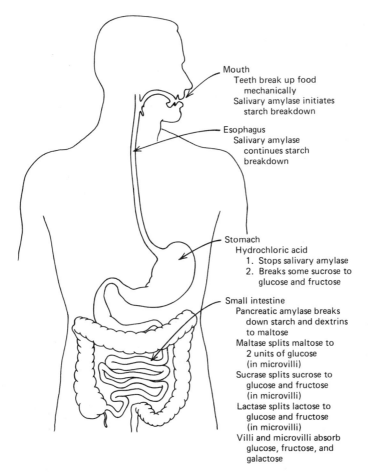

Mouth
 Teeth break up food
  mechanically
 Salivary amylase initiates
  starch breakdown

Esophagus
 Salivary amylase
 continues starch
 breakdown

Stomach
 Hydrochloric acid
  1. Stops salivary amylase
  2. Breaks some sucrose to
   glucose and fructose

Small intestine
 Pancreatic amylase breaks
  down starch and dextrins
  to maltose
 Maltase splits maltose to
  2 units of glucose
  (in microvilli)
 Sucrase splits sucrose to
  glucose and fructose
  (in microvilli)
 Lactase splits lactose to
  glucose and fructose
  (in microvilli)
 Villi and microvilli absorb
  glucose, fructose, and
  galactose

Fig. 1.1   Sites of digestion and absorption of digestible carbohydrates.

form glucose and fructose from sucrose, and lactase to cleave lactose into glucose and galactose.

Cellulose and other complex carbohydrates which constitute much of the fiber content of foods cannot be digested by people because we lack the appropriate enzymes to split out the monosaccharide components for absorption. Therefore, these substances move through the intestinal tract essentially unchanged, promoting the health of the body by speeding moevment of food residues through the tract for efficient excretion.

Monosaccharide molecules in the small intestine are small enough to pass through the intestinal wall, which is the

SUCRASE
Enzyme in the microvilli of the small intestine needed to split sucrose into glucose and fructose.

LACTASE
Enzyme in the microvilli of the small intestine that catalyzes the formation of glucose and galactose from lactose.

principal absorption site for carbohydrates and most other nutrients. The amount of surface area provided in the intestinal wall is of paramount importance for absorption, because each molecule must pass through individually. Unless molecules have an opportunity to be in direct contact with the intestinal wall when they are in the small intestine, they will continue their journey into the large intestine and ultimately be excreted without nourishing the body. Fortunately, the lining of the small intestine is made up of millions of tiny projections (called villi), which increase the surface area available for absorption to a remarkable degree. Augmenting the villi are microvilli, tiny projections on the surface of each of the villi. Because of the considerable surface area afforded by the villi and microvilli, monosaccharides are readily absorbed for ultimate use within the body.

TRANSPORT AND METABOLISM   As monosaccharide molecules pass through the intestinal wall, they enter the bloodstream for transport to the liver. Glucose is formed from other monosaccharides (notably fructose and galactose) in the liver; it is the form of carbohydrate the body uses. Glucose may be 1) used for energy, 2) converted into glycogen (the carbohydrate form in which reserve energy is stored), or 3) utilized to make fatty acids for forming fat in the adipose (fatty) tissues. Glycogen is stored in both the liver and in muscles until this readily-available energy is needed. The body's stores of liver glycogen and muscle glycogen are the first sources of energy used for activity, and this energy becomes available as the result of glycolysis, a series of complex chemical reactions. The final series of reactions is referred to as the Krebs cycle. Other names for these reactions are the citric acid cycle and the tricarboxylic acid cycle.

At various points in the Krebs cycle, carbon dioxide, water and energy are released. Glycogen can enter the Krebs cycle only by being split to release individual units of glucose, for it is the glucose molecules that ultimately feed into the cycle. The essential reactions of the Krebs cycle are shown in Fig. 1.2.

LIPIDS

Lipids are also organic compounds composed of carbon, oxygen, and hydrogen, but they contain considerably less oxygen than carbohydates. This difference imparts very different characteristics to this group of compounds.

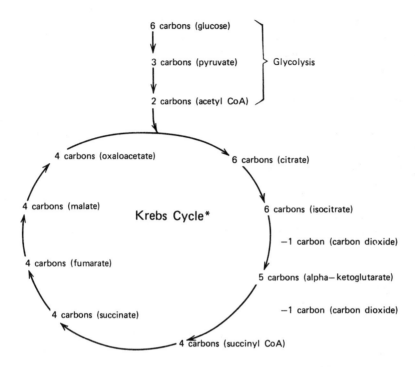

6 carbons (glucose)

↓

3 carbons (pyruvate) ⎫
⎬ Glycolysis
2 carbons (acetyl CoA) ⎭

↓

4 carbons (oxaloacetate) → 6 carbons (citrate)

4 carbons (malate)

Krebs Cycle*   6 carbons (isocitrate)

4 carbons (fumarate)   −1 carbon (carbon dioxide)

5 carbons (alpha−ketoglutarate)

4 carbons (succinate)   −1 carbon (carbon dioxide)

4 carbons (succinyl CoA)

*In addition to the carbon dioxide, metabolic water and energy are available as products of the Krebs Cycle.

Fig. 1.2 Outline of the Krebs cycle.

TYPES   A common way of categorizing lipids is on the basis of complexity, that is, as simple or complex. The simple lipids are either fats or waxes. The fats are of particular interest to nutrition. The simple fats have two components: glycerol and fatty acid(s). Glycerol is a very unusual alcohol, unique in its ability to link with up to three fatty acids to form fats. Fatty acids, the other component of simple fats, are organic acids of varying lengths containing varying amounts of hydrogen in relation to carbon. The different physical characteristics of such fats as butter and salad oils are the result of the fatty acids they contain.

Simple fats can be classified according to the number of fatty acids linked with glycerol (esterified). If only one fatty acid is esterified, the compound is called a monoglyceride. In simple fats containing two fatty acids linked with glycerol, the substance is designated a diglyceride. With three (the maximum number), the compound is a triglyceride. Triglycerides are the most common form of simple fats.

GLYCEROL
Alcohol found in all simple fats and capable of combining with a maximum of three fatty acids.

FATTY ACID
Organic acid composed primarily of carbon and hydrogen and frequently combined with glycerol.

MONOGLYCERIDES
Simple fats containing only one fatty acid combined with glycerol.

Fatty acids have a great influence over the physical characteristics of simple fats. Some fatty acids are short chains and some are long, differences which help explain why some fats are fluids and others are quite solid. Although this influence is important, the amount of hydrogen in a fatty acid is of even greater importance in nutrition. Fatty acids that cannot hold any more hydrogen than they already do are called saturated fatty acids. Conversely, those with less hydrogen than they can hold are unsaturated fatty acids. If a considerable amount of hydrogen can be added, the fatty acids are classified as polyunsaturated. Polyunsaturated fatty acids are of significance in nutrition. The various unsaturated fatty acids can be altered in their physical characteristics by hydrogenating them. Hydrogenation results in products like margarine and peanut butter in which the oil is hardened so it does not separate.

Phospholipids, lipoproteins, and sterols are rather complex lipid-related substances contained in foods. A familiar example of a phospholipid is lecithin, which is a very effective emulsifying agent. Lipoproteins are combinations of proteins with lipid materials. These are classified according to their density as 1) high-density lipoproteins (HDL), 2) low-density lipoproteins (LDL), and 3) very-low-density lipoproteins (VLDL). Lipoproteins, particularly VLDL and LDL, contain comparatively high amounts of cholesterol. Cholesterol is a sterol often associated with heart disease when serum cholesterol levels are comparatively high.

SOURCES Visible sources of fat include butter, fat surrounding the muscles in meat, and salad oils. In addition to these obvious sources, invisible fats are found in many places. Marbling in the muscles of properly fattened beef and pork, whipped cream, many cheeses, avocados, nuts, whole milk, and rich desserts are just some of the invisible sources. Chocolate, salad dressings, and fried foods are others.

FUNCTIONS Fats are the most concentrated source of energy (Table 1.2) in the diet, contributing nine kilocalories per gram — a figure more than double the amount of energy available from carbohydrates. This means that a large amount of energy can be supplied from a comparatively small quantity of food high in fat.

Another important function of fats is to provide satiety value. Because fats remain in the stomach longer than either carbohydrates or proteins, hunger is slow to return following a meal that is high in fat, and people often feel quite satisfied for up to four hours.

One of the polyunsaturated fatty acids is linoleic acid, a fatty acid abundant in some vegetable oils. Linoleic acid is classified as an essential fatty acid because it must be provided in the diet to maintain normal healthy skin. Although the body is capable of forming some fatty acids, it cannot make linoleic acid to meet the body's need.

Fats serve as the means of transporting the fat-soluble vitamins (A, D, E, and K). Besides acting as carriers for these key nutrients, fats make foods much more pleasing as a result of the richness of flavor they contribute.

Once in the body, fats may be used for energy, but they can be stored in the body as an energy reservoir. These fat deposits provide protection for the organs and contribute to beauty by softening the angularity of basic bone structure. Of course, this protective and beautifying padding can become a curse when excessive deposits of fat result from long periods of overeating. These fatty deposits also help regulate body temperature by insulating against cold.

LOW-DENSITY LIPOPROTEINS
Compounds of protein and lipids in the blood; protein levels are very low in relation to lipid and cholesterol content, which may be associated with some episodes of coronary heart disease.

CHOLESTEROL
A sterol, that is, an alcohol which is structurally similar to the sex hormones and is sometimes present in fairly high blood levels in cases of heart disease.

RECOMMENDED INTAKE   Recommendations regarding fat intake are based on the percentage of calories provided by fat in relation to those from carbohydrate and protein. The average American's fat intake appears to be somewhat too high for optimal health. Preferred fat intake is 30 percent of a day's total calories. Total

TABLE 1.2   Lipids: Types, Sources, and Functions

Types	Selected Sources	Functions
Simple Lipids Mono-, di-, and triglycerides	Butter, margarine, salad oils, fried foods, red meats, pastries, cheese, cream, nuts, avocado, chocolate, poultry with skin, fatty fish	Provide energy (9 kcal/g). Provide linoleic acid. Carry fat-soluble vitamins (A,D,E, and K). Satiety value. Deposits in body to protect organs and insulate.
Complex Lipids Phospholipids	Egg yolks	Emulsifiers.
Sterols	Crab, lobster, egg yolk	Formation of sterols and steroids.
Lipoproteins	Meats, milk	Transport of fatty compounds.

caloric intake should be limited to an appropriate level for achieving and maintaining a desirable weight. The desired reduction in fat intake can be accomplished by reducing the consumption of fried foods, controlling meat portions, and limiting the amount of salad dressing, butter, sour cream, and rich desserts in the diet. This requires some conscious change in many people's dietary habits.

Some salad oil rich in linoleic acid should be consumed as part of a day's recommended fat. This oil can be in such forms as salad dressings, margarines, or oil for frying, the preferred oils being corn, sunflower, safflower, and other plant oils (except tropical oils).

DIGESTION AND ABSORPTION   Enzymes are essential for the digestion of fats as well as carbohydrates, and enzyme action is dependent on intimate contact between enzymes and their substrates. Fats must be emulsified to obtain the very large surface area required for this contact. Processing begins in the mouth, where the fats are softened by chewing and warming (Fig. 1.3). The stomach continues softening the fat by liquefying it. Gastric lipase, an enzyme in the stomach, begins the process of splitting fatty acids from glycerol if the fats are in the emulsified form. Since digestion in the stomach is quite limited, the bulk of the fat consumed enters the small intestine as fluid, undigested fat. The bile, which has entered the small intestine from the liver via the gall bladder, immediately begins to emulsify the fat into extremely fine droplets. The emulsified state affords the contact surface necessary for pancreatic and intestinal lipases to digest fat molecules to their components, fatty acids and glycerol, which can be absorbed through the villi and microvilli in the walls of the small intestine. They are then joined together as fats once again.

TRANSPORT   Nutrients are transported in the body through the bloodstream, but lipids are not naturally miscible with blood, which is aqueous. Absorbed and reassembled fats enter the lymphatic system, where they are combined with protein to form chylomicrons. Chylomicrons are lipoprotein (lipid and protein) complexes capable of being carried in the aqueous medium of the blood. These chylomicrons enter the bloodstream just before the blood enters the heart.

METABOLISM   The reactions the body requires for energy to become available from fats begin with the release of free fatty acids from glycerol. Glycerol is metabolized in the pathways

LIPASE
Enzyme capable of splitting fatty acids from glycerol to digest fat.

GASTRIC LIPASE
Fat-splitting enzyme acting in the stomach.

PANCREATIC LIPASE
Fat-splitting enzyme made in the pancreas, but acting in the small intestine to digest fat.

INTESTINAL LIPASE
Enzyme produced in the small intestine and effecting the digestion of fats in this portion of the gastrointestinal tract.

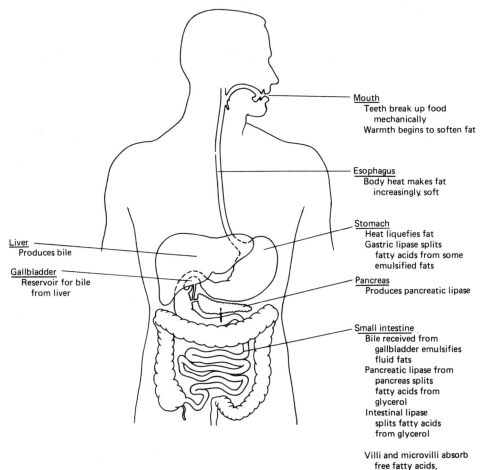

Mouth
Teeth break up food
mechanically
Warmth begins to soften fat

Esophagus
Body heat makes fat
increasingly soft

Stomach
Heat liquefies fat
Gastric lipase splits
fatty acids from some
emulsified fats

Liver
Produces bile

Pancreas
Produces pancreatic lipase

Gallbladder
Reservoir for bile
from liver

Small intestine
Bile received from
gallbladder emulsifies
fluid fats
Pancreatic lipase from
pancreas splits
fatty acids from
glycerol
Intestinal lipase
splits fatty acids
from glycerol

Villi and microvilli absorb
free fatty acids,
glycerol, and
monoglycerides

Fig. 1.3   Sites of digestion and absorption of fats.

described in the preceding discussion about carbohydrate metabolism. The free fatty acids undergo a progressive breakdown into two-carbon fragments by a process called beta oxidation. These two-carbon units can be used to synthesize sex hormones, cholesterol, other fatty acids, or other complex compounds. They may also enter the Krebs cycle by joining with the carbohydrate derivatives to form carbon dioxide and water and releasing energy. Without carbohydrates, two-carbon units from fatty acids will condense to ketone bodies, compounds

CHYLOMICRONS
Lipoproteins formed when absorbed components of digested fats have been reassembled and joined with protein for transport in the bloodstream.

BETA OXIDATION
Metabolism of fatty acids by breaking off two-carbon fragments.

KETONE BODIES
Chemical compounds formed by condensing two two-carbon fragments together.

RESEARCH INSIGHTS

Schatzkin, et al. Lack of effect of a low-fat, high-fiber diet on the recurrence of colorectal adenomas. *New England J. Med.: 342(16):* 1149. 2000.

Professional journals provide essential and timely communication between researchers and others working within the sciences. Original research articles contribute to basic knowledge regarding carefully defined and controlled studies. Review articles are written to draw together the results of related research articles and to interpret the summation or significance, according to the analysis of the author(s) of the research done by others.

An example of an original research article is the work reported by Dr. Schatzkin and 11 co-authors in 2000 by *The New England Journal of Medicine 342(16):* 1149 entitled "Lack of effect of a low-fat, high-fiber diet on the recurrence of colorectal adenomas." The hypothesis being tested was that dietary intervention can inhibit recurrent colorectal adenomas (precursors of most cancers of the large bowel). The subjects (2079 adults at least 35 years old who had had at least 1 colorectal adenoma removed and confirmed histologically no more than 6 months before entering the study) were randomly assigned into either the control or the intervention group. The intervention group (1037 men and women) received nutrition information, behavior-modification techniques, and optional counseling sessions (up to 50 hours, with 20 to be in the first year). The diet plan for the intervention group was to obtain 20 percent of the calories from fat, 18 grams of dietary fiber per 1000 kcal, and 3.5 servings of fruits and vegetables per 1000 kcal. Those in the control group (1042) were given the National Dairy Council's pamphlet on general dietary guidelines; no restrictions were placed on their diet patterns.

Data collected included height and weight at the beginning and at the 4 annual follow-up visits, background information such as demographics and various lifestyle choices (smoking, alcohol use, and supplements taken), and analysis of venous blood after overnight fasting. Colonoscopic examinations were done on all subjects 1 year and 4 years after the study began. Those performing colonoscopies and the pathologists who assessed the polyps removed during the course of the study were not informed whether subjects were in the control or in the intervention group. The end points were analyzed statistically using logistic-regression to determine the effect of intervention on recurrence and features of adenomas occurring during the course of the study.

The results of the study comparing the 958 intervention subjects with the 947 control subjects completing the 4-year project showed no significant difference in the recurrence of colorectal adenomas between the two groups. The findings of this study are in agreement with similar research conducted in Canada and Australia.

which are toxic to the body when they accumulate. To avoid ketosis, carbohydrates must be included in the diet.

PROTEINS

Proteins, like carbohydrates and fats, are made up of carbon, hydrogen, and oxygen, but they also contain nitrogen and, occasionally, other elements. All proteins are composed of amino acids, each of which possesses an organic acid group ($-COOH$) and an amino group ($-NH_2$). Although there are only 22 different amino acids commonly occurring in proteins, their sequence and frequency of occurrence result in a tremendous variety of proteins in nature.

CLASSIFICATION Some of the amino acids in proteins are required for life and growth and must be provided in the diet. These are called essential amino acids. The body needs other amino acids as well, but these can be synthesized in the body to meet the requirement. Amino acids which can be synthesized internally are therefore called nonessential amino acids. People require nine amino acids in their diets; the other amino acids are well used and important, but not absolutely essential. The nine essential amino acids for humans are histidine, methionine, threonine, tryptophan, isoleucine, leucine, lysine, valine, and phenylalanine.

Proteins containing all the essential amino acids are classified as complete proteins. From a nutritional standpoint, complete proteins are very important, for they provide a convenient and reliable way of obtaining all the necessary amino acids. They are, of course, a good source of nonessential amino acids as well. Animal proteins, with the exception of gelatin, are complete proteins and can be the sole source of protein. Plant proteins are incomplete and require careful combinations from different plant

KETOSIS
Potentially fatal condition caused by the accumulation of ketone bodies when inadequate carbohydrate is available for the two-carbon fragments from fatty acid metabolism to enter the Krebs cycle.

PROTEIN
Organic compound composed of carbon, hydrogen, oxygen, and nitrogen in the form of amino acids linked together into very large molecules.

ESSENTIAL AMINO ACID
Amino acid needed for life and growth, but which cannot be synthesized in the body.

NONESSENTIAL AMINO ACID
Amino acid which can be synthesized in the body.

COMPLETE PROTEIN
Protein containing all of the essential amino acids in amounts adequate to meet human requirements; animal proteins (except gelatin).

INCOMPLETE PROTEIN
Protein containing many of the essential amino acids in excellent amounts, yet too low in at least one of the essential amino acids to be used alone as a source of protein.

LIMITING AMINO ACID
Essential amino acid present in the least adequate amount in a protein.

LYSINE
Essential amino acid; limiting amino acid in cereals.

METHIONINE
Sulfur-containing essential amino acid; limiting amino acid in legumes.

COMPLEMENTARY PROTEINS
Two types of incomplete proteins that provide adequate amounts of the limiting amino acid in the other protein (e.g., cereals and legumes).

sources to obtain all the essential amino acids in adequate quantities.

Despite the fact that incomplete proteins may contain significant quantities of most of the essential amino acids, they lack adequate amounts of at least one. The one that is least adequate is called the limiting amino acid. In cereals, the amino acid present in the least adequate amount is lysine; the limiting amino acid in legumes is methionine. Fortunately, methionine levels in cereals are fairly high and lysine levels in legumes are excellent. When foods from the two categories are served together, the proteins complement each other and improve the usefulness of both foods as sources of protein. This situation is identified as the complementarity of proteins.

SOURCES   Beef, veal, pork, and lamb are red meats that provide excellent sources of complete proteins. Poultry, fish, eggs, milk, and cheese are other types of food providing complete proteins in important amounts that are used efficiently in the body. Particularly important plant sources are the various legumes, including soybeans, kidney beans, navy beans, lima beans, chick peas, and several other varieties of beans and peas. Soy protein's comparatively high nutritive value and its ability to be fabricated into a variety of forms, such as tofu and textured vegetable protein (TVP), have triggered extensive research to develop commercially viable soy protein products. Legumes contain about 20 percent protein, whereas cereals are significantly lower, but useful, protein sources. Cereals range from about 7 percent protein in rice to about 12 percent in wheat.

FUNCTIONS   The amino groups in amino acids are key groups in the formation of body tissues, which contain protein synthesized from amino acids provided by food. Growth and maintenance can occur only when protein intake is adequate (Table 1.3). Formation of the various hormones, enzymes, and antibodies is also dependent on the availability of protein.

Fluid levels in various compartments throughout the body are regulated, in part, by the presence of protein. The level of protein in blood plasma helps regulate the balance between fluid levels in the cells and in the bloodstream. The acidity or alkalinity in different parts of the body must be maintained within very narrow limits. Because proteins can function as either acids or bases, they play a major role in regulating acid-base balance.

TABLE 1.3   Classification, Food Sources, and Functions of Protein

Classification	Food Sources	Functions
Complete protein	Animal sources: beef, pork, veal, poultry, fish, eggs, cheese, milk	Promote growth and maintenance of tissues.
		Formation of hormones, enzymes, antibodies.
		Regulation of acid-base balance.
Incomplete protein	Plant sources: legumes (beans of all types, peas, soy, lentils), cereals (rice, corn, wheat, etc.), gelatin	Maintenance of proper osmotic pressure.
		Energy (4 kcal/g).

These functions are unique to proteins — carbohydrates and fats are unable to contribute to the body in these ways. However, proteins do share one function with these other nutrients: they provide energy.

DIETARY REQUIREMENTS   On the basis of need for protein per kilogram of body weight, newborns have the greatest requirement. They need 2.2 gm of protein per kilogram of body weight, in contrast to only 0.8 gm per kilogram for adults. Besides maintaining existing tissue, the high level needed in infancy and childhood corresponds to the dynamic growth of new tissue and maintenance of existing tissue, whereas adults no longer need protein for growth. Adult recommendations allow only for the protein needed to maintain tissue and form nitrogen-containing enzymes and other substances vital to the body's operation.

Protein needs are determined by studying the balance between the consumption and excretion of nitrogen. During periods of growth, people should be in positive nitrogen balance (retaining part of the nitrogen provided from the protein in foods eaten). Pregnant and lactating women, children, and people of any age who are recovering from surgery or burns should all be in positive nitrogen balance. Other adults should be in nitrogen equilibrium, that is, excreting the same amount of nitrogen they consume. Negative nitrogen balance, an undesirable situation, occurs in persons with fevers. As soon as the patient can tolerate

NITROGEN BALANCE Comparison of the amount of nitrogen consumed with that which is excreted; positive values are desired in periods of growth or repair of body tissues.

protein, intake should be increased to bring the person back into positive nitrogen balance or, at least, nitrogen equilibrium.

To ensure good utilization, protein can be consumed throughout the day, rather than at only one or two meals. This does not mean that meat must be served at every meal, for there are other foods capable of providing useful amounts of protein. For example, a glass of milk and a bowl of cereal at breakfast are perfectly suitable protein sources. A serving of meat or meat substitute (eggs, cheese, poultry, fish, or legumes) at each of the other two meals, accompanied by a glass of milk, will be sufficient to fulfill the need for protein. By being sure to eat breakfast and two other meals each day, people can readily include protein at appropriate intervals, ensuring excellent and efficient use of it in the body.

The choice of protein sources is also important. If animal protein sources are chosen in adequate amounts, protein needs will be met. However, vegetarian menus require considerable care to ensure that complementary proteins are provided at the same meal. Simply adding some cheese to refried beans or drinking a glass of milk while eating a bowl of split pea soup assures adequacy. Inclusion of legumes and cereals at the same meal is another inexpensive way to provide an appropriate complement of protein foods. In fact, special complete protein foods have been formulated and manufactured from plant protein sources to help meet dietary needs of children in some Third World countries. Scientifically developed mixtures like Incaparina, the protein food developed by the Institute of Nutrition for Central America and Panama (INCAP), eliminate the need for people to know how to mix plant proteins for good nutrition. The convenience and relatively low cost of such special plant protein mixtures have been of considerable importance in establishing them as an accepted part of the diet for children.

PEPSIN
Active protein-digesting enzyme splitting proteins into smaller polypeptide molecules in the stomach.

CHYMOTRYPSIN
Pancreatic protease digesting proteins and polypeptides into increasingly smaller fragments in the small intestine.

DIGESTION AND ABSORPTION Protein molecules must be broken down to their component amino acids to be absorbed efficiently without causing allergic responses. This digestive process does not begin until the chewed food has been swallowed and transported into the stomach (Fig. 1.4). Pepsin, a gastric protease (protein-digesting enzyme in the stomach), splits protein molecules into shorter fragments called polypeptides. These polypeptides then proceed to the small intestine.

The major part of digestion of proteins to individual amino acids occurs in the small intestine, where the pancreas delivers chymotrypsin and trypsin, proteolytic enzymes it produces.

These enzymes split proteins and polypeptides into smaller and smaller fragments. Carboxypeptidase, aminopeptidase, and dipeptidase also act in the small intestine to complete digestion begun by the pancreatic proteases. The names of these three intestinal enzymes indicate their actions: carboxypeptidase splits peptides from the acid end of the chain; aminopeptidase attacks at the opposite end. When only two amino acids are joined together, dipeptidase can finish the digestive process in the microvilli to release two free amino acids for absorption.

Individual amino acids and dipeptides are absorbed into the bloodstream through the microvilli without incident. Unfortunately, some individuals cannot break down specific proteins

TRYPSIN
A pancreatic protease acting on the acid group of methionine, tryptophan, tyrosine, and phenylalanine to digest proteins and polypeptides into shorter units in the small intestine.

CARBOXYPEPTIDASE
Intestinal enzyme splitting proteins and polypeptides from the acid end of the chain.

AMINOPEPTIDASE
Intestinal protease splitting proteins and polypeptides from the amino end of the chain.

DIPEPTIDASE
Protease in the microvilli in the small intestine that splits dipeptides into the two component free amino acids.

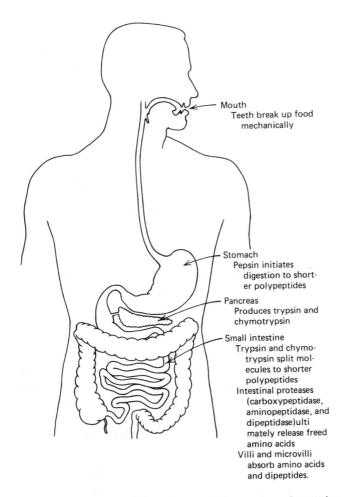

Mouth
Teeth break up food
mechanically

Stomach
Pepsin initiates
digestion to short-
er polypeptides

Pancreas
Produces trypsin and
chymotrypsin

Small intestine
Trypsin and chymo-
trypsin split mol-
ecules to shorter
polypeptides
Intestinal proteases
(carboxypeptidase,
aminopeptidase, and
dipeptidase)ulti
mately release freed
amino acids
Villi and microvilli
absorb amino acids
and dipeptides.

Fig. 1.4   Sites of digestion and absorption of proteins.

to their component amino acids, yet are able to absorb the molecules intact. When this happens, the foreign protein in the bloodstream triggers an allergic response.

TRANSPORT   Once amino acids enter the bloodstream, they are carried to the liver and added to its pool of amino acids. From this pool, they are carried to various tissues in the body and incorporated into proteins being synthesized for specific needs.

METABOLISM   The body needs to synthesize the specific proteins required to perform protein's many functions, which include the formation of tissues, enzymes, and hormones. These synthetic reactions are accomplished in the cells by a remarkable process in which nucleic acids provide the information needed to arrange individual amino acids into protein molecules comprised of the encoded sequence of building blocks. It is even possible for nonessential amino acids to be formed if they are needed in the synthesis of a particular protein. Unfortunately, protein synethsis is blocked if a necessary essential amino acid is lacking, because the body is incapable of forming it. This process of forming large molecules from small components in the body is called anabolism. Protein synthesis is therefore an example of the metabolic reactions termed anabolism. The liver's amino acid pool is an important source of many of the amino acids needed for protein synthesis.

ANABOLISM
Metabolic reaction resulting in the formation of a larger molecule; synthesis of proteins from amino acids is one example.

Catabolism, the degradation of large molecules, is an important aspect of protein metabolism in the body. Sometimes the acid group is split from an amino acid, whereas the amino group is removed in other instances; both are examples of catabolic reactions. When the amino group is removed, the catabolic process is called deamination. Transamination is the transfer of the amino group to another compound. Nonessential amino acids are formed by transamination.

CATABOLISM
Breakdown of complex molecules to simpler substances.

DEAMINATION
Catabolic reaction resulting in the removal of the amino group from an amino acid.

Two fragments remain from the deamination of an amino acid: the amino group and the remainder of the compound, which is now an organic acid. The amino group can enter the urea cycle and is ultimately excreted as urea in the urine. The nonnitrogenous portion of the amino acid is catabolized to yield carbon dioxide, water, and energy.

TRANSAMINATION
Transport of an amino group to a new substrate to form a new amino acid.

Metabolism of various amino acids follows a variety of rather complex routes requiring specialized enzymes for certain reactions. Some children lack the ability to metabolize phenylalanine normally. Consequently, this amino acid and its derivatives collect and are not catabolized normally. The result is severe mental retardation unless, with very early diagnosis, strict dietary control is promptly instituted. This condition is called phenylketonuria. Phenylketonuria is only one of the physical problems caused by the inability to metabolize an amino acid. Inborn errors of metabolism have been noted with not only phenylalanine, but also with histidine, leucine, and valine as well. Considerable research continues in this area of nutrition.

ENERGY

Energy is needed for three aspects of life: 1) basal metabolism, 2) physical activity, and 3) thermic effect. Carbohydrates, fats, and proteins are the substances in food that can provide the energy required for all of these purposes. Each person has different energy expenditures because of differences in such factors as sex, age, and physical activity. Individual expenditures, in fact, vary from day to day. Practical estimates of energy can be easily made; precise figures require use of special equipment and more time.

The values for energy expenditure and energy content in food are expressed in kilocalories. This unit is 1000 times larger than the calorie used in the physical sciences — the kilocalorie is accurate, if somewhat cumbersome. Energy in nutrition is often simply expressed as Calories or calories. Abbreviations used frequently are kcal, Cal, or cal. In discussions about nutrition, these terms are interchangeable.

BASAL METABOLISM The greatest need for energy is often that required for basal metabolism. Basal metabolism is the total of the various basic functions required for a person to stay alive. Breathing, the beating of the heart, maintenance of body temperature, and cellular functioning are examples of the basic nature of basal metabolism. Energy needs for basal metabolism are comparatively high. The basal metabolic rate (rate at which energy is expended for basal metabolism) is higher in infants and children than in adults. In fact, a 3-year-old child has nearly twice the need of a 75-year-old adult when computed on the basis of energy required per square meter of body surface. Males have a higher basal metabolic rate than females of the same age, and muscular individuals have a higher energy demand for basal metabolism than do those with less developed muscles.

The rate at which the body uses energy to maintain the basal processes is regulated by hormones, notably thyroxine (the hormone secreted by the thyroid gland). In normal individuals,

PHENYLKETONURIA
Accumulation of phenylalanine and its derivatives due to an incomplete enzyme system, leading to severe mental retardation unless treated promptly and carefully.

INBORN ERROR OF METABOLISM
Inability to metabolize a specific compound due to an incomplete metabolic enzyme system, the result of a hereditary defect.

BASAL METABOLISM
Energy-using reactions involved in breathing and maintaining other basic functions of the body at rest, but essential to survival.

THYROXINE
Hormone produced by the thyroid gland to regulate the rate at which basal metabolism occurs.

formation and secretion of thyroxine results in regulation at a level requiring from 1300 to 1600 kcal for basal metabolic needs. (A rough approximation of need can be made by multiplying weight in kilograms by 24.)

Individual energy requirements can be determined on the basis of body surface area, sex, age, and measurement of respiration while resting. If the thyroid gland is overactive (a condition called hyperthyroidism), the energy requirements for basal metabolism will be greater than normal. Conversely, low production of thyroxine (hypothyroidism) reduces the energy needed for maintaining body functions. Hyperthyroidism and hypothyroidism are not common, but they account for weight control problems in a small number of people.

PHYSICAL ACTIVITY   Individual energy needs vary considerably, and a person's activities can cause a change from day to day. Today, many people's lifestyles involve a considerable amount of time sitting, perhaps while driving a car or watching television. Many jobs often require only limited physical activity. The net result may be a surprisingly small amount of energy expended in moving the body throughout the day. On the other hand, the physical fitness fascination among some people of all ages has resulted in significant increases in caloric requirements for the physically active.

The actual amount of energy needed to offset the body's activities is determined by the weight of the person, the rate and amount of movement, and the time spent in the action. Two people who jog for 30 minutes would not use exactly the same amount of energy, even if they jogged the same length of time, because their weights and running speeds would probably differ. Although exact energy expenditure for physical activity is inconvenient for individuals to measure, there are tables that indicate approximate energy costs for typical activities. From such tables (see Table 1.4), approximate energy requirements for the day's activities can be calculated. Such calculations require careful logging of all activities and their duration. Lengths of time are multiplied by the energy value in the table and by the weight of the person in kilograms (obtained by dividing weight in pounds by 2.2).

THERMIC EFFECT   The last requirement for energy is that needed to derive energy from food. This includes energy needed for moving food through the gastrointestinal tract, digestion, absorption, and metabolic reactions. The sum of these various

HYPERTHYROIDISM
Excessive production of thyroxine and an accelerated basal metabolic rate, which may result in weight loss.

HYPOTHYROIDISM
Lower than normal production of thyroxine and a resulting slow basal metabolic rate, leading to overweight.

THERMIC EFFECT
The energy required for digestion, absorption, and metabolism of foods and their carbohydrate, lipid, and protein components; value approximated by calculating 10 percent of the calories required for activity and basal metabolism.

energy needs is called the thermic effect, a value requiring approximately 10 percent of the total figure obtained for basal metabolism and activity.

USING ENERGY INFORMATION   Approximate values for energy expenditures on a daily basis can be made by calculating basal metabolic needs, expenditures for activity, and thermic effect, and then totaling these values. A simple approximation of energy needs can be made by recording one day's activities and calculating the energy required, using the figures in Table 1.5. This table has been developed to include basal metabolism and thermic effect, as well as activity.

TABLE 1.4   Energy Required for Selected Activities[a]

Activity	Kcal/ kg/hr	Activity	Kcal/ kg/hr
Bicycling (rapidly)	7.6	Playing ping pong	4.4
Bicycling (moderately)	2.5	Reading aloud	0.4
Boxing	11.4	Rowing in race	16.0
Crocheting	0.4	Running	7.0
Dancing	3.8	Sawing wood	5.7
Dishwashing	1.0	Sewing, by hand	0.4
Dressing and undressing	0.7	Sewing, by machine	0.4
Driving	0.9	Singing loudly	0.8
Eating	0.4	Sitting quietly	0.4
Exercise		Skating	3.5
Very Light	0.9	Standing, relaxed	0.5
Light	1.4	Studying	0.4
Moderate	3.1	Sweeping with broom	1.4
Strenuous	5.4	Typing rapidly	1.0
Very strenuous	7.6	Vacuuming carpet	2.7
Fencing	7.3	Walking	
Horseback riding		3 miles/hour	2.0
Walk	1.4	4 miles/hour	3.4
Trot	4.3	5.3 miles/hour	8.3
Gallop	6.7	down stairs	—[b]
Laundry, light	1.3	up stairs	—[c]
Playing piano slowly	1.0	Washing floors	1.2
Playing piano rapidly	2.0	Writing	0.4

[a] Adapted from Taylor, MacLeod, and Rose, Foundations of Nutrition, Fifth Edition, MacMillan Co., New York, 1956.
[b] Allow 0.012 kcal per kilogram for an ordinary staircase with 15 steps, without regard to time.
[c] Allow 0.036 kcal per kilogram for an ordinary staircase with 15 steps, without regard to time

TABLE 1.5   Energy Required for Selected Activities[a] (Figures include energy for basal metabolism and thermic effect)

Activity	Men[b] Kcal/kg/hr	Women[b] Kcal/kg/hr
Sleeping	1.08	0.90
Typing	1.8	1.6
Sitting	1.39	1.15
Standing	1.75	1.37
Walking (3 mph)	3.7	3.0
Walking (22-lb pack)	4.0	3.4
Cooking	2.1	1.7
Regular housecleaning	3.1	2.5
Car repairing	4.1	2.5
Golfing	2.5–5.0	2.0–4.0
Dancing	5.0–7.5	4.0–6.0
Playing tennis	5.0–7.5	4.0–6.0

[a]Adapted from Durnin, J.V. and R. Passmore, Energy, work, and leisure, *Energy and Protein Requirements,* FAO/WHO Tech. Rept. No. 522, Geneva, 1973.
[b]Men assumed to be 65 kg (143 lb) and women assumed to be 55 kg (110 lb).

The estimated energy need can then be translated into a diet plan. Protein should contribute from 10 to 15 percent of the calories needed; fats should provide about 30 percent, and the remainder (55 to 60 percent) of the calories should be from carbohydrates. For a person who needs 2000 kcal, this translates to 200 to 300 kcal (50 to 75 gm) from protein, 600 kcal (67 gm) from fat, and 1100 to 1200 kcal (275 to 300 gm) of carbohydate daily.

MINERALS

Although energy and its sources are of prime importance in nutrition, there are other dietary essentials that do not undergo metabolic reactions to yield energy. Minerals, unlike carbohydrates, fats, and proteins, are not organic, that is, they do not contain carbon. Instead, these inorganic elements or compounds are non-carbon materials present in very small amounts in the body. Minerals are nonetheless vital, whether they are needed in small or somewhat larger quantities. Based on amounts found in the body, minerals are classified as macronutrient or micronutrient (trace) minerals. Macronutrient minerals include calcium, phosphorus, potassium, sulfur, sodium, chloride, and magnesium; micronutrient minerals include iron, manganese, copper, iodide, chromium, cobalt, fluoride, molybdenum, selenium, and zinc.

FUNCTIONS

Some generalizations can be made about actions of minerals, but specific minerals make unique contributions to the body and its operation. Collectively, minerals:

1. Control water balance.
2. Regulate acid-base balance.
3. Catalyze chemical reactions.
4. Provide structural foundations.
5. Act as key constitutents of essential substances (enzymes, hormones, and other unique compounds).

Water is found throughout the body in and between cells and in the bloodstream in varying concentrations. Mineral concentrations on either side of cell membranes determine osmotic pressure and water flow through the membranes separating the various body compartments. By helping to regulate osmotic pressure, minerals play an important role in determining the concentration of water in and between cells.

Acidity and alkalinity vary from one region of the body to another, yet the value is generally constant in specific areas. The concentration of some minerals helps maintain the slightly alkaline nature of the blood and the less alkaline reaction in the tissues, whereas other minerals are constitutents of acids. Organic phosphorus (phosphorus occurring in combination with organic compounds), chloride, and sulfur can form acids. Protein-containing foods (meat, poultry, eggs, fish, grains, and cereals) contain these acid-forming minerals and promote acid formation in the body. Calcium, iron, potassium, inorganic phosphate, magnesium, and sodium promote an alkaline reaction, thus opposing the acid-forming minerals. Fruits and vegetables, good sources of these alkaline-reacting minerals, are classified as base-formers (alkaline). Milk contains both acid and base-forming constituents and is therefore considered essentially neutral in its reaction within the body.

Some minerals are incorporated as parts of enzyme systems or can act simply as ions to catalyze various chemical

MACRONUTRIENT MINERALS
Inorganic, crystalline elements including calcium, phosphorus, potassium, sulfur, sodium, chloride, and magnesium.

MICRONUTRIENT MINERALS
Inorganic, crystalline elements present in extremely small amounts in the body; includes iron, manganese, copper, iodide, chromium, cobalt, fluoride, molybdenum, selenium, and zinc.

reactions in the body. Magnesium, calcium, potassium, manganese, zinc, and iron are essential minerals in a variety of metabolic reactions involving the utilization of carbohydrates, fats, and proteins. Minerals can even be involved in the process of absorption. For example, calcium aids in the absorption of the massive vitamin B_{12} molecule, and sodium and magnesium help in the absorption of simple sugars. Mineral ions (specfically calcium, potassium, magnesium, and sodium) are essential to the transmission of nerve impulses, including the messages involved in muscular contraction and relaxation.

Bones and teeth rely on calcium, phosphorus, fluoride, and magnesium for their growth and strength. Even in adulthood, the dynamic turnover of calcium and phosphorus in bones demands contant replacement of these minerals to maintain a strong framework. Potassium is a necessary component of soft tissues, and sulfur is a mineral found in the proteins of hair.

Among body compounds requiring minerals are two hormones: insulin, which contains zinc, and thyroxine, which contains iodide. Two vitamins contain an atom of mineral — vitamin B_{12} holds an atom of cobalt in its center, and sulfur is part of the structure of thiamin. Other compounds produced in the body also contain minerals. Hemoglobin in blood contains iron. Chloride combines in the stomach with hydrogen to form hydrochloric acid, which facilitates digestion. Cytochrome enzymes, needed for release of energy from carbohydrates, fats, and proteins, contain iron and copper. Two other enzymes, carbonic anhydrase and carboxypeptidase (needed respectively to release carbon dioxide from red blood cells and for protein metabolism), contain zinc; molybdenum is the mineral in xanthine oxidase, another enzyme.

Minerals perform their general and unique functions to regulate the body and its actions. Table 1.6 provides a summary of the functions and food sources of the individual minerals people need. In addition, a brief discussion of the various minerals follows as an overview of this important nutrient group.

CALCIUM

The most abundant mineral in the body is calcium, which constitutes about two percent of the body's total weight. It is stored in growing bones and teeth and continues to be deposited in mature bones to replace the calcium that is continually withdrawn throughout life. The dynamic nature of calcium in bones

TABLE 1.6   Minerals — Some of Their Sources and Functions

Mineral	Food Sources	Functions
Calcium	Milk and cheese, and milk-based foods (custards, puddings, hot chocolate) Tofu and soy milk Sardines, canned salmon, and other fish with bones Broccoli Greens	Tooth structure. Bone formation, maintenance, and growth. Muscle contraction. Aid in absorption of vitamin B_{12}. Activate pancreatic lipase. Blood clotting. Make acetylcholine (for transmitting nerve impulses).
Chloride	Table salt Eggs Meats Milk	Maintain proper osmotic pressure. Part of hydrochloric acid in stomach. Acid-base balance
Chromium	Whole-grain cereals Fruits and vegetables	Glucose into cells.
Cobalt	Organ meats Meats	Maturing of red blood cells (as part of vitamin B_{12}).
Copper	Cereals, legumes Meat, liver Nuts	Catalyze hemoglobin formation. Form connective tissue. Part of cytochrome enzyme system; used in energy release. Form phospholipids in myelin sheath lining nerves. Form dark pigment in hair and skin (melanin).
Fluoride	Fluoridated water	Add to strength of bones and teeth.
Iodine	Ocean fish Iodized salt	Part of thyroxine; regulate basal metabolism. Make some proteins. Aid in absorbing carbohydrates. Convert carotene to vitamin A.
Iron	Meats, organ meats Enriched and whole-grain cereals Greens Dried fruits Nuts Legumes	Transport oxygen and carbon dioxide (in hemoglobin and myoglobin). Red blood cell formation (hemoglobin). Aid in energy release (part of cytochromes). Part of myeloperoxidase, aid in killing bacteria

Mineral	Food Sources	Functions
Magnesium	Milk Breads and cereals Nuts Green vegetables	Catalyze conversion between ATP and ADP Calcium retention Conduct nerve messages. Relax contracted muscle. Aid in adjusting to cold.
Manganese	Legumes Cereals	Aid in amino acid metabolism. Bone development.
Molybdenum	Meats Legumes	Promote oxidation.
Nickel	Cereals	Associated with DNA and RNA
Phosphorus	Meats, poultry, fish Milk and cheese Cereals Legumes	Bone growth and maintenance. Tooth formation. Part of DNA, RNA, ADP, ATP, and TPP (compounds important in metabolic reactions).
Potassium	Meats Dried fruits Bananas, orange Peanut butter Potatoes	Transmit nerve impulses. Catalyze energy metabolism. Formation of proteins. Form glycogen. Acid-base balance. Maintain osmotic pressure
Selenium	Meats Ocean fish Wheat	Antioxidant (glutathionine peroxidase). Help to slow cancer growth at low levels.
Silicon	Whole-grain cereals	Collagen formation.
Sodium	Table salt Cured meats (ham) Olives, pickles Chips, crackers	Maintain osmotic pressure. Acid-base balance. Transmit nerve impulses. Muscle relaxation.
Sulfur	Meats Eggs Milk, cheese Legumes	Component of some structural proteins (hair, nails).
Zinc	Meats Whole-grain cereals Eggs Legumes	Part of carboxypeptidase (protein digestion).

is one of the primary reasons it is such a critical nutrient for adults as well as children.

Calcium is also a vital component of teeth, but teeth lose very little calcium once they have matured. Deciduous teeth, therefore, have their greatest need for calcium from the middle of pregnancy until they break through the gum. For permanent teeth, the critical period for calcium availability and deposition is from about three months of age until each one actually erupts.

Calcium is not confined only to bones and teeth. It triggers the release of thromboplastin from platelets in the blood and converts fibrinogen to fibrin, two key steps in the clotting of blood. Other functions of calcium in the body are: activation of pancreatic lipase (the enzyme needed for fat digestion in the small intestine), participation in the absorption of vitamin B_{12}, and transmission of nerve impulses (including muscular contraction).

To ensure the body has an adequate supply of calcium, milk and other dairy products should play a significant part in menus throughout life, not just in childhood. At least two glasses of milk daily are recommended to be certain adults are getting the calcium they require. Greens of various types are other useful sources. Tofu, a soybean product of Oriental origin, is a very good source of calcium and is gaining in general acceptance.

In addition to being sure the diet contains adequate calcium, factors influencing the rate of calcium absorption should be monitored to ensure that enough calcium will actually be available to the body. The efficiency of calcium absorption varies among individuals from one period of life to another. Calcium absorption, however, is favored by the presence of adequate vitamin D, ascorbic acid, protein, lactose, and phosphorus. People who have low calcium levels in the body will absorb dietary calcium more efficiently than someone who has had an adequate diet for an extended period.

*OSTEOPOROSIS
Reduction in bone mass, may be associated with inadequate calcium intake.*

An inadequate intake of calcium, frequently accompanied by an inadequate level of vitamin D, may result in poor tooth formation and stunting of growth. The bones not only grow poorly, but may also be malformed and evidenced as bowlegs or knock-knees. When calcium intake is inadequate over many months or years in adulthood, osteoporosis or osteomalacia may occur.

*OSTEOMALACIA
The adult counterpart of rickets, a weakening of bones associated with inadequate calcium intake.*

RESEARCH INSIGHTS

Bronner, F. and D. Pansu, Nutritional aspects of calcium absorption. *J. Nutr. 129:* 9. 1999.

Bronner and Pansu's work is a review article that draws upon approximately 50 research papers as the authors present a very detailed and methodical examination of calcium in human nutrition, including elaboration of the roles of calcium in the body and mechanisms involved in the pathways from consumption, absorption, and utilization to excretion. Factors cited as influencing calcium absorption include pH (acidity promotes solubility and absorption), source of calcium (fiber tends to impede solubilization of calcium, while calcium in milk is absorbed readily because of the presence of lactose, vitamin D, phosphopeptides, and amino acids), and the level of calcium in the diet. Active and passive transepithelial calcium transport and calcium absorption in the colon are also discussed. This paper provides a convenient source and compilation of information that otherwise can only be found through a prolonged and extensive search in pertinent professional journals. From time to time review articles fulfilling this function appear in the literature to consider many different topics of particular interest.

IRON

HEMOGLOBIN
Protein compound containing iron and capable of carrying oxygen or carbon dioxide in the blood.

IRON-DEFICIENCY ANEMIA
Blood condition characterized by low hemoglobin level and fatigue due to limited hemoglobin formation, the result of inadequate iron.

Iron, although classified as a micronutrient, is the mineral of particular concern among women of childbearing age. The potential for lack of iron among this group results from a combination of regular menstrual iron losses and inadequate intake. Iron is a structural part of hemoglobin, the iron-containing compound in the blood that carries oxygen to the tissues and carbon dioxide from the tissues to the lungs for excretion. With insufficient iron, hemoglobin formation drops, accompanied by decreased oxygen-carrying capacity in the blood. The result is iron-deficiency anemia, a condition characterized by fatigue and low hemoglobin.

Another iron-containing compound, myoglobin, is the pigment occurring in muscle tissue. Like hemoglobin, myoglobin can only be made when iron is available. In hemoglobin and myoglobin, as well as in certain other iron-containing compounds, the ability of iron to be oxidized and reduced is responsible for the unique behavior of these compounds in the body. Oxidative enzymes (including the cytochromes, cytochrome oxidase, peroxidase, and catalase) are essential for the release of energy from carbohydrates, fats, and proteins because of their ability to undergo oxidation and reduction reactions.

To meet these needs, iron can be provided from meats (particularly organ meats, such as liver and heart), clams, oysters, spinach, dried fruits, lima beans, and nuts, as well as whole grain or enriched cereal products. Even when attention is paid to eating these foods regularly, iron intake is likely to be inadequate among people eating fewer than 2000 kcal daily.

Part of the problem with iron deficiency may be difficulty in absorbing the mineral, even when it is provided in reasonable amounts. Ascorbic acid and other organic acids favor absorption; moreover, animal sources are absorbed better than plant sources. People who are low in iron absorb this mineral better than those who are well supplied with it.

Because of difficulty in absorbing iron and the limited availability of iron in many diets, enrichment is a common practice in the processing of refined cereal products. These are wise choices for people who prefer refined cereals to the somewhat more nutritious whole grains. The level of iron enrichment in refined cereals is set by the Federal government at 13 to 16.5 mg per pound of flour. Some debate has ensued over the level of enrichment deemed to be appropriate. Elevated iron intake is not recommended because of the possibility of developing a toxic condition called hemosiderosis. Extensive use of iron cooking pots can have a similar effect. Excessive levels in the body cause high concentrations of iron in the liver and spleen and may also increase the incidence of infections. Hemochromatosis is also characterized by unusually high levels of iron in the body, but it is due to a genetic defect in limiting iron absorption. High levels of iron in the diet aggravate hemochromatosis.

COPPER

Copper, like iron, has the ability to be oxidized and reduced by chemical reactions. This property is used in catalyzing oxidation-reduction reactions in the cytochrome system during the release of energy from carbohydrates, fats, and proteins. Copper is also a catalyst in the formation of hemoglobin, although it does not get bound into the molecule. As a part of the enzyme tyrosinase, copper is involved in the formation of melanin (a dark pigment in skin and hair) from tyrosine (an

HEMOSIDEROSIS
Abnormal condition characterized by too much iron being absorbed into the body as a result of excessive intake; high levels of iron in the liver and spleen and increased infections are symptoms.

HEMOCHROMATOSIS
Genetic defect causing iron to be absorbed too readily; high iron intakes compound the problem.

MELANIN
Dark pigment in skin and hair formed with the aid of tyrosinase, a copper-containing enzyme, from tyrosine.

amino acid). Phospholipids needed to form the myelin sheath lining nerve fibers are synthesized with the aid of copper.

Adequate amounts of copper can be obtained from a diet containing cereals, cereal products, nuts, and legumes. Liver is also an excellent source of this mineral.

FLUORIDE

FLUORIDATION
Control of the level of fluoride in a water supply, usually at a level of about 1 part per million (1 ppm).

Fluoride may have created more arguments and controversy than any other mineral. This began with the finding that fluoride in drinking water is quite effective in preventing dental caries. When fluoridated water is drunk throughout the period when teeth are forming, fluoride is deposited in the matrix of the teeth in the form of fluorapatite, a hard crystalline material that is much more resistant to bacterial decay than the normally present hydroxyapatite. The protection provided by fluoridated water ensures continuing resistance to dental caries throughout the adult years as well. Fluoride is also deposited in bones, a process which continues into the adult years if fluoridated water is drunk. The dynamic nature of bones, as opposed to that of teeth, points out the importance of fluoride in teeth during childhood.

Fluoridated water in city water supplies is the most effective means of ensuring that all children in a city will have an adequate fluoride intake during their formative years to ensure optimal protection against dental caries. Opponents of this public health measure have been effective in blocking fluoridation of water in some cities. Topical applications of stannous fluoride by dentists, use of fluoridated toothpastes, sodium fluoride tablets, and bottled fluoridated water are alternatives for obtaining the fluoride needed during the growing years in these cities. Unfortunately, these measures are more costly than simply fluoridating the water supply and are somewhat less effective.

IODIDE

Regulation of basal metabolic rate is achieved in large measure from the level of thyroxine available from the thyroid gland. Sufficient iodide must be consumed to manufacture the thyroxine required to supply energy for the body's basic operations. Iodide is a structural component of each molecule of thyroxine. If too little iodide is available through the diet, the thyroid gland will make a futile effort to produce sufficient thyroxine, causing a swelling of the thyroid gland near the base of the throat. This condition is called goiter.

Goiter, a problem endemic in the Midwest many years ago, has been virtually erased as a public health problem because of the common practice of using iodized salt, which is salt with added potassium iodide. Such salt is the main source of iodide in the diet. Salt containing iodide must be labeled as iodized salt with the indication: "This salt supplies iodide, a necessary nutrient." The wise shopper will be careful to select salt labeled in this manner to ensure adequate iodide intake.

ZINC

Poor taste perception, limited growth, and delayed sexual maturation are symptoms associated with an inadequate intake of zinc. Although most people's zinc is adequate, those eating diets very high in whole grain cereals and low in meats have occasionally developed zinc deficiencies. Zinc is a necessary

GOITER
Swelling of the thyroid gland at the base of the throat due to an iodide deficiency; symptoms include weight gain, lethargy, and irritability.

IODIZED SALT
Table salt to which potassium iodide has been added as a protection against endemic goiter.

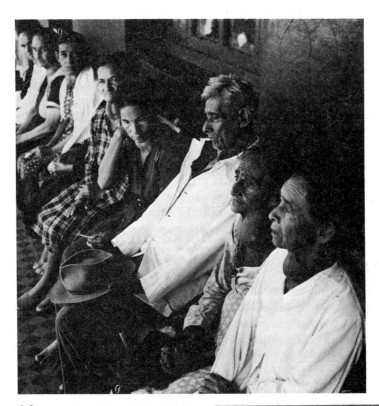

Goiter, a condition caused by an inadequate iodine intake, is characterized by swelling of the thyroid gland in the neck. In land-locked areas with iodine-deficient soil and little seafood or other food sources of iodine, such as in the remote Asuncion region of Paraguay, goiter is a common problem.

component of carboxypeptidase and alkaline phosphatase, enzymes required for digestion of protein and for bones, respectively.

DIETARY APPLICATIONS

Because minerals are contained in varying amounts in different foods, variety in the diet is important in ensuring an adequate intake of the many essential minerals. Emphasis on milk, a wide variety of fruits and vegetables, moderate portions of meats and other protein-rich foods, and enriched or whole grain breads and cereals is an effective way of obtaining the quantity and variety of minerals needed for good health. Some women may need an iron supplement to provide the necessary level, but a well-planned diet should provide the other minerals adequately, if drinking water is fluoridated.

TOXICITY

Although it is important to obtain enough of the various minerals to meet the body's need, too much of some minerals can be toxic. Excess iron and its toxicity were discussed in the section on iron and hemosiderosis. Similarly, too much fluoride (about 9 ppm) can disfigure a growing child's teeth by causing discoloration and mottling. Elevated blood pressure can be associated with high intakes of sodium chloride; elimination of added salt at the table and less salt in cooking are effective means of curbing sodium and chloride excesses.

Other minerals are known to be toxic when consumption is particularly high. For example, molybdenum levels in the soil are high enough in some locations to cause grazing animals to develop bone abnormalitites and low hemoglobin levels. People who have comparatively high intakes of selenium (0.2 mg daily is the maximum recommended intake) may develop brittle nails and hair loss. Both symptoms appear to be the result of selenium replacing sulfur in hair and nail proteins.

Heavy metals may be contaminants in foods and can cause toxicity. Bone meal and dolomite, for example, sometimes contain small amounts of lead, which gradually accumulate in the body. This is why these two products are not recommended as sources of calcium. Mercury is another heavy metal which sometimes finds its way into the food supply when fish are caught in waters contaminated with it.

VITAMINS

Of the various types of nutrients, vitamins are generally needed in the smallest quantity, yet they are frequently touted as being miracle nutrients. Certainly, they are necessary for life, but so are the other nutrients. These popular substances are divided into two categories — fat-soluble and water-soluble vitamins. The fat-soluble vitamins are vitamins A, D, E, and K. The water-soluble vitamins include the B vitamins (thiamin, riboflavin, niacin, pantothenic acid, pyridoxine, folacin, biotin, vitamin B_{12}) and vitamin C.

Vitamins of both categories are defined as organic substances which must be included in the diet in very small amounts to maintain life and promote growth. This definition distinguishes vitamins from minerals, because minerals are inorganic. The fact that vitamins are required in very small amounts separates these substances from carbohydrates, fats, and proteins. The stipulation that vitamins must be provided in the diet eliminates all compounds that can be formed in the body at levels adequate to maintain life and promote growth. Vitamins, in short, are unique.

FAT-SOLUBLE VITAMINS

VITAMIN A In 1912, the vitamin era erupted with simultaneous discoveries of vitamin A by researchers at Yale (Osborne and Mendel) and the University of Wisconsin (McCollum and Davis). Laboratory animals that were given a diet with no milk fat developed eye problems and eventually died. However, animals given the same diet until the eye abnormality developed and then given butter fat or egg yolk regained their health. Vitamin A was discovered, and the vitamin era was launched. Later experiments showed that dark green, leafy, or yellow vegetables could be used in place of butter fat or egg yolk to achieve similar results.

Vitamin research proved to be quite complex. Enthusiastic researchers required about 20 years just to confirm the structure of the compound known as vitamin A. After another 15 years of research, synthetic vitamin A was made in 1946.

Vitamin A is involved in the health of the eye; it is best known for promoting vision in dim light. Adequate vitamin A in the diet helps form rhodopsin in the rods of the retina. Rhodopsin is a key material in the generation of electrical impulses that send visual messages to the brain. If rhodopsin is

RHODOPSIN
Key compound in the visual cycle in the rods; vitamin A is necessary for its formation.

not formed in the visual cycle, night blindness results. This is an early sign of inadequate intake of vitamin A.

Bone growth in children is promoted by vitamin A. The stunting that occurs from a vitamin A deficiency sometimes leads to such limited skull growth that there may even be a pinching of the optic nerve, causing blindness.

The eyes are vulnerable to change when vitamin A is deficient; the surface of the eye can get dry and harden. Gradually, Bitot's spots form and xerophthalmia develops, causing blindness if the vitamin A shortage continues.

Ordinarily, vitamin A is present in quantities sufficient to produce the body's mucus secretions, notably in the nasal passages. When vitamin A intake is low, less mucus will be secreted, and the nasal passages will become dry and susceptible to bacteria. This reduces resistance to bacterial invasion and increases the likelihood of illness. Resistance to infection is definitely enhanced when vitamin A intake is returned to recommended levels. In a vitamin A deficiency, the skin develops a rough, somewhat thorny texture resembling the "goose bumps" that rise when a person is chilly.

The vitamin A needed by the body to avoid these deficiency symptoms can be obtained from a variety of foods. Vitamin A itself is available in whole milk, butter, cheese, and liver, as well as in vitamin A-fortified skim milk. Many dark green, leafy, and yellow vegetables are rich sources of carotenes, which are pigments readily converted in the body into active vitamin A. Spinach, broccoli, carrots, and sweet potatoes are a few of the good sources of provitamin A (carotenes).

Vitamin A is a good example of a substance that does not fit the philosophy, "if a little bit is good, more is better." People taking capsules that provide daily doses of about 50,000 IU (International Units) gradually build toxic levels of vitamin A in their bodies. Their symptoms include loss of appetite, blurred vision, irritability, headaches, diarrhea, nausea, drying and cracking skin, and hair loss. This condition is called hypervitaminosis A. If the capsules are discontinued, this problem can be reversed.

VITAMIN D Strong bones and teeth require a matrix containing calcium and phosphorus, minerals which are absorbed efficiently if the body has enough vitamin D. With inadequate vitamin A over a period of time, growing children develop rickets. This fat-soluble vitamin is unique because it can be formed in the body when the skin is exposed to bright sunlight for some time. Skin contains cholesterol, and direct sunlight converts cholesterol into vitamin D. Despite this potential synthesis, vitamin D is still considered a vitamin because most people do not get enough sunlight to produce the amount they need. The presence of smog in urban areas interferes with vitamin D synthesis, and warm clothes worn in cold climates prevent vitamin D synthesis much of the time.

Because the body's production of vitamin D will probably be inadequate, a dietary source is important for people of all ages, particularly growing children. In the past, children were plagued with a daily spoonful of cod liver oil to provide the vitamin D they needed. Today, milk is usually fortified with 400 IU (10 mg) of vitamin D per quart, fulfilling the daily need for vitamin D.

Hypervitaminosis D can develop when large supplements of vitamin D are taken. Although the amount of vitamin D causing toxic symptoms varies among individuals, children may exhibit problems with daily doses of 1800 IU (4.5 times the recommended intake). Adults may have symptoms at 5 times the RDA. Among these symptoms are vomiting, loss of appetite, excessive thirst, irritability, and high blood calcium levels.

RICKETS
Condition in which bones are soft enough to bend (bowlegs) due to inadequate absorption of calcium and phosphorus; caused by too little vitamin D.

HYPERVITAMINOSIS D
Condition caused by gross excesses of vitamin D, causing too much calcium to be absorbed and resulting in death unless vitamin D intake is reduced.

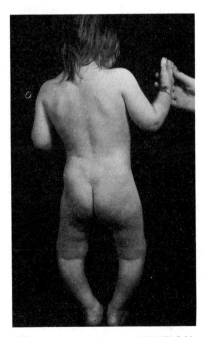

Poor calcification of bones due to a lack of vitamin D causes misshaping, evidenced in the load-bearing bones by bending of the shafts and swelling at the joints where two bones press against each other.

Finally, calcium can be deposited in the blood vessels, kidneys, and lungs, ultimately resulting in death. It is not possible to develop these symptoms simply from food sources of vitamin D.

VITAMIN E   Among some people, vitamin E is considered to be the "sexy" vitamin (a truly inaccurate description). This idea apparently developed when early vitamin E research, using rats as experimental animals, demonstrated that reproductive capability was lost in a vitamin E deficiency. This finding was interesting, but research has failed to demonstrate this among people. People do need vitamin E, however, as an antioxidant to help spare vitamin C, vitamin A, and polyunsaturated fatty acids for their unique functions. Otherwise, these essential nutrients could combine with oxygen and lose their functional ability.

The scientific designation for vitamin E compounds is tocopherol, which commonly occurs in three forms: alpha, beta, and gamma tocopherols. These are found naturally in plant seeds that provide the edible vegetable oils commonly used in cooking and in salad dressings. The food industry relies on tocopherols to serve as antioxidants during marketing and storage periods before the foods are eaten.

Although vitamin E is essential as an antioxidant in the body, no one has yet identified a physical problem caused by a deficiency of vitamin E. Because people will generally eat enough of the green vegetables, meats, and vegetable oils that provide vitamin E in the diet, a supplement is not needed. To date, toxic conditions arising from too much vitamin E have not been detected.

VITAMIN K   Blood clotting depends on the presence of vitamin K, which is why it is sometime referred to as the antihemorrhagic vitamin. Dietary sources include egg yolks, liver, and dark green, leafy vegetables. In early infancy however, babies acquire bacteria in the intestinal tract that are capable of synthesizing vitamin K. Because this ability to manufacture enough vitamin K is usually retained throughout life, it is not surprising that a vitamin K deficiency is of little concern to most people.

WATER-SOLUBLE VITAMINS

THIAMIN   Early in the twentieth century, when vitamin research was new, vitamins were designated in alphabetic order, beginning with vitamin A. Logically, the second substance being studied was named vitamin B, soon followed by vitamin C. All went well until subsequent investigations revealed that vitamin B was not a single substance, but several different substances that gradually evolved into the eight B vitamins we now recognize. The sensible solution to the naming problem that arose was simply to add a subscript to the particular B vitamin. The first of these was vitamin B_1, usually referred to as thiamin. This word indicates the presence of sulfur (thi-) and an amino (-amin) group in its molecule.

Energy needed by the body is released during metabolic reactions in cells. Enzymes and coenzymes are essential to catalyze various chemical changes, and several of the B vitamins are components of specific enzyme systems or coenzymes. Thiamin is part of thiamin pyrophosphate (TPP), a coenzyme functioning in the Krebs cycle to facilitate carbohydrate metabolism and resultant energy release. Because fragments of fats and proteins also proceed through the Krebs cycle, thiamin (in TPP) is necessary for metabolism of these potential energy sources, too.

THIAMIN PYROPHOS-PHATE (TPP) Coenzyme containing thiamin; essential as a catalyst in energy release from carbohydrates, fats, and proteins in the Krebs cycle.

Formation of ribose, the 5-carbon sugar incorporated into DNA (deoxyribonucleic acid) and RNA (ribonucleic acid), requires the presence of thiamin. DNA and RNA are crucial compounds involved in protein synethesis.

RIBOSE Five-carbon sugar in DNA and RNA that requires thiamin for its synthesis in the body.

When people have too little thiamin in their diets, they will develop symptoms of beriberi, the deficiency condition. These include nausea, vomiting, loss of appetite, depression, and irritability, as well as an awkward, careful walk. Sometimes edema (a bloated appearance) develops, whereas other patients may appear emaciated. The condition with edema is called wet berberi; the emaciated form is dry beriberi. Unless the diet is corrected and thiamin levels are adequate, beriberi results in death. Children with inadequate thiamin in their diets are susceptible to a very fast-moving beriberi, with death occurring quite rapidly.

DNA Deoxyribonucleic acid; nucleic acid essential to protein synthesis and containing ribose derivative.

RNA Ribonucleic acid; ribose–containing nucleic acid involved in protein synthesis.

Whole-grain or enriched breads and cereals, meats, eggs, legumes, milk, and potatoes are very good sources of thiamin. Because thiamin activity is quickly lost when food is cooked in an alkaline medium or in excess water, cooking conditions should be controlled to minimize losses of this water-soluble vitamin.

BERIBERI Deficiency condition characterized by vomiting, nausea, nervous disturbances, and edema or emaciation prior to death; caused by lack of thiamin.

RIBOFLAVIN The second member of the B vitamin group is riboflavin. The coenzymes in which riboflavin is found are flavin mononucleotide (FMN) and flavin adenine dinucleotide (FAD). Their specific catalytic roles are involved with the Krebs cycle and release of energy from carbohydrates, fats, and proteins, yet their involvement is different from that of thiamin-containing TPP.

Milk is a particularly good source of riboflavin, although much of the riboflavin activity is lost if the milk is exposed to sunlight or ultraviolet light for more than a short time. Riboflavin is also present in green vegetables, fish, meats, and eggs. Some of this vitamin is lost when these foods are cooked in water.

Even with this wide array of food sources, people sometimes do not eat sufficient quantities of riboflavin. Lesions then develop, particularly at the corners of the mouth; the tongue becomes a magenta color, and the surface of the tongue becomes glossy. These problems, caused by a lack of riboflavin, are symptoms of ariboflavinosis. By adding good sources of riboflavin to the diet, ariboflavinosis can be corrected.

NIACIN   Niacin is the B vitamin related to a vitamin deficiency condition of particular concern in this country a century ago. At that time, an alarming number of poor people were dying of pellagra. Symptoms of diarrhea, symmetrical dermatitis, and dementia formed a pattern that eventually resulted in death. Finally, in 1917, Dr. Joseph Goldberger (a physician and member of the U.S. Public Health Service) proved that pellagra was a result of the limited diet typical to the South, where people had very limited means to purchase food. From that time, 20 years elapsed before niacin was identified as the missing nutrient.

Nicotinamide adenine dinucleotide and nicotinamide adenine dinucleotide phosphate (NAD and NADP) are the two energy-releasing coenzymes containing niacin (in the form of nicotinamide). These coenzymes are important in oxidation-reduction reactions involving the cytochrome system and intertwined with Krebs cycle reactions. Niacin is therefore essential to the regulation of energy release from carbohydrates, fats, and proteins. The breakdown of glycogen (the storage form of carbohydrate in the body) and the synthesis of fatty acids also require niacin.

The high incidence of pellagra a century ago is evidence that levels of the vitamin niacin can be low enough to threaten health unless particular attention is given to eating enough niacin sources. Meats, poultry, and fish are especially good sources. Enriched and whole-grain breads and cereals are also of value because of their quantity in some diets. Potatoes, legumes, broccoli, other vegetables, and fruits add to the day's intake. Milk is also important in meeting niacin needs. Animal sources of niacin add to the diet because they are good sources of tryptophan, an amino acid that can be converted to niacin. In fact, about half of the body's need for niacin is satisfied by the conversion of tryptophan to niacin.

VITAMIN B_6   Vitamin B_6, also called pyridoxine, is of particular importance in protein metabolism. In the form of pyridoxal phosphate, this vitamin serves as a coenzyme with enzymes like transaminases and deaminases to synthesize new nonessential amino acids needed in protein synthesis and to initiate the breakdown needed for the release of energy from amino acids. The conversion of tryptophan to niacin specifically requires vitamin B_6. Pyridoxine is also part of glycogen phosphorylase, the enzyme system needed for breaking down glycogen to release energy. Although vitamin B_6 joined the ranks of the B vitamins after thiamin, riboflavin, and niacin had been well defined, it is now attracting considerable interest among researchers and is clearly of great importance in nutrition.

Symptoms of a vitamin B_6 deficiency include excessive irritability, convulsions, mental changes such as confusion and depression, and weight loss. Rarely is a frank deficiency of vitamin B_6 diagnosed, but women taking oral contraceptives appear to have an increased need for this particular vitamin. In a few cases, some of these women may need a vitamin B_6 supplement. A mixed diet that includes the usual quantities of meats, milk, whole-grain cereals, bananas, potatoes, cabbage, and other vegetables, will usually provide an adequate amount of vitamin B_6.

PANTOTHENIC ACID   The Greek word from which pantothenic acid got its name means "everywhere," and that says practically all there is to say about sources of this B vitamin. Pantothenic acid is found in almost all foods; organ meats, breads, and cereals are particularly outstanding sources. This broad availability explains why deficiency symptoms are not found among the world's people. When an experimental diet was devised to explore the symptoms that might occur in a deficiency, the problems were fatigue, headache, poor coordination and leg cramps, abdominal discomfort, and a retarded rate of antibody formation.

Pantothenic acid is combined with adenine and phosphate to form a coenzyme called coenzyme A (CoA). This coenzyme is vital to the breakdown of fat molecules so they can enter the Krebs cycle for energy release. Many other reactions

NICOTINAMIDE ADENINE DINUCLEOTIDE PHOSPHATE (NADP)
Niacin-containing coenzyme which includes a phosphate group; essential to energy release from carbohydrates, fats, and proteins.

TRYPTOPHAN
Amino acid capable of being transformed in the body into niacin; 60 mg of tryptophan will yield about 1 mg of niacin.

PYRIDOXINE
A common name for vitamin B_6.

COENZYME A (Co A)
Coenzyme consisting of pantothenic acid, adenine, and phosphate; functions in energy-producing metabolic reactions and in the synthesis of cholesterol, sex hormones, and fatty acids.

involving energy release in metabolism also require CoA. CoA combines with two-carbon fragments to facilitate the formation of cholesterol, sex hormones, and fatty acids.

BIOTIN   Biotin is officially classified as a B vitamin by most nutritionists despite the fact that it does not actually fit the definition of a vitamin. The classification problem stems from the fact that this compound is synthesized in the intestinal tract and is absorbed into the body, apparently in adequate amounts. A biotin deficiency never seems to be a problem for most people.

Biotin functions in the body in several different ways. The metabolism of carbohydrates, fats, and proteins involves biotin. Biotin, for instance, is involved in the removal of the amino group from amino acids (deamination) and in carboxylation. Fatty acid oxidation is dependent on biotin, and carbohydrate metabolism to release energy also utilizes biotin.

FOLATE
B vitamin of particular importance in pregnancy.

MEGALOBLASTIC ANEMIA
Blood abnormality in which the red blood cells fail to mature to their smaller size, resulting in an accumulation of large, immature erythrocytes.

FOLATE   Folate, sometimes called folic acid or folacin, is one of the B vitamins increasingly noted as one that may be inadequate in some people's diets. The original interest in this vitamin centered around the search for a cure for pernicious anemia, an anemia that caused deaths in the United States up until earlier in this century. Although folate did not solve the problem of pernicious anemia, it did prove to be an important factor in megaloblastic anemia (anemia in which red blood cells do not mature normally). A folate deficiency is evidenced by a disproportionate number of large, immature red blood cells in comparison with the number of smaller, mature erythrocytes. This situation is sometimes seen in late pregnancy when fetal demands added to maternal needs raise the requirement for folate.

SINGLE CARBON UNIT
One carbon atom and its hydrogen, that can be transported from one compound to another with the aid of folate to make new compounds.

The transfer of single carbon units from one compound to another is a key function of folate. By transferring this "building block" to another group, folate is able to promote synthesis of compounds needed to build nucleic acids, formation of nonessential amino acids, and production of porphyrin (the basic structure in such compounds as hemoglobin and myoglobin).

PORPHYRIN
Ring structure of carbon and hydrogen that can be complexed with iron and/or other atoms to make hemoglobin and other key molecules in the body.

This vitamin's name suggests the types of food in which folacin is particularly abundant. Spinach and other dark green, foliage-type greens are high in folate. Since storage causes some loss of folate, these foods should be used soon after purchase. Other fruits and vegetables also contain folate. Mushrooms and liver are very rich sources, too. Since 1998, grain products (including all types of flour) must be fortified with folate at the level of 140 µg/100 g.

VITAMIN B$_{12}$ Although folate did not prove to be the solution to pernicious anemia, researchers fortunately discovered that another of the B vitamins, vitamin B$_{12}$, was effective against this potentially fatal anemia. Pernicious anemia is characterized by macrocytic (abnormally large) red blood cells and by changes in the nervous system. Vitamin B$_{12}$ (also called cobalamin) was able to correct both of these conditions, whereas folate was ineffective in treating problems with the nerves.

Vitamin B$_{12}$ is needed in coenzyme forms to make DNA, which is essential for the maturation of red blood cells. This vitamin is also involved in carbohydrate metabolism and in the production of single carbon units. Single carbon units are provided by the action of vitamin B$_{12}$ and are transferred by folate to synthesize cholesterol and other related compounds. In fact, folate and vitamin B$_{12}$ perform in several complementary ways.

Most people who eat a mixed diet receive adequate vitamin B$_{12}$, because all animal foods are sources. A few people are limited in their ability to pass the very large molecules of vitamin B$_{12}$ through the intestinal wall. Consequently, they become deficient in this essential vitamin even though their diet is adequate. Their problem stems from lack of intrinsic factor, a substance normally available in the intestinal tract that binds the molecule and facilitates absorption. By injecting vitamin B$_{12}$ at appropriate intervals, physicians are able to circumvent the absorption problem and provide the necessary vitamin directly into the body.

Strict vegetarians who eliminate all animal products from their diets eventually develop generalized fatigue, muscle weakness, and smooth tongue (glossitis), symptoms of a vitamin B$_{12}$ deficiency. However, several years may elapse before these symptoms become evident if the vegetarian eats a general diet for a period of years and builds good body stores of vitamin B$_{12}$ before becoming a vegetarian. Ovo- and ovolactovegetarians will obtain enough vitamin B$_{12}$ in their diets to avoid this problem.

VITAMIN C   Long ago the Indians knew that a brew made with spruce bark would cure people who were suffering from a dietary problem later identified as scurvy. On the other side of the ocean, research on sailors in the British navy showed that scurvy could be cured or prevented by providing a diet containing daily sources of citrus fruits. Eventually, the identity of the substance in these foods was established, and ascorbic acid or vitamin C was found to be an essential vitamin.

PERNICIOUS ANEMIA
Condition characterized by macrocytic red blood cells and nervous system changes.

COBALAMIN
Another name for vitamin B$_{12}$.

ASCORBIC ACID
Another name for vitamin C, one of the water-soluble vitamins.

SCURVY
Condition characterized by swollen gums, loose teeth, muscle weakness, and poor appetite; caused by an inadequate intake of vitamin C.

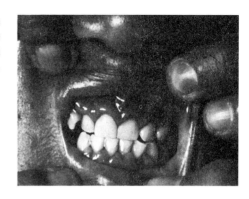

Inflamed and swollen gums are evidence of scurvy, the condition caused by a deficiency of vitamin C.

Vitamin C is necessary for the formation of collagen, the connective tissue that holds tissues together throughout the body. This function means that vitamin C is important for maintaining the matrix of bones and teeth as well as for healing cuts and other wounds requiring the closure of tissues. Inadequate vitamin C leads to fragile capillary walls and ready bruising under the skin. Swollen gums, loosening of teeth, inability to heal when cut, poor appetite, and muscle weakness are some of the more apparent symptoms of a lack of vitamin C. This condition is called scurvy, and this problem can be promptly relieved by adding vitamin C to the diet.

Sometimes megadoses of vitamin C are touted as being the way to prevent and cure colds, a claim which has yet to be proven despite a number of experiments. Nevertheless, colds are such an omnipresent problem that many people have flocked to drug stores to buy vitamin C capsules. Prolonged ingestion of large doses of vitamin C can lead to kidney and bladder stones and possibly to a deficiency of vitamin B_{12}. Infants whose mothers had taken massive doses of vitamin C during pregnancy developed scurvy after birth because they had become dependent on high doses in the fetal stage. By first giving these infants high doses of vitamin C and then gradually reducing the dosage, they can be returned to normal vitamin C levels without developing scurvy.

A summary of vitamins, their sources, and their functions is provided in Table 1.7.

TABLE 1.7   Vitamins — Their Sources, Functions, and Deficiency Conditions

Mineral	Food Sources	Functions	Deficiency
Fat Soluble:			
Vitamin A	Margarine, butter, liver, egg yolk; milk; provitamin A sources include broccoli, carrots, sweet potatoes, leafy green vegetables	Vision in dim light, normal skin, optimum growth	Xerophthalmia, night blindness, hyperkeratosis
Vitamin D	Vitamin D-fortified milk, eggs, cheese	Absorption and utilization of calcium and phosphorus, optimum growth, calcification of bones and teeth	Rickets, osteomalacia
Vitamin E	Vegetable oils, leafy green vegetables	Antioxidant to spare unsaturated fatty acids, vitamin A and ascorbic acid	
Vitamin K	Dark green, leafy vegetables, liver, egg yolks	Blood clotting	Hemorrhage
Water Soluble:			
Thiamin	Meats, eggs, legumes, enriched and whole-grain cereals and breads	Coenzyme (TPP) to release energy from carbohydrates, fats, and proteins; aids in formation of ribose for DNA and RNA	Beriberi
Riboflavin	Milk, meats, fish, poultry, asparagus, broccoli, legumes, whole-grain and enriched breads	Flavoprotein (FMN and FAD) enzymes for cellular respiration and releasing energy, conversion of tryptophan to niacin	Ariboflavinosis
Niacin	Meats, poultry, peanut butter, whole-grain and enriched cereals	Coenzyme needed to release energy from carbohydrates, fats, and protein; coenzyme involved in fatty acid synthesis	Pellagra
Vitamin B_6	Meats, bananas, beans, spinach, cabbage, potatoes	Metabolism of fats and carbohydrates; formation of nonessential amino acids; release of energy from protein; production of antibodies	
Pantothenic Acid	Organ meats, whole-grain cereals, and most foods	Component of coenzyme A; releases energy from carbohydrates, fats, and proteins; synthesis of cholesterol, fatty acids, and hemoglobin	

Mineral	Food Sources	Functions	Deficiency
Biotin	Egg yolks, milk, organ meats, legumes, nuts	Deamination of proteins; release of energy from carbohydrates, fats, and amino acids; production of antibodies; carboxylation	
Folacin	Dark green, leafy vegetables, mushrooms, liver, kidney, fruits, vegetables	Transfer single carbon units to synthesize new non-essential amino acids, nucleic acids and hemoglobin; cell growth; normal maturation of red blood cells	Macrocytic anemia
Vitamin B_{12}	Meat, poultry, fish, milk, eggs	Maturation of red blood cells; maintain health of nervous tissues	Pernicious anemia
Vitamin C	Citrus fruits, strawberries, tomatoes, cantaloupe, broccoli, potatoes, cabbage, tropical fruits	Formation of collagen, normal strength of blood vessels, protection against infections, promotes calcification of teeth and bones, utilization of some amino acids	Scurvy

WATER

INTRACELLULAR WATER
Water contained within the cells.

EXTRACELLULAR WATER
Water in the body held outside the cells.

INTRAVASCULAR WATER
Water in the blood-stream.

Water is such a common part of life that it is easy to forget how important it is. The fact is that people will die far more quickly from lack of water than from lack of food. When we examine the composition of the body, we find that between 55 and 65 percent of its total weight is water. The significance of water is obvious. Within the body, water is found in the cells (intracellular water), outside the cells (extracellular water), and in the bloodstream (intravascular water). Because of its capacity as a solvent and its ability to move in and out of cells, water can transport nutrients to cells and remove waste products from metabolism within the cells. It also serves as a lubricant, facilitating movement of the joints and transport of the food mass through the digestive tract. Chemical reactions in the body are aided by water. Water that passes through the skin and evaporates on the surface is extremely important in keeping the body at normal temperature. In one sense, water serves as a structural component because its presence in cells helps them remain properly extended.

Water is a major component of many foods, particularly fruits and vegetables. Large amounts are also available when juices, other beverages, and soups are consumed. To meet the need for water in the body, people should drink at least six glasses of water or other beverage daily. Hot weather increases the need for water because of an increased perspiration loss.

RECOMMENDED DIETARY ALLOWANCES

As a result of past studies and continuing research, considerable understanding of nutrition and the need for individual nutrients has been gained. The Food and Nutrition Board of the National Academy of Sciences — National Research Council is a prestigious body of nutrition scientists responsible for recommending necessary and appropriate levels of essential nutrients to meet the body's daily needs, based on the needs of groups of people. These values have been reviewed and updated in the light of new research approximately every five years and published, along with the rationale for the recommendations. The 1989 revision of the Recommended Dietary Allowances is utilized now in an abridged version (Table 1.8 and 1.9) and includes 8 nutrients (phosphorus, magnesium, thiamin, riboflavin, niacin, vitamin B_6, and folate) which are presented as recommended dietary allowances (RDA) for persons age 1 or older. The values for calcium, vitamin D, fluoride, pantothenic acid, biotin, and choline are stated as adequate intakes (AI) for all ages. The recommendations for the other 9 nutrients in the table are indicated as AI for infants up to age 1.

RDA
Abbreviation for Recommended Dietary Allowances, values identified by the Food and Nutrition Board of the National Academy of Sciences — National Research Council.

AI
Adequate Intake; stated when knowledge is not sufficient to state as RDA.

Table 1.10 suggests recommended energy levels for reference individuals who are about average in their energy expenditure for activities. These figures do not include a margin of safety, because this might lead to overweight. Maintenance of a desirable weight is the individual's best gauge for appropriate caloric intake.

Table 1.11 indicates the upper limit of intake considered to be safe; this limit includes the intake both from food and from any supplements. The nine nutrients for which upper intake levels (UL) were designated in 1998 are calcium, phosphorus, magnesium, vitamin D, fluoride, niacin, vitamin B_6, synthetic folic acid, and choline. Additional listings are being studied and will be made available when the values have been established.

UL
Tolerable Upper Intake Level; value warning of potential risk level.

TABLE 1.8 Food and Nutrition Board, National Academy of Sciences — National Research Council Recommended Dietary Allowances[a], Revised 1989 (Abridged)

Designed for the maintenance of good nutrition of practically all healthy people in the United States

Category Age (yrs) or Condition	Weight[b] (kg)	(lb)	Height[b] (cm)	(in)	Protein (g)	Vitamin A (µg RE)[c]	Vitamin K (µg)	Iron (mg)	Zinc (mg)	Iodine (µg)
Infants 0.0–0.5	6	13	60	24	13	375	5	6	5	40
0.5–1.0	9	20	71	28	14	375	10	10	5	50
Children 1–3	13	20	90	35	16	400	15	10	10	70
4–6	20	44	112	44	24	500	20	10	10	90
7–10	28	62	132	52	28	700	30	10	10	120
Males 11–14	45	99	157	62	45	1,000	45	12	15	150
15–18	66	145	176	69	59	1,000	65	12	15	150
19–24	72	160	177	70	58	1,000	70	10	15	150
25–50	79	174	176	70	63	1,000	80	10	15	150
51+	77	170	173	68	63	1,000	80	10	15	150
Females 11–14	46	101	157	62	46	800	45	15	12	150
15–18	55	120	163	64	44	800	55	15	12	150
19–24	58	128	164	65	46	800	60	15	12	150
25–50	63	138	164	64	50	800	65	15	12	150
51+	65	143	160	63	50	800	65	10	12	150
Pregnant					60	800	65	30	15	175
Lactating 1st 6 months					65	1,300	65	15	19	200
2nd 6 months					62	1,200	65	15	16	200

Note: This table does not include nutrients for which Dietary Reference Intakes have recently been established (see Dietary Reference Intakes for Calcium, Phosphorus, Magnesium, Vitamin D, and Fluoride [1997] and Dietary Reference Intakes for Thiamin, Riboflavin, Niacin, Vitamin B6, Folate Vitamin B12, Pantothenic Acid, Biotin, and Choline [1998].)

[a] The allowances, expressed as average daily intakes over time, are intended to provide for individual variations among most normal persons as they live in the United States under usual environmental stresses. Diets should be based on a variety of common foods in order to provide other nutrients for which human requirements have been less well defined.

[b] Weights and heights of Reference Adults are actual medians for the U.S. population of the designated age, as reported by NHANES II. The median weights and heights of those under 19 years of age were taken from Hamill et al. (1979). The use of these figures does not imply that the height-to-weight ratios are ideal.

[c] Retinol equivalents. 1 retinol equivalent = 1 µg retinol or 6 µg β-carotene.

TABLE 1.9 Food and Nutrition Board, National Academy of Sciences — National Research Council Dietary Reference Intakes; recommended intakes for individuals, Revised 2000

Life stage group	Calcium (mg/d)	Phosphorus (mg/d)	Magnesium (mg/d)	Vit. D (μg/d)[a,b]	Fluoride (mg/d)	Thiamin (mg/d)	Riboflavin (mg/d)	Niacin (mg/d)[c]	Vit. B6 (mg/d)	Folate (μg/d)[d]	Vit. B12 (μg/d)	Pantothenic Acid (mg/d)	Biotin (μg/d)	Choline[e] (mg/d)	Vit. C (mg/d)	Vit. E[f] (mg/d)	Selenium (μg/d)
Infants																	
0–6 mo.	210*	100*	30*	5*	0.01*	0.2*	0.3*	2*	0.1*	65*	0.4*	1.7	5*	125*	40*	4*	15*
7–12 mo.	270*	275*	75*	5*	0.6*	0.3*	0.4*	4*	0.3*	80*	0.5*	1.8*	6*	150*	50*	6*	20*
Children																	
1–3 yrs.	500*	460	80	5*	0.7*	0.5	0.5	6	0.5	150	0.9	2*	8*	200*	15	6	20
4–8 yrs.	800*	500	130	5*	1*	0.6	0.6	8	0.6	200	1.2	3*	12*	250*	25	7	30
Males																	
9–13 yrs.	1,300*	1,250	240	5*	2*	0.9	0.9	12	1.0	300	1.8	4*	20*	375*	45	11	40
14–18 yrs.	1,300*	1,250	410	5*	3*	1.2	1.3	16	1.3	400	2.4	5*	25*	550*	75	15	55
19–30 yrs.	1,000*	700	400	5*	4*	1.2	1.3	16	1.3	400	2.4	5*	30*	550*	90	15	55
31–50 yrs.	1,000*	700	420	5*	4*	1.2	1.3	16	1.3	400	2.4	5*	30*	550*	90	15	55
51–70 yrs.	1,200*	700	420	10*	4*	1.2	1.3	16	1.7	400	2.4[g]	5*	30*	550*	90	15	55
>70 yrs.	1,200*	700	420	15*	4*	1.2	1.3	16	1.7	400	2.4[g]	5*	30*	550*	90	15	55
Females																	
9–13 yrs.	1,300*	1,250	240	5*	2*	0.9	0.9	12	1.0	300	1.8	4*	20*	375*	45	11	40
14–18 yrs.	1,300*	1,250	360	5*	3*	1.0	1.0	14	1.2	400[h]	2.4	5*	25*	400*	65	15	55
19–30 yrs.	1,000*	700	310	5*	3*	1.1	1.1	14	1.3	400[h]	2.4	5*	30*	425*	75	15	55
31–50 yrs.	1,000*	700	320	5*	3*	1.1	1.1	14	1.3	400[h]	2.4	5*	30*	425*	75	15	55
51–70 yrs.	1,200*	700	320	10*	3*	1.1	1.1	14	1.5	400	2.4[g]	5*	30*	425*	75	15	55
>70 yrs.	1,200*	700	320	15*	3*	1.1	1.1	14	1.5	400	2.4[g]	5*	30*	425*	75	15	55
Pregnancy																	
≤18 yrs.	1,300*	1,250	400	5*	3*	1.4	1.4	18	1.9	600[h]	2.6	6*	30*	450*	80	15	60
19–30 yrs.	1,000*	700	350	5*	3*	1.4	1.4	18	1.9	600[h]	2.6	6*	30*	450*	65	15	60
31–50 yrs.	1,000*	700	360	5*	3*	1.4	1.4	18	1.9	600[h]	2.6	6*	30*	450*	65	15	60
Lactation																	
≤18 yrs.	1,300*	1,250	360	5*	3*	1.4	1.6	17	2.0	500	2.6	7*	35*	550*	115	19	70
19–30 yrs.	1,000*	700	310	5*	3*	1.4	1.6	17	2.0	500	2.6	7*	35*	550*	120	19	70
31–50 yrs.	1,000*	700	320	5*	3*	1.4	1.6	17	2.0	500	2.6	7*	35*	550*	120	19	70

Note: This table presents Recommended Dietary Allowances (RDAs) in bold type and Adequate Intakes (AIs) in ordinary type followed by an asterisk (*). RDAs and AIs may both be used as goals for individual intake. RDAs are set to meet the needs of almost all (97 to 98 percent) individuals in a group. For healthy breastfed infants, the AI is the mean intake. The AI for other life-stage and gender groups is believed to cover needs of all individuals in the group, but lack of data or uncertainty in the data prevent being able to specify with confidence the percentage of individuals covered by this intake.

[a] As cholecalciferol. 1 μg cholecalciferol = 40 IU vitamin D.
[b] In the absence of adequate exposure to sunlight.
[c] As niacin equivalents (NE). 1 mg of niacin = 60 mg of tryptophan; 0–6 months = preformed niacin (not NE).

[d] As dietary folate equivalents (DFE). 1 DFE = 1 μg food folate = 0.5 μg of folic acid from fortified food or supplement consumed with food = 0.5 μg of synthetic (supplemental) folic acid taken on an empty stomach.

[e] Although AIs have been set for choline, there are few data to assess whether a dietary supply of choline is needed at all stages of life.

(cont. on next page)

TABLE 1.10   Median Heights and Weights and Recommended Energy Intake

Category/ Age (yrs)	Weight (kg)	(lb)	Height (cm)	(in)	REE[a] (kcal/day)	Average Energy Allowance (kcal)[b] Multiples REE	(per kg)	(per day)[c]
Infants								
0.0–0.5	6	13	60	24	320		108	650
0.5–1.0	9	20	71	28	500		98	850
Children								
1–3	13	29	90	35	740		102	1,300
4–6	20	44	112	44	950		90	1,800
7–10	28	62	132	52	1,130		70	2,000
Males								
11–14	45	99	157	62	1,440	1.70	55	2,500
15–18	66	145	176	69	1,760	1.67	45	3,000
19–24	72	160	177	70	1,780	1.67	40	2,900
25–50	79	174	176	70	1,800	1.60	37	2,900
51+	77	170	173	68	1,530	1.50	30	2,300
Females								
11–14	46	101	157	62	1,310	1.67	47	2,200
15–18	55	120	163	64	1,370	1.60	40	2,200
19–24	58	128	164	65	1,350	1.60	38	2,200
25–50	63	138	163	64	1,380	1.55	36	2,200
51+	65	143	160	63	1,280	1.50	30	1,900
Pregnancy								
1st trimester								+0
2nd trimester								+300
3rd trimester								+300
Lactating								
1st 6 months								+500
2nd 6 months								+500

[a]Calculation based on FAO equations, then rounded.
[b]In the range of light to moderate activity, the coefficient of variation is ±20%.
[c]Figure is rounded.
Reprinted with permission from *Recommended Dietary Allowances*, 10th ed., © copyright 1989 by the National Academy of Sciences, published by the National Academy Press, Washington, D.C.

(cont. from previous page) of the life cycle, and it may be that the choline equivalent can be met by endogenous synthesis at some of these stages.
[f]As α-Tocopherol. α-Tocopherol includes RRR-α-tocopherol, the only form of α-tocopherol that occurs naturally in foods, and the 2R-stereoisomeric forms of a-tocopherol (RRR-, RSR-, RRS-, and RSS-α-tocopherol that occur in fortified foods and supplements. It does not include the 2S-stereoisomeric forms of α-tocopherol (SRR-, SSR-, SRS- and SSS-α-tocopherol), also found in fortified foods and supplements.
[g]Because 10 to 30% of older people may malabsorb food-bound Vitamin B-12, it is advisable for those older than 50 years to meet their RDA mainly by consuming foods fortified with Vitamin B-12 or a supplement containing Vitamin B-12.
[h]In view of evidence linking folate intake with neural-tube defects in the fetus, it is recommended that all women capable of becoming pregnant consume 400 μg from supplements or fortified foods in addition to intake of food folate from a varied diet. It is assumed that women will continue to consume 400 μg from supplements or fortified food until their pregnancy is confirmed and they enter prenatal care which ordinarily occurs after the end of the periconceptional period — the critical time for formation of the neural tube.

© 2000 by the National Academy of Sciences. Reprinted courtesy of the National Academy Press, Washington, D.C.

TABLE 1.11 Dietary Reference Intakes: Tolerable Upper Intake Levels (UL[a]) for Certain Nutrients and Food Components

Food and Nutrition Board, Institute of Medicine — National Academy of Sciences

Life-Stage Group	Calcium (g/day)	Phosphorus (g/day)	Magnesium (mg/day)[b]	Vitamin D (µg/day)	Fluoride (mg/day)	Niacin (mg/day)[c]	Vitamin B_6 (mg/day)	Synthetic Folic Acid (µg/day)[c]	Choline (g/day)
0–6 months	ND[d]	ND	ND	25	0.7	ND	ND	ND	ND
7–12 months	ND	ND	ND	25	0.9	ND	ND	ND	ND
1–3 years	2.5	3	65	50	1.3	10	30	300	1.0
4–8 years	2.5	3	110	50	2.2	15	40	400	1.0
9–13 years	2.5	4	350	50	10	20	60	600	2.0
14–18 years	2.5	4	350	50	10	30	80	800	3.0
19–70 years	2.5	4	350	50	10	35	100	1,000	3.5
>70 years	2.5	3	350	50	10	35	100	1,000	3.5
Pregnancy									
≤18 years	2.5	3.5	350	50	10	30	80	800	3.0
19–50 years	2.5	3.5	350	50	10	35	100	1,000	3.5
Lactation									
≤18 years	2.5	4	350	50	10	30	80	800	3.0
19–50 years	2.5	4	350	50	10	35	100	1,000	3.5

[a]UL = the maximum levl of daily nutrient intake that is likely to pose no risk of adverse effects. Unless otherwise specified, the UL represents total intake from food, water, and supplements. Due to lack of suitable data, ULs could not be established for thiamin, riboflavin, vitamin B_{12}, pantothenic acid, or biotin. In the absence of ULs, extra caution may be warranted in consuming levels above recommended intakes.

[b]The UL for magnesium represents intake from a pharmacological agent only and does not include intake from food and water.

[c]The ULs for niacin and synthetic folic acid apply to forms obtained from supplements, fortified foods, or a combination of the two.

[d]ND: Not determinable due to lack of data of adverse effects in this age group and concern with regard to lack of ability to handle excess amounts. Source of intake should be from food only to prevent high levels of intake.

Reprinted with permission. © copyright 1989 by the National Academy of Sciences, published by the National Academy Press, Washington, D.C.

PLANNING ADEQUATE DIETS

Tables of values that identify the necessary amounts of each nutrient to be well nourished are impressive, but they also are overwhelming for anyone other than a professional dietitian to apply. RDA and AI values are utilized by professionals in their work as they develop plans for feeding groups of people and also individuals. However, all people have to feed themselves healthfully on a daily basis even though they may have had little or no training in nutrition. Practical guidelines are now available to help everyone in menu planning for good health.

The 2000 Dietary Guidelines for Americans (5th edition) is the most recent public statement that has been presented to outline appropriate dietary and lifestyle choices for good nutrition and optimal health. These guidelines were developed by the Dietary Guidelines Advisory Committee, whose members were appointed by the U.S. Department of Agriculture (USDA) and the U.S. Department of Health and Human Services (USDHHS).

The seven guidelines included in the 2000 Dietary Guidelines for Healthy Americans age 2 and older are:

1) Aim for fitness
   —Aim for a healthy weight
   —Be physically active each day

2) Build a healthy base
   —Let the Pyramid guide your food choices
   —Eat a variety of grains daily, especially whole grains
   —Eat a variety of fruits and vegetables daily.
   —Keep foods safe to eat

3) Choose sensibly
   —Choose a diet that is low in saturated fat and cholesterol and moderate in total fat
   —Choose beverages and foods to moderate your intake of sugars
   —Choose and prepare foods with less salt
   —If you drink alcoholic bevereages, do so in moderation

The Food Guide Pyramid, a visual presentation of a good diet, was developed jointly by USDA and USDHHS to serve as the focal point of the nation's nutrition education message. The base or foundation of the pyramid is the bread, cereal, rice, and pasta group. Resting above this base are two groups: the vegetable group and the fruit group. A still smaller higher level of the pyramid is comprised of the milk, yogurt, and cheese group and the meat, poultry, fish, dry beans, eggs, and nuts group. At the apex of the Food Guide Pyramid is a small pyramid, the fats, oils, and sweets.

With the exception of the top category, the numbers of servings recommended daily are indicated for each group. However, the admonition accompanying the fats, oils, and sweets is to use sparingly. The recommended numbers of servings daily for the various groups are:

Bread, cereal, rice, and pasta	6–11 servings
Vegetables	3–5 servings
Fruits	2–4 servings
Milk, yogurt, and cheese	2–3 servings
Meat, poultry, fish, dry beans, eggs, and nuts	2–3 servings

The total amount of food needed by a person each day is determined by several factors, including age, sex, and activity level. Obviously, an active young male adult will require more food than a 3-year-old girl needs. Table 1.12 indicates the numbers of servings for various groups to help individuals apply the Food Guide Pyramid to their own daily food needs.

Serving sizes need to be defined and respected if the above recommendations are to result in a healthy diet for a person. The Food Guide Pyramid serving sizes are:

Bread, cereal, rice, pasta
    1 slice bread; 1 ounce ready-to-eat cereal;
    1/2 cup cooked cereal, rice, or pasta

Vegetable
    1 cup raw, leafy; 1/2 cup cooked or chopped raw;
    3/4 cup juice

Fruit
    1 medium apple, banana, orange;
    1/2 cup chopped, cooked, or canned;
    3/4 cup juice

Milk
    1 cup milk or yogurt; 1 1/2 ounce natural cheese;
    2 ounces process cheese

Meat
    2–3 ounces lean meat, poultry, or fish;
    1/2 cup cooked dry beans;
    1 egg or 2 tablespoons peanut butter equals
        1 ounce lean meat

TABLE 1.12 Numbers of Servings Recommended for Various American Population Groups

Group	Many women, older adults	Children, teen girls, active women, most men	Teen boys, active men
Calorie level[a]	1600	2200	2800
Bread	6	9	11
Vegetable	3	4	5
Fruit	2	3	4
Milk	2–3[b]	2–3[b]	2–3[b]
Meat	2	2	3
	(5 oz total)	(6 oz total)	(7 oz total)
Total fat (grams)	53	73	93
Added sugar (teaspoons)	6	12	18

[a]Based on diet using low-fat, lean foods and only using fats, oils and sweets sparingly.
[b]Women who are breast-feeding, teenagers, and young adults (to age 24) need 3 servings daily.

Within each food group defined by the Food Guide Pyramid there are many potential choices. Depending on the choices made, the calorie intake can be quite variable. Also, the other nutrients will be influenced by the selections that are made. Variety of choices should be emphasized, for this variety also brings a wide range of the needed nutrients. Brief overviews of the food groups defined by the Food Guide Pyramid follow.

BREADS, CEREALS, RICE, PASTA The grains that are common sources of breads and cereal products include wheat, corn, rice, oats, rye, and barley. Whole-grain cereals and cereal products provide important amounts of thiamin, riboflavin, niacin, protein, starch, and fiber, as well as useful levels of other vitamins and minerals. Often, cereals are refined, a process which removes significant amounts of vitamins, minerals, and fiber. Fortunately, thiamin, riboflavin, niacin, and iron are returned when refined products are enriched. Enriched products, nevertheless, lack some of the trace minerals and fiber provided in whole grain products. Despite some differences in nutritive content, enriched cereals are an adequate choice in this group if people do not like whole-grain breads and cereals.

VEGETABLES Vegetables also are high in vitamins, minerals, carbohydrate, and fiber. Of particular importance in this group are the dark green, leafy and yellow vegetables, which are rich

REFINED CEREAL Wheat or other cereal that has had germ and bran portions removed from individual grains, a process which reduces fiber, vitamin, and mineral content but extends shelf life.

WHOLE GRAIN CEREAL Cereal containing bran and germ, as well as the endosperm of the grain.

ENRICHED CEREAL Refined cereal with thiamin, riboflavin, niacin, iron, and sometimes calcium added to replace some of the nutrients removed by the refining process.

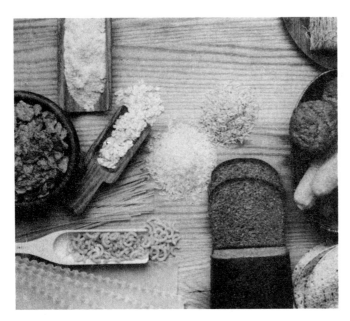

Enriched and whole-grain cereal products of many varieties can be used to provide the B vitamins and iron that are expected to be provided by the bread and cereal group in the Daily Food Guide.

sources of carotenes (pigments that are converted to active vitamin A in the body). Crucifers (cabbage, cauliflower, kale,

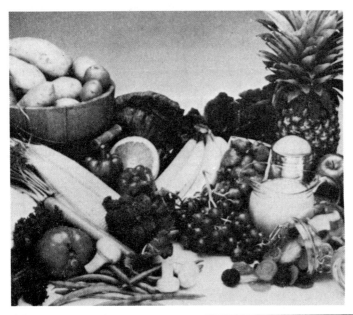

Considerable variety should be chosen in the fruit and vegetable groups of the Daily Food Guide to ensure good sources of the various vitamins and minerals needed in the diet and to provide fiber.

broccoli, brussels sprouts, and other vegetables with a "cabbage-like" flavor) may be somewhat protective against cancer.

FRUITS All fruits are excellent sources of carbohydrate and fiber. They also contribute various vitamins and minerals, depending upon the particular fruit being eaten. Citrus and tropical fruits and berries are especially valuable sources of vitamin C and should be eaten frequently, preferably at least one serving daily.

MILK, YOGURT, CHEESE Milk may be whole, reduced fat, lowfat, or nonfat (fat free), and it should be fortified with vitamin D. The recommendation is for 2 to 3 servings, but adolescents may have more. Eight-ounce servings are assumed, although individual glasses of milk can be less as long as the final total is reached.

LACTOSE INTOLERANCE Inability to digest lactose efficiently, due to inadequate lactase in the small intestine; condition character- ized by abdominal discomfort and gas following consumption of milk.

Some people have discomfort if they drink a whole glass of milk at one sitting. This is caused by lactose intolerance. Sometimes this problem can be avoided by drinking a smaller glass of milk or by serving milk which has had much of the lactose (milk sugar) either enzymatically treated to break down the lactose or fermented by bacteria (sweet acidophilus milk, for example).

Considerable variety is available within this group, even though this category is based on a single food — milk. In addition to the fluid milks with varying levels of fat, there are cultured buttermilk, milk with added lactose, and sweet acidophilus milk, as well as yogurt, cheese, and ice cream. Such items as cream

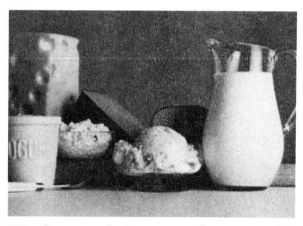

Milk, cheese, yogurt, and ice cream afford a variety of choices to provide the recommended servings in the milk group at different energy levels.

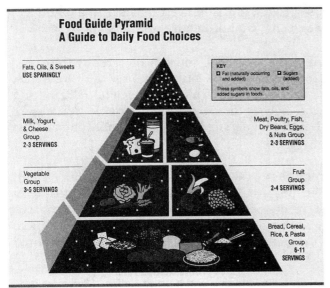

Food Guide Pyramid

soups and baked custards provide valuable sources of milk, too. Generous use of cheese or ice cream to provide necessary calcium intake from the milk group can lead to a weight problem because of their high calorie content. For people watching their weight, nonfat milk is a particularly wise choice for this group.

MEATS, POULTRY, DRY BEANS AND PEAS, EGGS, AND NUTS

This group is included to ensure adequate protein intake, but it also provides excellent amounts of iron, thiamin, and niacin, as well as useful quantities of several other minerals and vitamins. Pork, beef, veal, and lamb are categorized specifically as meats. Poultry, eggs, fish, and other seafood belong to this group. Plant sources of protein are useful, but incomplete in their amino acid content. However, various nuts and legumes (lima beans, pinto beans, split peas, chick peas, navy beans, and other beans) can be used generously in meeting protein requirements, especially if they are served with a bit of cheese or accompanied by a glass of milk to round out the amino acid pattern.

Two 3-ounce portions of cooked meat or meat alternative are recommended daily. For many people, emphasis in this category needs to be given to reducing portion size rather than increasing intake. This recommendation is based on the fact that overweight is a frequent problem among Americans, and the fat content of meats contributes significantly to caloric intake when large portions are eaten.

SUMMARY

Food is the source of nutrients needed by the body to promote growth, maintain life, and fuel activities. These nutrients are categorized according to their chemical nature and amounts that are required in the diet. Three groups of nutrients — carbohydrates, lipids, and proteins — are referred to as energy nutrients, for they provide the total amount of energy available to the body. Mono-, di-, and polysaccharides are groupings indicating complexity of carbohydrates. Many of the carbohydrate compounds are broken down by digestive enzymes in the gastrointestinal tract to their component monosaccharides for absorption through the villi in the small intestine. A few serve as roughage or fiber, increasing motility in the gastrointestinal tract. Absorbed monosaccharides undergo many chemical changes to provide energy via the Krebs cycle and the electron transport system.

Lipids are important sources of energy when there is sufficient carbohydrate available for their metabolism in the body. They are also necessary in the diet as a source of linoleic acid and as a carrier of fat-soluble vitamins. For absorption, fats are usually split into their components — fatty acids and glycerol.

The other energy nutrient is protein, a complex organic compound containing nitrogen. Hundreds of amino acids, the building blocks of proteins, are combined in a single protein by using unique sequences of amino acids. These amino acids may be essential amino acids (those needed for life but not made in the body) or nonessential. Humans need nine essential amino acids (histidine, methionine, threonine, tryptophan, isoleucine, leucine, lysine, valine, and phenylalanine). Animal proteins, with the exception of gelatin, are excellent sources of complete protein. By mixing plant proteins from different sources (legumes, cereals, and nuts), adequate protein can be obtained in vegetarian meals. Adequate protein is vital for normal growth and the formation of antibodies, hormones, enzymes, and the many tissue proteins.

Energy requirements are based on the amount of energy needed to keep a resting body operating (basal metabolism), the amount necessary for all body movements and activities, and the energy expended in releasing energy from food (thermic effect).

The balance between caloric intake and expenditure determines whether weight is gained, maintained, or lost.

Several inorganic materials are essential for such functions as controlling water balance, regulating acid-base balance, catalyzing chemical reactions, providing structure, and forming key constituents of such essential substances as enzymes and hormones. Calcium is a crucial component of bones and teeth, and a deficiency may lead to osteoporosis or osteomalacia. Iron is the mineral contained in hemoglobin, the compound in the blood responsible for oxygen transport and waste elimination. An iron deficiency causes iron-deficiency anemia. Copper serves as a catalyst in such reactions as the formation of hemoglobin and in the cytochrome system reactions in the release of energy. Fluoride, because of its ability to strengthen the matrix of bones and teeth during tooth formation, is an important mineral for children and is recommended as fluoridated water in the diet. Goiter, an enlargement of the thyroid gland in the throat caused by inadequate iodine in the diet, is rarely seen in the United States today because of the use of iodized salt. Although not common in the United States, a zinc deficiency can occur and is evidenced by poor taste perception and delayed sexual maturation. Excessive amounts of some minerals may present problems, such as elevated blood pressure from excessive salt intake and hemosiderosis from too much iron. Heavy metals, such as lead and mercury, should not be included in the food consumed.

Vitamins, categorized as either fat-soluble or water-soluble, are needed in extremely small amounts in the body. Vitamin A is a fat-soluble vitamin needed for night vision, normal skin, and growth. Vitamin A deficiencies can cause night blindness, xerophthalmia, and hyperkeratosis. The other fat-soluble vitamins include vitamin D, which is important for the absorption of calcium, vitamin E, and vitamin K. The vitamin D deficiency leads to rickets; vitamin E serves as an antioxidant, but no known physical problems result from a deficiency. In very young infants, a vitamin K deficiency can result in hemorrhaging.

Vitamin C is a widely-publicized water-soluble vitamin needed to form connective tissue, protect against infections, and promote bone growth. Scurvy develops when vitamin C is inadequate in the diet. The B vitamins (thiamin, riboflavin, niacin, vitamin B_6, pantothentic acid, biotin, folate, and vitamin B_{12}) perform a wide variety of functions. Several of them serve as coenzymes in reactions involved in energy release. Folacin and vitamin B_{12} are needed for maturation of red blood cells. A thiamin deficiency causes beriberi; ariboflavinosis is the result of a riboflavin deficiency, and pellagra is caused by lack of niacin.

Water is also a nutrient. Its importance is due to its function as a solvent and transport medium essential for carrying nutrients to cells and removing waste products. Another contribution of water is its role as a lubricant in helping the food mass move through the gastrointestinal tract and in lubricating joints and other parts of the body.

The amounts of nutrients needed for good health on a daily basis have been identified by the Food and Nutrition Board with the Institute of Medicine at the National Academy of Sciences. These are presented in the tables of Recommended Dietary Allowances (RDA), Adequate Intake (AIs), and Tolerable Upper Intake Level (ULs).

These values are interpreted in practical terms via the 2000 Dietary Guidelines for Americans and the Food Guide Pyramid. The Food Guide Pyramid is based on 5 recommended groups (bread, cereal, rice, and pasta; vegetable; fruit; milk, yogurt, and cheese; and meat, poultry, fish, dry beans, eggs, and nuts). The amounts recommended in each group are based on age, sex, and activity level of the person. Serving sizes and numbers of servings recommended for each group are presented in this chapter. Fats, oils, and sweets are to be eaten only sparingly.

BIBLIOGRAPHY

FOOD AND NUTRITION BOARD *Recommended Dietary Allowances* 10th ed. National Academy Press. Washington, D.C. 1989. Revised 1998.

FOOD AND NUTRITION BOARD Dietary Reference Intakes (DRIs) for calcium, phosphorus, magnesium, vitamin D, and fluoride. *Nutrition Today 32(5):* 182. 1997.

FOOD AND NUTRITION BOARD Most frequently asked questions. . . about 1997 Dietary Reference Intakes (DRIs). *Nutrition Today 32(5):* 189. 1997.

JOHNSON, R.K. AND E. KENNEDY The 2000 Dietary Guidelines for Americans: what are the changes and why were they made? *J. Am. Dietet. Assoc. 100(7):* 769. 2000.

MONSEN, E.R. New Dietary Reference Intakes proposed to replace the Recommended Dietary Allowances. *J. Am. Dietet. Assoc. 86(8):* 754.

WELSH, S., ET AL Development of the Food Guide Pyramid. *Nutrition Today 27(6):* 12. 1992.

CHAPTER TWO

Physical Development

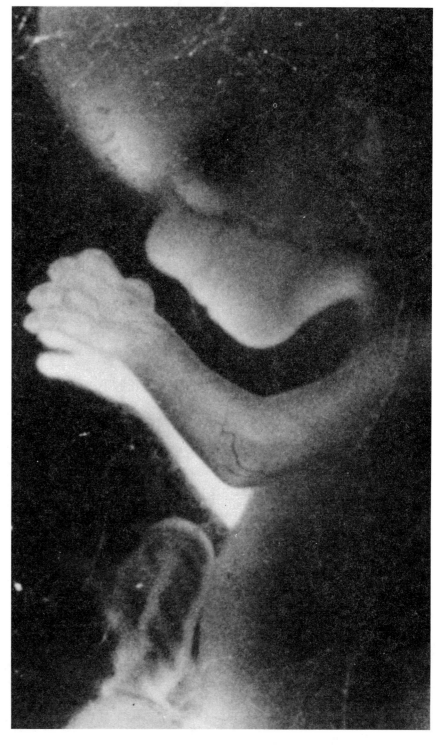

OVERVIEW

ANTENATAL
Period from conception to birth; also often termed prenatal.

POSTNATAL
Period from birth throughout life.

ZYGOTE STAGE
First 2 weeks of pregnancy.

EMBRYONIC STAGE
Weeks 3–8 of pregnancy.

FETAL STAGE
Week 9 until birth.

As the nation's history is often divided into antebellum and postbellum periods, so the study of human growth is ordinarily divided into two periods — antenatal and postnatal. The antenatal, or prenatal, period is marked by spectacular growth, in both size and function. Yet despite the fantastic changes prior to birth, considerable growth must be accomplished between birth and the end of adolescence. To achieve growth potential by adulthood, a tremendous amount of nutrients must be isolated from available foods and incorporated into the innumerable complex substances comprising the total body. When you consider the figures for height, weight, and other aspects during growth, keep in mind the body's wonderful ability to process food into functional physical structures.

The antenatal period begins with the zygote stage, which leads to implantation in a two-week period, the embryonic stage is from the third week through the eighth week of pregnancy, and the fetal stage extends from the ninth week to birth. In contrast to the three distinct stages identified in

61

the antenatal phase of growth, postnatal stages are not clearly defined. However, in the first year of life attention is often focused on growth. The beginning of the second year until age five is a period of continued, but slower growth, and rather unremarkable growth remains the pattern until the impressive spurt and final tapering off of growth in adolescence.

PRENATAL DEVELOPMENT

THE FIRST PHASE

Initially, the ovum is fertilized by the male sperm, which leads to the formation of a zygote. The zygote is a fertilized ovum containing a nucleus and cytoplasm enclosed in a membrane. Within the zygote, cell division occurs rapidly, resulting in 16 cells by the end of the first 72 hours. These cells, considerably smaller than the original ovum, are called blastomeres. The result is formation of a cluster of cells, the morula, by the time the developing being enters the uterus. Usually, the morula reaches the uterus within five days of fertilization. The tight clustering of cells changes to an arrangement in which the cells form a single layer around a fluid-filled hollow. All the cells within this blastocyst need to be present so that cell division and differentiation can proceed normally.

The ring of outer cells in the blastocyst is differentiated and destined to become the supporting organs of the pregnancy. These cells, called the trophoblastic cells, will develop into four important structures: 1) the amnion (fluid-containing sac or membrane in which the organism develops), 2) the yolk sac, 3) the chorion (protective covering), and 4) the placenta (vital link for exchange between maternal and fetal systems). It is the inner cell mass that becomes the embryo.

About eight days after fertilization, the blastocyst begins to attach itself to the endometrium lining the uterus. Attachment of the tiny blastocyst (about 0.01 inch in diameter) occurs with the trophoblastic cells oriented toward the interior of the uterine cavity and the fluid-filled portion (the inner cell mass) adjacent to the uterine wall. Implantation is a very important step nutritionally, for this attachment with the maternal tissues intitiates development of the avenue that will provide for exchange of nutrients and waste between the two systems.

ZYGOTE
Fertilized ovum; consists of nucleus, cytoplasm, and a surrounding membrane.

BLASTOMERES
Small cells resulting from the division of the ovum in the early phase of pregnancy.

MORULA
Cluster of blastomeres (cells) traversing the fallopian tube and entering the uterus.

BLASTOCYST
A spherical collection of cells resulting from the repeated division of cells from a fertilized ovum and consisting of a single layer of cells surrounding a fluid-filled hollow.

TROPHOBLASTIC CELLS
Cells destined to form the external cover of the embryo and the supporting organs (amnion, yolk sac, chorion, and placenta) of pregnancy.

AMNION
Fluid-containing sac enclosing the developing being.

YOLK SAC
Sac connecting with the embryonic tissue until the placenta is developed, becoming part of the umbilical cord.

Outer embryonic membrane involved in the formation of the placenta and surrounding the amnion.

THE EMBRYONIC PHASE

From implantation until the end of the second month of pregnancy, remarkable developments occur as the developing being (now called an embryo) undergoes key changes. The inner cell mass differentiates into three germinal layers — the ectoderm, the mesoderm, and the endoderm. The ectoderm primary germ layer will develop into the outer layer of skin, tooth enamel, nerve tissues, the epithelial lining of the mouth, nose, and similar regions, hair, and nails (Table 2.1). The mesoderm will be the source of the various types of muscles, including heart, smooth, and skeletal muscles. The mesoderm is also the

TABLE 2.1 Approximate Timetable for Growth and Development During the Antenatal Period

Stage	Age (weeks)	Approximate Size	Development
Ovum	0	0.004"	

Zygote	0–2	0.007"	Subdivision
			  Trophoblastic cells (external)
			  Embryo (internal cells)

Embryo	3–8	0.007–1.18"
		0.01 lb
			Three layers:
			  Ectoderm (brain, nervous system, hair, skin, nails)
			  Mesoderm (voluntary muscles, excretory system, circulatory system, heart, bones, inner skin)
			  Endosperm (inner lining of digestive and respiratory tracts, glands)
			Protein synthesis

	3	0.007"	Forebrain, midbrain, hindbrain
	4	0.16"	Heart beats, neural fold for central nervous system; digestive system forming; beginning of budding of arms and legs
	5	0.21"	Central nervous system; intestinal tract; lungs, liver, skin
	6	0.43"	Umbilical cord and beginning of placenta Arm buds; bones
	7	0.75"	Teeth germs; lining of esophagus and intestine
	8	1.2"	Digits well formed; tail-like process disappears; face and features forming; internal organs developing Placenta complete

origin of kidneys, bones, gonads, connective tissue, and blood. The endoderm forms the digestive tract and associated structures, including glands and the epithelial tissues of the respiratory and digestive tract.

Prospective parents are usually on tenterhooks until they know whether their child is a boy or a girl. Resolution of this question actually starts during the embryonic period in about the seventh week when sexual differentiation begins. This differentiation requires a little over two weeks to complete.

Development of the nervous system is given priority in the embryonic stage, with the primitive streak (a fold in the ectoderm)

PLACENTA
Somewhat flat structure responsible for the exchange of nutrients and waste between the mother and embryo in the second and third trimesters of pregnancy.

TABLE 2.1 Approximate Timetable for Growth and Development During the Antenatal Period (cont.)

Stage	Age (weeks)	Approximate Size	Development
Fetus	9–40	1.2–2.0" 0.01–7.7 lb	Protein production; continuing maturation in preparation for birth
	9	1.2–2.4" 0.01 lb	Connective tissue, cartilage, and bone
	12	2.8–3.5" 0.06 lb	Bone calcification; sex readily determined; nails developing; eyes almost developed; blood formation beginning in bone marrow; adipose tissue
	16	3.9–6.7" 0.26 lb	Maximum rate of growth; strong heart-beat; hair on head; muscles active; myelination beginning
	20	7.1–10.6" 0.73 lb	Brain is 13 percent of total weight; enamel and dentin depositing in teeth; creamy coating developing; heart-beat discernible
	24	11.0–13.4" 1.32 lb	Eyebrows and eyelashes; calcification of teeth; lungs developing, but not able to function; eyelids separate
	28	13.8–15.0" 2.2 lb	Wrinkled skin; lungs and intestines immature
	32	16.5–17.7" 3.5 lb	Subcutaneous fat deposits; fair chance of survival
	36	18.5" 5.5 lb	Fine hair disappearing; skin still has creamy coating
	40	20" 7.7 lb	Birth

becoming evident when the developing organism is about 2 1/2 weeks old. The primitive streak continues to develop until the fourth week, when the neural folds fuse together, forming the neural tube. This tube serves as the foundation for the development of the central nervous system. Through differentiation, the anterior of the neural tube develops into the brain; its posterior forms the spinal column. The significant spinal and cranial nerves evolve from the cells at the crest of the neural tube. Development of this crucial system results from differentiation which occurs during the first three weeks of pregnancy, a sobering fact that emphasizes the importance of optimal physical condition in the early period, when a woman may not know she is pregnant. Of course, considerable refinement occurs during the remainder of pregnancy, but the areas that will become the brain, nervous system, and spinal cord are identifiable within three weeks.

After the nervous system has become established and the rudiments of the brain have been defined, growth is directed toward developing the heart and circulatory system (Fig. 2.1). The heart develops from the mesoderm, assuming an S-shaped appearance before its final shape. The development of this vital structure is so rapid that there is actually a heartbeat within 28 days of conception! The blood supply is generated by the embryo itself.

Concurrently, the respiratory and digestive systems develop as a result of changes in the tube in the endoderm. The lungs, liver, and digestive tract develop from the dorsal part of the yolk sac. Toward the end of the embryonic period (around the eighth week), the epithelial linings of the intestine and esophagus also develop rapidly. Meanwhile, the respiratory system is also differentiating, with the buds of the lungs, the trachea, and bronchi being evident at about six weeks of gestation. The developing lungs move into the thoracic cavity slowly during the early fetal period.

By the end of the first month of gestation, the ear canal, eustachian tube, and eardrum are evident, and much of the differentiation is completed within six weeks of conception. The arm buds appear, and the bones begin to develop within the sixth week. The appearance of the clavicle is soon followed by the long bones of the arms and those of the legs. The teeth germs, derived from both the ectoderm and the mesoderm, begin to develop into teeth at about seven weeks of gestation. The ectoderm in the

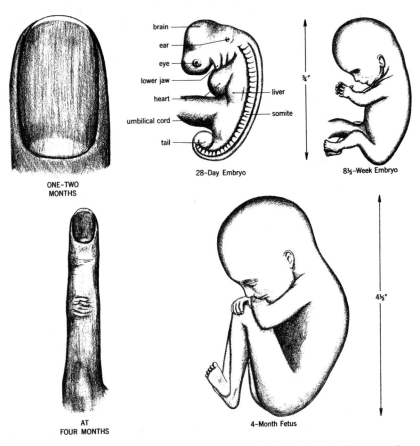

brain
ear
eye
lower jaw
heart
umbilical cord
tail
liver
somite

28-Day Embryo

¾"

8½-Week Embryo

ONE-TWO
MONTHS

AT
FOUR MONTHS

4½"

4-Month Fetus

Fig. 2.1   Embryonic and fetal development during the first four months.

germs will form the enamel of the developing teeth; the mesoderm will evolve into dentin and pulp.

The embryonic period, lasting through the eighth week of pregnancy, is a key time for establishing the various systems comprising the body. In fact, all the systems are defined by the end of the eighth week.

THE FETAL PERIOD

Differentiation is the significant achievement of the embryonic period. In contrast, the fetal period is distinguished by remarkable cellular growth — a growth measured by multiplication in the number of cells and by the increased cell size. The significance of this growth during the ninth week through birth at about 40 weeks is apparent when we note the increased length (from 1.2 inches at nine weeks to about 20 inches at birth) and weight gain during the same period (from 0.01 lb to more than 7.5 lb). Increased cellular content is accompanied by formation of necessary intercellular substances.

Protein synethesis continues to be vital to the fetal period, just as it played an important part in the embryonic stage. However, the focus of this synthesis is on the continued production of comparatively large quantities of the types of proteins that were first synthesized during the embryonic period. Production of both DNA (deoxyribonucleic acid) and necessary proteins in the cells results in an increase in individual cell size during this phase of pregnancy, where emphasis is on growth.

HYPERPLASIA
Unusually rapid cell division; in the case of brain development, hyperplasia is normal in the first stage.

The importance of protein synthesis is emphasized in the brain, where growth is particularly rapid during this period. In the first stage of brain development, the cells divide very rapidly (a process called hyperplasia), increasing the weight of the brain and raising the protein content. Soon the rate of cell division is reduced, although the number of cells continues to increase somewhat. In fact, at 20 weeks of gestation, the brain represents 13 percent of the total weight of the fetus, a value that persists through birth. This is quite a contrast to adults, whose brains represent only 2 percent of total weight. For this remarkable brain growth to occur, a considerable amount of protein must be synthesized. Myelination (formation of the protective coating) of the brain is quite limited at the time of birth. Much of the increase in brain weight occurring after birth is the result of completion of the myelin covering.

MYELIN
Protective covering of the brain and other parts of the nervous system.

The heart begins beating during the fourth week of gestation, and its chemical composition remains relatively constant. By the time the fetus is 20 weeks old, the heart represents about 0.6 percent of the total weight in contrast to about 0.4 percent in adults. Clearly, the growth of the heart parallels the growth of the body far more closely than does the brain, with its remarkably accelerated development during gestation.

Structural parts of the body — bones, connective tissue, and cartilage — become significant during the third month. The calcification process begins in about the eighth week. During calcification and development of the bones, there is a gradual and continuing loss of water, accompanied by an increase in both total nitrogen and connective tissue nitrogen, calcium, and phosphorus. The ratio of calcium to phosphorus shows an increase throughout the fetal period. Protein increase in the body during the 32 weeks of the fetal stage occurs at a much faster rate than during the embryonic period. Only about 0.4 gm of protein are present at the end of eight weeks, but the average protein content is about 362 gm at birth.

Fatty deposits (adipose tissue) usually begin to appear in the fetus in the fourth month of gestation. The last two months of pregnancy are the period when deposition occurs most rapidly. The combination of growth of the various systems and fatty deposits results in a fairly constant rate of weight gain in the fetus from about the 19th week to the 32nd week, when the rate of gain is slowed. Once the fetus reaches about 6.6 lb, the weight gain rate decreases sharply, as shown in Fig. 2.2. Related to this weight gain pattern is the fact that the relative proportion of water in the muscles decreases appreciably as completion of gestation approaches. Accompanying this drop in muscle water content is a drop in sodium and chloride levels.

DEVELOPMENT OF THE PLACENTA

A key development during pregnancy is the formation of a specialized organ, the placenta, which is the means of providing nutrients and oxygen to the embryo and fetus, as well as the means of removing waste products. Not only is the placenta essential for these transport functions, it is also the site where

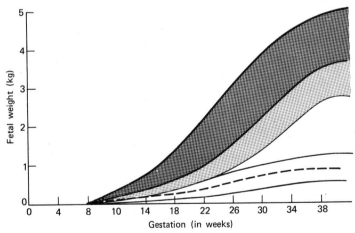

Fig. 2.2   Mean weight of the human fetus (solid line), mean weight of the placenta (dotted line), and range of fetal weight (shaded area). Adapted from R. Greenhill. *Obstetrics*. Thirteenth Edition. Saunders. Philadelphia. 1965.

some maternal hormones are produced. Gonadotropic hormones, estrogens, and gestagens are hormones important in stimulating development during pregnancy. The placenta's key roles explain why there is a positive correlation between placental size and the outcome of pregnancy.

Placental development begins with a small group of cells multiplying so rapidly that within three weeks of conception the placenta extends over 20 percent of the uterus. In fact, by the end of the first week, the blastocyst is able to penetrate the uterine mucosa. The trophoblast promptly begins to appear in the lacunae at about the 12th day, but circulation does not begin until approximately one week later (19 days).

LACUNAE
Small spaces in the trophoblast in which maternal blood is found by the twelfth day of pregnancy.

The reticulum, or network, of the placenta develops into a somewhat regular form, best described as being root-like in appearance, with roots radiating from the chorion of the placenta. The chorion is the membrane providing connection to the fetal blood supply, while another layer, the decidua vera, performs this role on the maternal side. Chorionic villi (Fig. 2.3) form and are penetrated by capillaries that are ultimately extensions of the two arteries from the embryo to the umbilical cord and return. Thus, the villi provide the route by which fetal blood supply is brought into close proximity with maternal blood, for maternal blood circulates in the intervillous spaces surrounding the villi. The umbilical cord also houses a vein bringing nutrients to the fetus. Although there is no actual merging of maternal and fetal blood supplies, the large surface area provided by the villi admirably promotes exchange between the two.

UMBILICAL CORD
Structure containing the vein that brings nutrients and oxygen to the embryo or fetus and the two arteries that remove waste products from the fetus to the mother.

Around the fourth week of pregnancy, the embryonic heart starts to pump blood, and the placenta starts to perform in its transport mode. By the seventh week, the placenta begins to serve as protection, blocking the transfer of some drugs, viruses, or other undesirable substances to the embryo. The growth of the placenta is even more rapid than the embryo (and fetus) for almost the first four months of pregnancy. Gradually, the growth rate of the fetus overtakes that of the placenta, and the placenta stops growing at 36 weeks of gestation. In fact, there may be a small decrease in size during the final phase of pregnancy. The placenta usually weighs about one-seventh as much as the infant at birth, or about 500 gm (a little over 1 lb) for an infant weighing 3500 gm (almost 7 1/4 lb).

The role of the placenta in the transport of oxygen, as well as nutrients, is central to normal fetal development. Development of the fetal vascular system and adequacy of maternal

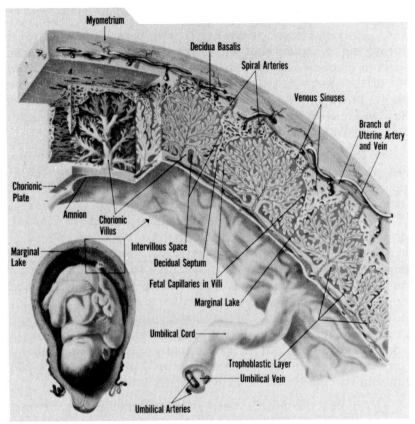

Fig. 2.3   Diagram of the Placenta.

Labels in figure:
Myometrium
Decidua Basalis
Spiral Arteries
Venous Sinuses
Branch of Uterine Artery and Vein
Chorionic Plate
Amnion
Chorionic Villus
Marginal Lake
Intervillous Space
Decidual Septum
Fetal Capillaries in Villi
Marginal Lake
Umbilical Cord
Trophoblastic Layer
Umbilical Vein
Umbilical Arteries

blood circulation are essential to meeting fetal needs. In women who smoke during pregnancy, smoking appears to limit circulation and constrict the uterine arteries, which is detrimental to normal growth during the fetal period. The consequence well may be birth of a small-for-date baby.

The procedures involved in exchanging nutrients, oxygen, and waste materials between mother and fetus are complex. Actually, there are four different mechanisms which may be involved in accomplishing these exchanges: active transport,

SMALL-FOR-DATE BABY
Baby that is lighter than the normal weight of a newborn of the same gestational age.

pinocytosis, simple diffusion, and facilitated diffusion. One or more of these mechanisms may be involved at any time.

ACTIVE TRANSPORT
Energy-consuming transport of some nutrients bound to protein carriers allowing these nutrients to pass through the barrier separating maternal blood from the fetal supply.

Active transport is an absorption mechanism involving energy derived from adenosine triphosphate (ATP). Amino acids, glucose (and fructose to a very limited extent), vitamin C, the B vitamins, and some minerals (calcium, iron, and sodium) are transferred from the maternal blood supply to the fetus by an energy-expending process. Active transport occurs when a nutrient bound to a carrier protein has enough energy available from ATP to traverse the electrochemical barrier between the maternal and fetal circulatory systems.

CALCITONIN
Hormone helping to regulate calcium levels in the blood by favoring deposit of calcium in bones when blood calcium levels are above normal.

Fortunately, for the deposition of calcium in the fetus, active transport can establish a higher concentration of a nutrient on one side of the placenta than on the other. Fetal calcium levels are higher than those on the maternal side of the placenta. This high level of calcium in the fetal blood stimulates production of calcitonin (hormone promoting removal of calcium from the blood) in the fetus. This calcitonin supply favors removal of calcium from the blood by depositing it in the body's storage reservoirs, the bones — exactly what is needed for optimal growth and development of the fetus! The situation is enhanced by an opposite reaction that occurs simultaneously in the mother. Since the active transport of calcium in the maternal

PARATHYROID HORMONE
Hormone promoting withdrawal of calcium from bones to restore normal blood calcium levels.

blood is accompanied by a corresponding loss of calcium in the maternal blood, production of the parathyroid hormone is stimulated in her body. Parathyroid hormone causes the mother's bones to give up calcium to help reach the normal level of calcium in her blood. The additional calcium resulting from stimulation of the production of parathyroid hormone makes still more calcium available to undergo active transport to the fetus. In this way, the nutrient transfer cycle is perpetuated to the benefit of the infant's skeletal development.

PINOCYTOSIS
Transfer of certain polypeptide units by surrounding them with fluid, folding the fluid and polypeptide into the cell, and pinching off from the maternal side of the placenta.

Amino acids are transferred from the mother to the fetus by active transport to provide the building blocks of protein needed for growth and development. However, some much larger protein units of immunological importance, as well as hormonal polypeptides, need to be transferred intact to the fetus from the mother, a task which cannot be accomplished by active transport. Pinocytosis is the transfer mechanism making this movement possible. A comparatively large protein molecule surrounded by fluid can be folded into a cell and then pinched off from the maternal side of the placenta to be received into the fetal system. Immunoglobulin (IgG), an important protective substance that provides resistance to infections during gestation and for more than six months after birth, is transferred to the fetus by pinocytosis.

Diffusion permits some minerals to pass between the maternal and fetal sides without added energy and without the need for a carrier protein. Sodium, chloride, magnesium, and potassium are all examples of minerals entering the fetus by simple diffusion. Oxygen is also shifted by simple diffusion.

The fetus needs to synthesize its own fats, generally making the component fatty acids from acetate and other precursors that are easily transferred from the mother. Linoleic acid, the essential fatty acid, can apparently be transferred, because it cannot be synthesized by the fetus. Free cholesterol apparently can also be transferred directly to the fetal supply, although slowly. In the chorionic tissue of the placenta, phospholipids are split; the free phosphate ion is then transferred to the fetus for incorporation in fetal phospholipids.

The ability of two-carbon fragments, resulting from the metabolism of fats, to pass to the fetus can present a hazard to a fetus if the mother is trying to lose weight. Ordinarily, two-carbon fragments that are split from fatty acids enter the Krebs cycle for ultimate breakdown to carbon dioxide, water, and energy. However, this process proceeds normally only when there is sufficient carbohydrate to combine with these fragments, a situation which may not be true in people on severe diets. Ketone bodies begin to build up in the mother as some of her fatty deposits are used for energy, and these ketone bodies can be transferred to the fetus, causing impaired neuropsychological development. Clearly, weight reduction diets during pregnancy represent an unnecessary hazard to the fetus.

Not only must nutrients be transferred to the fetus, but waste products must also be removed. For instance, urea, uric acid, creatinine, and possibly some amino acids have to be returned to the maternal side of the placenta for excretion. Carbon dioxide is held in combination with fetal hemoglobin until the transfer can be made with oxygen from maternal hemoglobin. This exchange provides the fetus with necessary oxygen while eliminating waste carbon dioxide. The increasing blood flow and expanding area for maternal blood in the intervillous spaces of the placenta favor the exchange of oxygen for carbon dioxide, as well as the delivery of adequate quantities of nutrients during the demanding latter phases of pregnancy.

IMMUNOGLOBULIN (IgG)
Protective protein transferred from maternal side to fetal system by pinocytosis to provide resistance to infections during the fetal period and through at least the first six months of life.

DIFFUSION
Passage of an ion or other simple substance between the fetal and maternal systems without the need for a carrier or additional energy.

RESEARCH INSIGHTS

Godfrey, K.M. and D.J.P. Barker, Fetal nutrition and adult disease. *Am. J. Clin. Nutr. 71(suppl):* 1344S. 2000.

In this paper, Godfrey and Barker examine numerous longitudinal research studies exploring possible relationships between intrauterine growth and development and health risks in adulthood. Data from the United Kingdom, Norway, the United States, South Wales, and South India have shown an association between low birth weight and adult coronary heart disease. Death rates in adults from coronary heart disease decreased as birth weights rose from <2.2 kg to 4.3 kg; low fetal growth rate appeared to be associated with cardiovascular disease in adulthood. People who were thin or short at birth also were found to have increased likelihood of high blood pressure, elevated cholesterol values, and/or altered glucose metabolism and type 2 diabetes in their adult years.

These longitudinal effects of possible nutritional shortcomings during the intrauterine period remain the subject of study. The type of inadequacy, its duration and time during the pregnancy are of significance. Animal studies have indicated that fetal adaptations to nutritional stresses occur in an attempt to promote development and ultimate birth. However, physiological adaptations during the fetal period can result in permanent alterations in metabolism. Low-birth-weight infants who subsequently develop type 2 diabetes as adults provide an illustration of probable fetal adaptations. Undernutrition in the early part of pregnancy leads to development of small, but normally proportioned infants. In contrast, inadequate nutrition in the latter part of pregnancy may have little impact on birth weight, but may result in newborns that are disproportionate or short at birth.

Fetal tissue adaptations triggered by inadequate nutrition may be the result of changes in substrate availability and possibly hormonal influences. The intrauterine environment programs the development of systems and tissues such as the cardiovascular, respiratory, endocrine, immune, and central nervous systems, as well as muscles, bone, kidney, and the liver. Intrauterine programming appears to have an influence on health in the adult years for people with inadequate nutrition from the maternoplacental supply at some period prenatally.

Recognition of the potential influence of nutritional adequacy during the intrauterine period on health risks in adulthood is creating a need for more research to identify the optimal dietary plan for women during pregnancy. At the present level of knowledge, changes from current recommendations are not warranted. However, pregnant women who are not consuming a diet that meets the suggested intakes of all nutrients will need to make appropriate dietary changes if they are to promote optimal health for their developing fetuses and the adults ultimately resulting from their pregnancies.

POSTNATAL DEVELOPMENT

HEIGHT

Individuals vary in their growth rates, but they all grow at a decelerating rate the first year after birth. During the intrauterine period, growth is so rapid that most infants are almost 20 inches long at birth! If that remarkable growth were to continue during the first year, a one-year-old baby would be over 40 inches tall! Instead, the average height at one year is just under 30 in., representing an increase of about 50 percent over birth length; the rate of gain drops, on the average, from almost 5 in. during the first four months to about 2 in. in the last third of the first year (Table 2.2).

In contrast to the usual first-year growth of about 10 in., growth in the second year decelerates (Figs. 2.4 and 2.5) to a total

TABLE 2.2   Mean Heights (inches) of Boys and Girls from Birth to 36 Months[a]

Age	Percentile, Boys			Percentile, Girls		
	10th	50th	90th	10th	50th	90th
Birth	18.7	19.9	21.0	18.3	19.6	20.5
4 months	23.7	25.1	26.4	23.1	24.4	25.7
8 months	26.7	28.0	29.3	25.9	27.2	28.6
12 months	28.7	30.0	31.4	27.9	29.3	30.7
18 months	31.0	32.4	34.1	30.4	31.9	33.5
24 months	32.9	34.5	36.3	32.5	34.0	35.7
30 months	34.7	36.3	38.2	34.3	35.9	37.6
36 months	36.4	38.0	39.9	35.8	37.6	39.4

[a]Adapted from National Center for Health Statistics, Health Resources Administration, Dept. of Health and Welfare, Hyattsville, MD 20782.

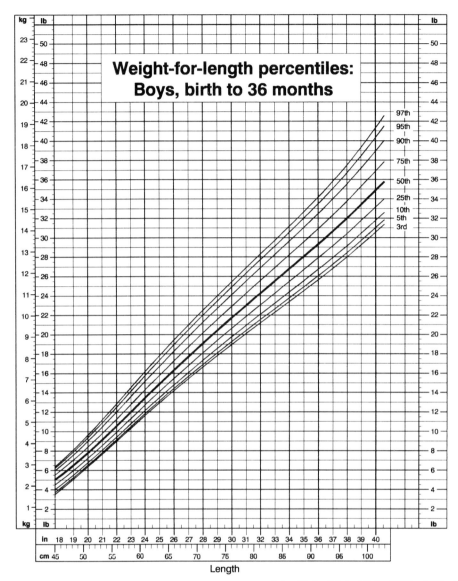

**Weight-for-length percentiles:
Boys, birth to 36 months**

Fig. 2.4   Weight-for-length percentiles (5th, 10th, 25th, 50th, 75th, 90th, 95th) for boys from birth to 36 months (National Center for Health Statistics in collaboration with the National Center for Chronic Disease Prevention and Health Promotion). 2000.

increase of approximately 5 in. between the first and second birthdays. After the second year, the growth rate levels off to a rate resulting in an increase of about 1 1/2 in. each year until the

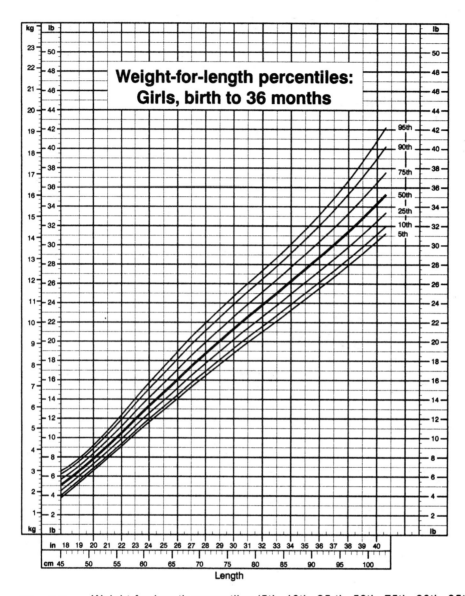

Fig. 2.5 Weight-for-length percentiles (5th, 10th, 25,th, 50th, 75th, 90th, 95th) for girls from birth to 36 months (National Center for Health Statistics in collaboration with the National Center for Chronic Disease Prevention and Health Promotion). 2000.

child reaches the adolescent growth spurt. If the growth rate remained as rapid throughout childhood as it is in the first year, height would increase by half each year, leading to some truly remarkable giants!

TABLE 2.3   Mean Heights (inches) of Boys and Girls, Ages 4 to 18[a]

Age (years)	Percentile, Boys			Percentile, Girls		
	10th	50th	90th	10th	50th	90th
4	38.3	40.5	42.6	38.0	40.0	41.8
5	40.8	43.3	45.4	40.4	42.7	44.8
6	42.4	45.7	48.0	42.0	45.1	47.6
7	45.3	47.9	50.4	44.7	47.5	50.2
8	46.5	50.0	52.6	46.7	49.8	52.8
9	49.3	52.0	54.9	48.8	52.0	55.4
10	51.2	54.1	57.3	51.0	54.4	58.0
11	53.2	56.4	59.9	53.4	57.0	60.5
12	55.2	58.9	62.8	56.0	59.6	63.0
13	57.4	61.6	65.7	58.3	61.9	65.1
14	58.6	64.2	68.4	59.6	63.1	66.4
15	62.3	66.5	70.4	60.3	63.7	67.1
16	64.5	68.3	71.8	60.7	63.9	67.4
17	66.0	69.4	72.6	61.1	64.2	67.4
18	66.4	69.6	73.0	61.4	64.4	68.3

[a]Adapted from National Center for Health Statistics, Health Resources Administration, Dept. of Health and Welfare, Hyattsville, MD 20782.

Boys are usually longer than girls at birth, and their small lead in height continues until puberty. The earlier onset of puberty for girls results in their being taller than boys during the early teens (Table 2.3). However, the range between the 10th and 90th percentiles means that many girls in the upper percentiles for height will be at least as tall or taller than boys in the lower percentiles for the same age, particularly in the years before the boys enter puberty.

When looking at the total person (including genetic, dietary, and environmental influences), growth rates vary somewhat among races, as well as between sexes. The mean birth length of an Afro-American is somewhat shorter than that of a White. However, this difference is countered during the first two years of life, when Afro-Americans catch up to and surpass White infants in height. In contrast, Oriental infants average less at birth in terms of height and weight, and, in general, tend to remain smaller than the averages for Whites. *Average* is stressed here as there is a great variation among individuals of any race.

The steady increase in height during the early years of childhood continues until the adolescent growth spurt is triggered. The age at which children enter puberty varies considerably, and girls ordinarily reach this point at a younger age than boys. Girls usually begin their rapid growth period between 10 1/2 and 11 years of age. Peak growth rate is reached at about 12 years of age, followed by a decreased rate between the ages of 13 and 14. The total period of rapid growth usually lasts from 2 to 2 1/2 years, resulting in an increase in height of about 6 1/3 in. By about age 15, girls will have reached 99 percent of their adult height (Table 2.4). Their growth usually ceases by the time they are 17 years old.

TABLE 2.4   Percentage of Mature Height Attained at Different Ages[a]

Chronological Age (years)	Percentage of Eventual Height	
	Boys	Girls
1	42.2	44.7
2	49.5	52.8
3	53.8	57.0
4	58.0	61.8
5	61.8	66.2
6	65.2	70.3
7	69.0	74.0
8	72.0	77.5
9	75.0	80.7
10	78.0	84.4
11	81.1	88.4
12	84.2	92.9
13	87.3	96.5
14	91.5	98.3
15	96.1	99.1
16	98.3	99.6
17	99.3	100.0
18	99.8	100.0

[a]From Bayley's longitudinal study of 150 boys and girls in California. *J. Pediat. 48:* 187, 1956.

Boys grow according to a pattern somewhat delayed in comparison to girls. The period of rapid growth for boys begins between ages 12 1/2 and 13, with the maximum rate occurring at 14 for most boys. Height increase during the approximately 2 1/2 years of rapid growth is remarkable — about 8 in. No wonder clothes never seem to fit during this period. Growth rate decelerates after this impressive spurt, but continues at least until the age of 18. Physical growth for boys and girls between the ages of 2 and 18 is charted in Figs. 2.6 and 2.7, respectively.

WEIGHT

Weight increases vary considerably from one person to another and are definitely less predictable than height. Nevertheless, general patterns of growth, as shown by weight, are interesting and useful in charting development in children. Increases in weight are more spectacular than increases in height during the growing years. Height usually increases about 3 1/2 times from birth to maturity, but adult weight normally is about 20 times birth weight!

The birth weight of girls averages about a third of a pound (approximately 140 gm) lighter than that of boys. First-born infants are generally lighter than those born later in the family sequence. If mothers are small themselves or of comparatively low socioeconomic backgrounds, their babies' birth weights will tend to be lighter than average.

Weight gain should be consistent with increases in height and should not be considered as the sole criterion of growth during infancy and early childhood. The normal infant will double its birth weight at about four months. Usually, birth weight is tripled by the first birthday. However, the rate of gain drops significantly during the second year, consistent with the slowing growth in stature. At the age of two, most toddlers will weigh about four times more than their birth weight. After the second birthday, the gain in weight settles down to a fairly constant gain of about five to six pounds a year until the adolescent growth spurt begins.

The adolescent spurt in height precedes accelerated weight gain by about three months. Then, increase in weight begins to parallel increase in height. The usual weight increase in the growth spurt is between 35 and 44 pounds in about 30 months, when growth is at a maximum.

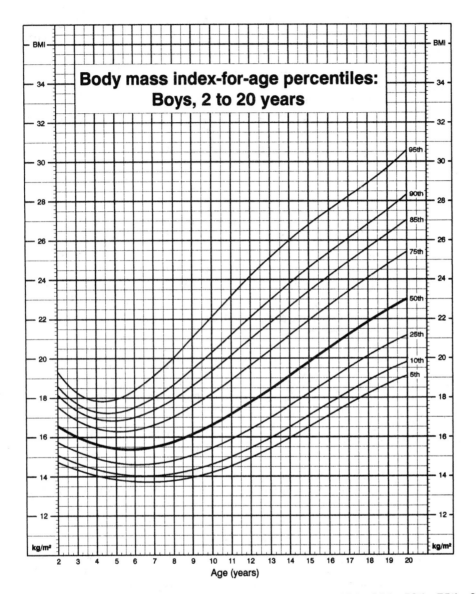

Fig. 2.6   Body mass index-for-age percentiles (5th, 10th, 25th, 50th, 75th, 90th, and 95th) for boys ages 2 to 20 (National Center for Health Statistics in collaboration with the National Center for Chronic Disease Prevention and Health Promotion). 2000.

The dramatic periods of growth in infancy and puberty are sometimes referred to as critical periods because of their importance in achieving desirable physical characteristics resulting from normal growth. The phenomenon of growth occurs in three distinct stages. Hyperplasia is the first phase, when the number

HYPERPLASIA AND HYPERTROPHY Intermediate phase of growth, marked by both an increase in cell number and cell size.

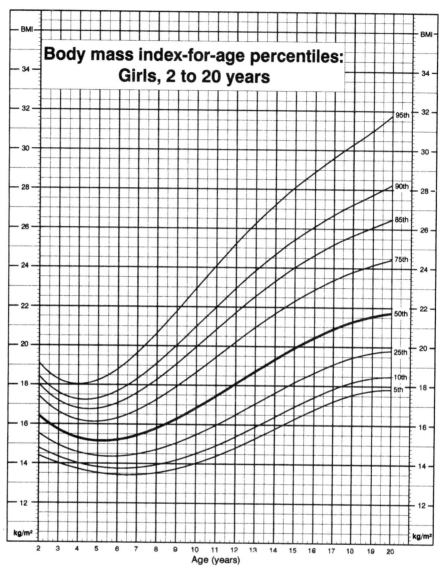

Body mass index-for-age percentiles: Girls, 2 to 20 years

Fig. 2.7   Body mass index-for-age percentiles (5th, 10th, 25th, 50th, 75th, 90th, and 95th) for girls ages 2 to 20 (National Center for Health Statistics in collaboration with the National Center for Chronic Disease Prevention and Health Promotion). 2000.

of cells increases significantly. Nutrition is particularly important for the organs during hyperplasia. Nutrient inadequacies may result in the formation of fewer cells than normal in the brain or other parts of the body, and supplemental nutrients after hyperplasia cannot overcome the reduction in the number of cells during the critical period.

In the second phase, while continuing to increase in number, cells also start to increase in size. This combination of growth in both number and in size is called hyperplasia and hypertrophy. The third stage is one of hypertrophy, that is, the cells are increasing in size only.

HYPERTROPHY
Intermediate phase of growth, marked by an increase in cell size only.

SKELETAL GROWTH

Not all parts of the body grow at the same rate after birth. As can be seen in Fig. 2.8, there is a noticeable change in the proportion of the head to the rest of the body. The head, which represents about one-fourth of the body length at birth, is ultimately only about one-eighth of the adult height. On the other hand, the legs increase from less than 40 percent of total length at birth to about 50 percent of adult height. These differences in growth during childhood cause gradual transitions in the way a person walks because of the shift in the center of gravity. In fact, the child just learning to walk is actually quite top-heavy due to the mass of the head. The arms, like the legs, are comparatively shorter at birth than in adulthood. Another interesting change can be seen by comparing the circumference of the chest and the head at birth and in adulthood. At birth, the two are about the

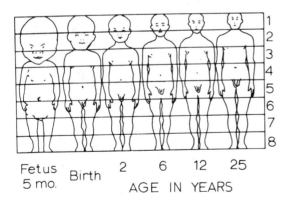

Fig. 2.8   Changes in body proportions during growth, keeping height constant. (Adapted from *The Development and Growth of the External Dimensions of the Human Body in the Fetal Period.* Scammon, R.E. and L.A. Calkins. Copyright 1929 by the University of Minnesota. University of Minnesota Press, Minneapolis.)

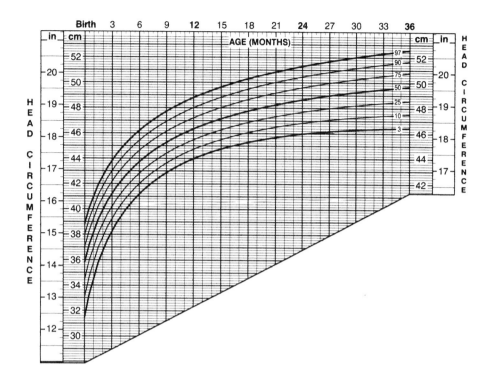

Fig. 2.9 Head circumference-for-age percentiles (5th, 10th, 25th, 50th, 75th, 90th, 95th) for boys from birth to 36 months (National Center for Health Statistics in collaboration with the National Center for Chronic Disease Prevention and Health Promotion). 2000.

same, but the circumference of the chest in adulthood clearly exceeds that of the head.

These various comparisons emphasize the point that the head is much closer in size to maturity at birth than are the other parts of the body. Furthermore, the head, which is already about 70 percent of its adult size at birth, continues to grow rapidly for the first six months of life (Figs. 2.9 and 2.10). The trunk grows faster than any other region of the body during the first year,

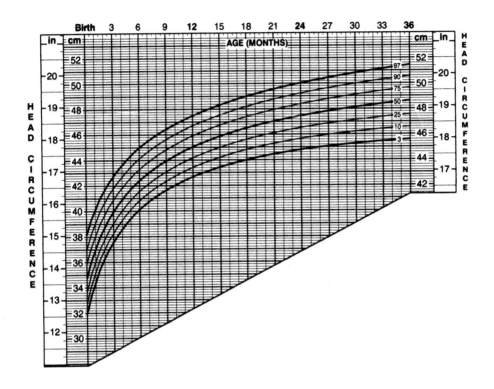

Fig. 2.10   Head circumference-for-age percentiles (5th, 10th, 25th, 50th, 75th, 90th, 95th) for girls from birth to 36 months (National Center for Health Statistics in collaboration with the National Center for Chronic Disease Prevention and Health Promotion). 2000.

usually reaching about 60 percent of its final length in this period. From the age of one year until the adolescent growth spurt, the legs are the region of the greatest growth, developing faster at the extremities than near the trunk. By the time of adolescence, the legs will have reached about two-thirds of their final length.

Several changes occur during the adolescent growth spurt. Growth in the trunk becomes a prominent feature. First, the hips and chest begin to grow at an increased rate, followed by the shoulders. The trunk lengthens, and finally the chest expands. Remarkably, these many changes occur in the space of about a year during the teenage growth spurt.

The skeleton is the source of considerable information about the state of maturation, for all skeletons follow a set maturational sequence. The first phase is development of bony centers; ultimately, 806 bony centers will be formed. In the second phase, the bony centers are modified in shape and subsequently fused into groups. In the final stage, there are orderly changes in the texture and composition of the bony centers. This sequence can be noted in the development of the jawbone and collarbone, which appear as bony centers in the first six weeks of prenatal development, and in a ridge at the top of the hipbone, which begins to develop as a bony center during puberty. When ossification begins, the first hard bony tissue is deposited in the bony center. As the bones begin to grow and touch each other, this contact changes and shapes the bony centers. The time the bony centers fuse varies with each portion of the skeleton. Some bony centers at the base of the skull fuse before birth, whereas certain bones in the wrists and ankles do not fuse during life.

Bone composition changes from the coarse and irregular tissues of early childhood to the more uniform secondary bony tissue of mature bones. These changes can be clearly noted in the development of any of the long bones in the arm or leg. First, differentiation from tissue into a white, rubbery substance (cartilage) occurs. This cartilage is gradually extended into the shape of a long bone, which is encircled by a ring of actual bone tissue at the center of the long cartilage. Growing in both directions, the ring of bone extends slowly along the length of the shaft until only the ends of the cartilage extend beyond this bone tissue

OSSEOUS
Bony

sleeve. As the sleeve develops, interior cartilage is being replaced by bony (osseous) tissue, which is rather spongy.

EPIPHYSIS
Bony end of the long bones.

As cartilage is extended at both ends, the bone continues to lengthen until the bony epiphysis (end of the long bone) appears in the cartilage at both ends. Beginning in the center of the cartilage, the epiphysis grows ever wider until only a thin disk of cartilage remains between the epiphysis and the bone shaft. This remaining disk of cartilage accomplishes the growth in bone length noted during childhood. Eventually, active growth of the cartilage disk stops, and cartilage is replaced by the hard bone of the sleeve and by spongy bone on the inside. When this transition is completed, the bony epiphysis and shaft are fused together, and growth is no longer possible.

As noted, bone length is accomplished as a result of cartilage growth. Fortunately, bones are also able to grow in circumference, which is important for strength in the lengthening bones. Increase in circumference is achieved by depositing new layers of bone on the exterior of existing bone. At the same time, older layers are being removed inside. During the growing years, the inner region of the bone is filled with spongy bone only in the ends of the bones. The dynamic nature of bone even in the adult years influences nutritional requirements throughout life, not just in childhood.

Height and bone maturation do not always proceed at an average rate. Skeletal maturity can be observed by studying X-rays of a child's wrist and hands. Atlases of X-rays of many children have been compiled to permit detailed study of growth and maturation rates. Some children are significantly smaller than an average child of the same age, and skeletal age may also be behind the average child of the same age. On the other hand, some small children have skeletal maturity consistent with their chronological age. When skeletal maturity and growth are both lagging, there is reason to anticipate that the child will continue to grow after other children have reached skeletal maturity, which will eliminate the discrepancy in height. However, it is predicted that small children who are on target with skeletal maturation will be shorter than normal.

Not all bones in the body mature at the same time. Differences can be noted simply by looking at the hand and wrist bones of 1-year-old infants. Three of the 28 bones will already be completely ossified, whereas some of the remaining bones will not become ossified and stop growing until much later. A similar circumstance is seen in the skull. There are six soft spots (the fontanelles) in the skull at birth, but gradual ossification ordinarily results in a completely ossified, rigid skull by the time the child is two. The unusually rapid rate of bone growth in the entire skull during the first nine months of life has been noted previously.

FONTANELLES Soft, membrane-covered areas in the skull that are present at birth, but are usually eliminated by growing skull bones by the age of two.

TEETH

CALCIFICATION Not all teeth begin to form at the same time, but they all follow the same developmental sequence in forming and preparing to erupt through the gums. For instance, the primary central incisor will begin to undergo calcification of the crown at a fetal age of 4 to 4 1/2 months and will be fully calcified when the infant is about 6 to 10 weeks old. Actual eruption usually occurs at about 6 months of age. At the opposite end of the developmental calendar is the third molar of the permanent teeth, which starts to calcify when the child is between 7 and 10 years old (Fig. 2.11).

ENAMEL
The hard protective layer covering the surface of a tooth.

DENTIN
The rather hard, dense substance comprising the main interior of the tooth under the enamel.

Teeth all begin to develop according to a pattern (Figs. 2.12 and 2.13) defined at the dentino-enamel junction. The matrix of enamel builds outward from this junction, layer upon layer. Dentin is also deposited in layers, but it builds inward toward the pulp cavity. When enamel deposits reach the size of the mature tooth, the cells needed for enamel deposition vanish. Enamel formation cannot occur after this point, even if tooth enamel is damaged. In contrast, dentin can be formed along the surface of the pulp if dental caries are causing erosion, but dentin's regeneration rate is rather slow, generally not adequate to compensate for the action of developing caries.

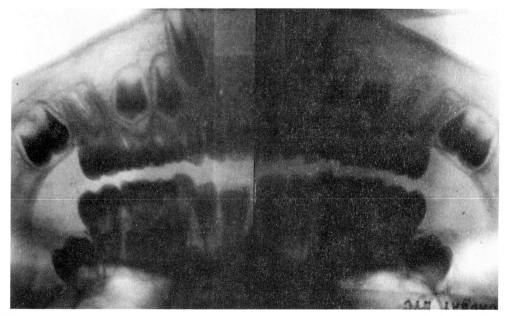

Fig. 2.11   Development of the permanent teeth continues over an extended period while the deciduous teeth are serving their functions. This X-ray shows the teeth of a nine-year-old.

Incremental lines in teeth form when calcification is interrupted. Normally, teeth develop rings or incremental lines at birth, 3 months, 10 months, 2 1/2 years, and 5 years. The trauma of birth and the adjustment from a parasitic to an independent existence are reflected in the ring that develops in teeth at that time. The next line develops at 3 months. The rationale for this line is the depletion of mineral stores that were deposited during the fetal period. Optimum calcification occurs in primary and permanent teeth between the fourth month of pregnancy and delivery, whereas the poorest calcification period is from birth to 10 months of age. Poor, but slightly better calcification periods are found between ages 2 1/2 and 5 and between ages 10 and 13. From 10 months until 2 1/2 years, the calcification process is

INCREMENTAL LINES
Apparent ring in enamel of teeth due to physical events that interrupt the calcification process.

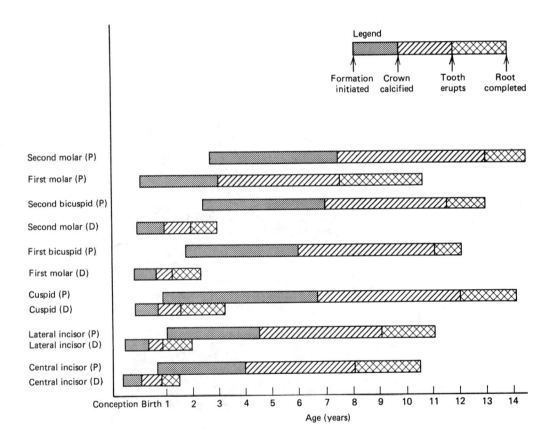

Fig. 2.12   Development of upper deciduous (D) and permanent (P) teeth.

only moderately favorable, whereas between the ages of 6 and 10 years calcification is good.

ERUPTION   The sequence in which primary teeth erupt through the gums is somewhat different from the eruption of permanent teeth. The first primary tooth is the central incisor, which comes through the gum at about six months of age, and the other primary teeth usually appear within the next 18 months. At about six years, the maximum number of teeth are contained, for the permanent ones are present (but not erupted), and and the primary teeth have not yet been lost. Gradually, the primary (deciduous) teeth are lost and replaced by the permanent teeth. Eruption of the permanent teeth usually occurs over a period of

DECIDUOUS TEETH
The primary teeth;
teeth that will fall out
to make room for
permanent teeth.

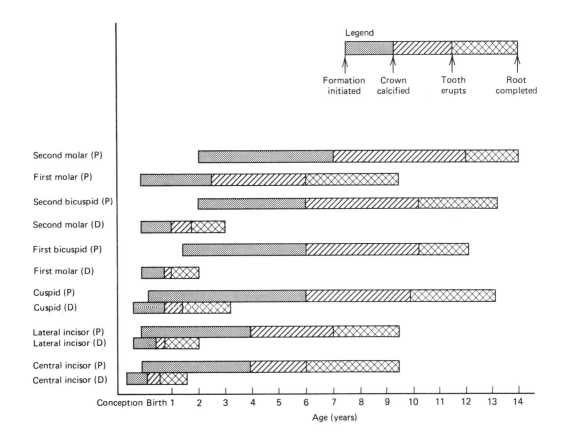

Fig. 2.13   Development of lower deciduous (D) and permanent (P) teeth.

at least nine years, beginning with the first molar at about age 6 and continuing well into the teens. Often, the third molar does not erupt until after age 15.

NERVOUS SYSTEM

The tremendous diversity in growth occurring in the various parts of the body following birth can be markedly contrasted by comparing the remarkable increase in the weight of the genital system, the muscles, and the pancreas from birth to maturity (an increase of approximately 30 to 40 times birth weight) with the growth of the nervous system (a modest 5 times)! The basic features of the nervous system are present at birth, although the brain doubles its birth weight during the first year, and the spinal cord continues to mature. An important stage in maturation after birth is the development of the myelin sheath, the protective covering on many nerve fibers of the brain and spinal cord. The motor pathways need to develop the myelin sheath after birth, whereas the pathways of transmission in the sensory tracts are fairly well myelinated at birth. New nerve cells stop developing at a fetal age of about six months, but existing nerve fibers continue to grow in length and diameter even after the myelin sheath has formed.

MYELIN SHEATH Protective covering or insulation surrounding nerve fibers, an important development for transmission of nerve impulses.

CARDIOVASCULAR SYSTEM

Birth represents a dramatic moment when the transition from dependent to independent being must occur, and this makes dramatic demands on the cardiovascular system. Oxygenation of the blood can no longer occur in the placenta. The lungs were bypassed during the fetal period, but they must now oxygenate the infant's blood supply, and the fetal bypass has to be terminated. At birth, the heart is somewhat larger in proportion to the rest of the body than it will be at maturity. The heart represents about 0.75 percent of total body weight at birth, but only about 0.4 percent of the body weight of a normal, mature person. This difference is possible because the lungs occupy less space in the rib cage at birth than they do as they expand later. During growth, the left ventricle walls of the heart thicken considerably more than those of the right ventricle because of the difference in work load. Growth of the heart, arteries, and veins parallels the growth of the child, with a significant increase occurring in the size of the heart during the rapid growth period of adolescence. Actually, the heart increases in weight from birth through the growing years at a slightly slower rate than the overall rate of increase for the entire body.

VENTRICLE Cavity or compartment in the heart.

Ordinarily, the newborn infant has an abundance of white blood cells at birth, and the number drops somewhat during adolescence. Red blood cells are at normal, adequate levels at birth, particularly when the infant's mother had sufficient iron in her diet during pregnancy. However, the red blood cell count drops during the first three months of life until the ability to form red blood cells is well established in the infant. A substantial increase in red blood cells occurs during adolescence, particularly in males, if the diet provides adequate levels of iron.

RESPIRATORY SYSTEM

As soon as breathing begins, the lungs increase rapidly in size, and air passages begin to change. The respiratory surface increases as additional alveoli (air cells in the lungs) and modifications of the respiratory bronchioles (tubes in the passageway of the trachea) develop. The diameters of the tubes also increase. The larynx grows rapidly at puberty, a change that is particularly noticeable in boys, who undergo a distinct change in voice. These developments result in a mature respiratory system weighing 20 to 25 times as much as it did at birth, a change roughly comparable to the change in skeletal weight.

DIGESTIVE SYSTEM

The capacity of the stomach actually triples in the first two weeks of life! The average capacity of a newborn is between 30 and 90 cc (2–3 tablespoons). It rises to between 90 and 150 cc at one month, to between 210 and 360 cc at one year, to about 500 cc at two years of age, and may increase to 900 cc just before puberty. As the infant grows, the stomach will gradually shift its position and part of the stomach may sometimes extend into the pelvic region. The small intestine, which reaches the pelvic region by maturity, is ordinarily between 300 and 350 cm (centimeters) long at birth, but it doubles in length by the onset of puberty.

Because the liver is important in blood formation during the fetal period, it is approximately 5 percent of body weight at birth. Although the liver continues to grow during childhood, the rate of growth is somewhat slower than other parts of the body; total body weight represented by the liver of an adult is only about 2.5 percent. The gall bladder, yet another important component of the digestive system, grows rapidly during the first two years of life.

The feeding response is vital to survival. Fortunately, newborns ordinarily develop the sucking response very quickly after birth, although premature infants take a bit longer, even a few days. Sucking triggers related contractions of the esophagus and peristalsis (involuntary contractions of the intestine that help move the food mass through the gastrointestinal tract).

EXCRETORY SYSTEM

Newborn infants have about twice the percentage of body weight from extracellular fluid as adults. Ordinarily, newborns will derive about 43 percent of their total body weight from extracellular fluid, as opposed to about 25 percent for adults. From this very high value at birth, there is a decrease in extracellular fluid, particularly during infancy, with a somewhat smaller decrease occurring during adolescence. The exchange of extracellular water in infants is very dynamic, for they ordinarily exchange about half of their extracellular water daily. Considerable loss can be attributed to fecal excretions. Infants have very limited ability to control water exchange, which makes them more susceptible to dehydration than adults.

The kidneys increase rather slowly in weight during gestation until the latter stage, when they begin to grow a bit more rapidly. They continue fairly rapid weight gain during the first year after birth, with a slower gain continuing into adolescence. Total weight gain of the kidneys from birth to maturity is from 10 to 15 times their birth weight. Urine excreted by infants is relatively acidic. Disturbances, such as those caused by diarrhea, can quickly lead to acidosis and abnormal fluid balance, with edema or dehydration being the result.

ENDOCRINE SYSTEM

Normal growth processes are masterminded by the pituitary gland and the hormones it produces. The anterior lobe of the pituitary gland produces several hormones: growth hormone, thyrotropin, corticotropin, two gonadotropins, and prolactin. Growth hormone facilitates hormone synthesis by promoting the transport of amino acids across cell walls. The breakdown of fatty acids and cartilage formation are also regulated by growth hormone. Giantism or dwarfism can be the result if the anterior lobe of the pituitary gland fails to function properly.

The thyroid gland is significant because of its role in producing thyroxine, which in turn influences basal metabolism. The functioning of the adrenals and the gonads is influenced

PERISTALSIS
Automatic contraction and relaxation of various muscles in the digestive tract to aid in moving the food mass through the gastrointestinal tract.

ENDOCRINE SYSTEM
Various ductless glands producing and secreting hormones into the bloodstream; includes the pituitary, thyroid, parathyroids, adrenal, thymus, pancreas, and ovaries or testes.

PITUITARY GLAND
Small endocrine gland associated with the gray matter of the brain that produces several hormones in its anterior lobe.

THYROID GLAND
Endocrine gland in the neck; produces thyroxine, the hormone regulating basal metabolic rate.

significantly by the thyroid gland. Normal growth and development, including bone growth and sexual development, are dependent upon normal functioning of the thyroid gland. Calcitonin is another hormone produced by the thyroid gland; it regulates calcium metabolism.

ADRENAL GLANDS
A pair of endocrine glands located adjacent to the kidneys; source of some steroid hormones and adrenaline.

ADRENALINE
Hormone produced by the adrenals; also called epinephrine.

PARATHYROID GLANDS
Endocrine glands in the neck that produce parathormone.

PARATHORMONE
Hormone produced by the parathyroid glands to trigger release of calcium from bones to maintain blood calcium levels.

The adrenal glands undergo an unusual pattern of development after birth. First, they lose about half their birth weight during the first three weeks of life. This loss is followed by a slow regaining of weight until they achieve their original weight by the age of three. Steroid hormones produced in the adrenal cortex are: 1) aldosterone, which regulates water balance and sodium and potassium excretion; 2) corticoids, which influence growth and help regulate carbohydrate-protein balance; and 3) androgens, which promote maleness and retention of nitrogen. Adrenaline is another product of the adrenals.

Regulation of calcium and phosphorus metabolism in the body is essential to normal body functioning, and the parathyroid glands play a vital role in this regulation by producing parathormone, the hormone triggering removal of calcium from bones when blood calcium levels are low. Normally, checks and balances provided by the thyroid and parathyroid glands will be effective in promoting optimal growth and bone formation. Hyperparathyroidism can lead to bone malformations.

The testes in males and the ovaries in females grow rapidly during early infancy and again in adolescence. The ovaries actually double their birth weight during the first six months of life, and they double again during adolescence. In contrast, the uterus in a female baby decreases in infancy to about half the weight it had at birth, a loss that is not counteracted until about 11 years later.

DEVELOPMENTAL MILESTONES

Not surprisingly, infants develop in their musculature and physical coordination at individual rates. Nevertheless, they proceed through the same developmental sequence, even though the age of occurrence varies from one infant to another. Careful research has been conducted to establish approximate timetables for achieving various milestones. Table 2.5 summarizes the ages at which 50 percent of the infants studied by Frankenberg and Dodds were able to do the activity indicated. Other researchers have found somewhat different ages for the various feats, but the sequence of development always remains the same. The various activities are important not only becuase they reveal physical development, but also because they begin to influence the nutrient need. Differences in persistence at various activities and vigor exercised in motor movements are key factors in determining the energy requirements for physical activity during infancy.

Clarke-Stewart and Koch (1983) cite a similar sequence of development, although the developmental tasks performed are identified on a monthly basis and are expanded beyond the list reported by Frankenberg and Dodds (1967). The tasks are noted on a monthly basis up to the age of one year, followed by an annual list to age five. Selected tasks are reported in Table 2.6. Whole body movements, such as scooting or crawling, usually begin at about seven months of age, with considerable individual variation expected. As mobility increases, energy needs increase for doing these activities. This need is partially offset by the slowing growth rate as infants approach their first birthday.

TABLE 2.5   Median Age for Performing Selected Developmental Tasks[a]

Developmental task	Age at which 50% can perform task (months)
Lift head when lying on stomach	2.2
Roll over from stomach to back	2.8
Sit up when propped	2.9
Sit without being supported	5.5
Stand while holding on	5.8
Walk while holding on	9.2
Stand momentarily before falling	9.8
Stand alone	11.5
Walk alone	12.1
Walk backward	14.3
Walk up steps	17.1
Kick ball forward	20.0

[a]Adapted from Frankenberg, W.K. and J.D. Dodds, Denver Developmental Screening Test. *J. Ped. 71:* 181. 1967.

TABLE 2.6 Approximate Age for Performing Selected
Developmental Tasks[a]

Developmental task	Age at which 50% can perform task (months)
Lift chin when resting on stomach	1
Lift chest and shoulders when resting on stomach	2
Reach for object while lying on back, but miss	3
Sit with support and head erect	4
Roll over from stomach to back; grasp at objects unsuccessfully; sit on lap	5
Sit in high chair; grasp dangling objects	6
Sit alone a short time; wriggle or scoot	7
Stand with help	8
Stand and hang onto furniture; roll over from back to stomach	9
Creep; sit a fairly long time	10
Walk when led; stand alone	11
Pull up to stand by furniture; take step and fall	12
Climb stairs; walk alone	13
Run	<2 years
Unlace shoes; pick up and stack blocks	2 years
Trace a circle	3 years
Trace a cross (+); button own cloths	4 years
Lace shoes; trace diamond easily and triangle slowly	5 years

[a]Clarke-Stewart and Koch. *Children — Development through Adolescence.* Wiley. New York. 1993.

SUMMARY

Development begins with the zygote stage for the first two weeks following conception and is succeeded by the embryonic stage from the third through the eighth week of pregnancy. The fetal stage is the point from the ninth week through birth. From the original cell mass, the ectoderm is differentiated to develop into the outer skin, nerve tissues, tooth enamel, hair, nails, and the linings of the mouth, nose, and similar regions. The mesoderm evolves into the voluntary muscles, excretory system, circulatory system, heart, bones, and inner skin. The endoderm becomes the digestive system, the respiratory tract, and the glands.

The remarkable differentiation occurring during the embryonic stage is followed by the amazing growth of the fetal period. Cell formation and growth result in the birth of infants averaging about 20 inches in length and weighing about 7.5 lb. The development of the placenta is an essential aspect of pregnancy, for this organ provides the route for the developing being to obtain nutrients and excrete waste.

Following birth, there is about a 50 percent increase in height in the first year. By the end of the second year, growth rate has slowed to about 2.5 inches a year; this holds until the adolescent growth spurt begins. On the average, boys are taller than girls of the same age. Girls pass boys for a short time at the beginning of adolescence because they reach their pubertal period about two years earlier than boys.

Weight gains are much more variable than height increases; normal infants double their birth weight at about four months of age and triple their weight by the first birthday. They gain another seven or more pounds during the second year, but the rate usually drops to five to six pounds annually after the age of two.

The different parts of the body develop at different rates, which changes the physical proportions observed at various ages. At birth, the head represents about one-fourth of body length, whereas it is only about one-eighth the height of an adult. Legs grow to about half the total body height by the time adulthood is reached. Bones undergo slow developmental changes resulting in the evolution of mature bone from the original cartilage. Although growth processes, including the maturation of bone and development of teeth, always follow a specific sequence, the time required varies from one individual to another. Chronological age and maturational age do not always coincide. The development and functioning of the various systems in the body are essential to the growing child, and hormones produced in the child's body will have a major influence on various aspects of growth.

Developmental milestones have been studied to establish norms for accomplishing various physical tasks. Many children can sit up before six months, and they can usually walk while holding onto something when they are just over nine months old. By age one, many can walk. Even when a child does not achieve specific abilities at the prescribed time, the achievements that do occur follow a predictable developmental sequence.

BIBLIOGRAPHY

BAER, M.J. *Growth and Maturation.* H.A. Doyle, Cambridge, MA. 1973.

CHEEK, D.M. *Fetal and Postnatal Cellular Growth.* Wiley, New York. 1975.

CLARKE-STEWART AND KOCH. *Children — Development through Adolescence.* Wiley, New York. 1983.

CRUISE, M.O. Longitudinal study of growth of low birth weight infants. 1. Velocity and distance growth, birth to 3 years. *Ped. 51:* 620. 1973.

FALKNER, F. Normal growth and development. *Postgrad. Med. 62:* 58. 1977.

FANCOURT, R., ET AL Follow-up study of small-for-date babies. *Br. Med. J. 1:* 1435. 1976.

FRANKENBERG, W.K. AND J.B. DODDS. Denver Developmental Screening Test. *J. Ped. 71:* 181. 1967.

FRISANCHO, A.R., ET AL Influence of growth status and placental function on birth weight of infants born to young still-growing teenagers. *Am. J. Clin. Nutr. 40:* 801. 1984.

GARDNER, D. AND J. PEARSON. Growth chart for premature and other infants. *Arch. Dis. Child. 46:* 783. 1971.

GARN, S.M., ET AL Growth, body composition and development of obese and lean children. In Winick, M. ed. *Childhood Obesity.* Wiley. New York. 1975. p. 23.

GRAHAM, G.C. Environmental factors affecting the growth of children. *Am. J. Clin. Nutr. 25:* 1184. 1972.

GRAHAM, G.C., ET AL Growth standards for poor urban children in nutrition studies. *Am. J. Clin. Nutr. 32:* 703. 1979.

HAMILL, P.V., ET AL Physical growth. National Center for Health Statistics, percentiles. *Am. J. Clin. Nutr. 32:* 607. 1979.

KAFTOS, A.F. AND P. ZEE. Nutritional benefits from Federal food assistance. *Am. J. Dis. Child. 131:* 265. 1977.

KORSLUND, M.K., ET AL Anthropometric measurements of white and black southen adolescent girls. *J. Am. Diet. Assoc. 90(3):* 394. 1990.

MARTONELL, R., ET AL Genetic and environmental determinants of growth in Mexican-Americans. *Ped. 84:* 864. 1989.

MUSSEN, P.H., ET AL *Child Development and Peronality.* Harper & Row. New York, 5th ed. 1979.

NATIONAL CENTER FOR HEALTH STATISTICS. NCHS growth charts, 1976, *Monthly vital statistics report 25 (3, suppl. HRA):* 76-1120. Rockville, MD. 1976.

NEUMANN, C.G. AND M. ALPAUGH. Birthweight doubling time: fresh look. *Ped. 57:* 469. 1976.

NEWELL, G., ET AL Physical measurements of 9- to 12-year-old children in Kansas. *J. Am. Diet. Assoc. 84:* 1445. 1984.

O'CONNELL, J.M., ET AL Growth of vegetarian children. *Ped. 84:* 475. 1989.

REED, R.B. AND H.C. Stuart. Patterns of growth in height and weight from birth to eighteen years of age. *Ped. 24 (suppl):* 904. 1959.

ROBECK, M.C. *Infants and Children: Their Development and Learning.* McGraw-Hill. New York. 1978.

SMITH, D.W. *Growth and Its Disorders.* W.B. Saunders. Philadelphia. 1977.

STOCH, M.B. AND P.M. SMYTHE. 15-year developmental study on effect of severe undernutrition on subsequent physical growth and intellectual functioning. *Arch. Dis. Child. 51:* 327. 1976.

TANNER, J.M. AND R.H. WHITEHOUSE. Clinical longitudinal standards for height, weight, height velocity, and stages of puberty. *Arch. Dis. Child. 51:* 170. 1976.

WINGERD, J. AND E.J. SCHOEN. Factors influencing length at birth and height at five years. *Ped. 53:* 737. 1974.

WINICK, M., ED. *Nutrition and Development.* Wiley, New York. 1972.

WINICK, M., ED. *Nutrition and Fetal Development.* Wiley, New York. 1974.

WINICK, M. *Malnutrition and Brain Development.* Oxford University Press. New York. 1976.

CHAPTER THREE

Mental Development

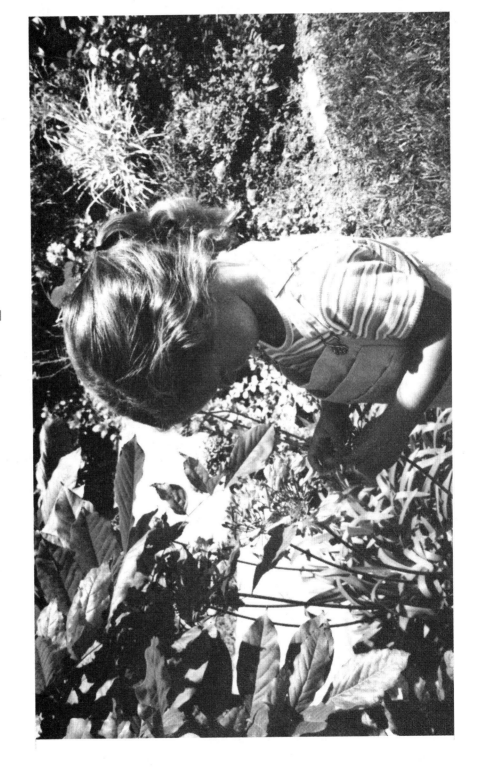

OVERVIEW

From the point of differentiation in the third week of gestation to birth, the brain grows at a remarkable rate and constitutes about 13 percent of the body's weight at birth. It is clear that physical brain development is of high priority. Despite this degree of development at birth, much myelination of the brain remains to be completed during the first few months after birth. Brain cell size increases, and the brain nearly doubles its weight during the first year. These physical developments have been well studied and documented. The problem, from the perspective of nutrition, is to determine the effect of nutrition on mental development, a person's use of the brain.

MENTAL DEVELOPMENT

BRAIN GROWTH

Parents are concerned about how bright their children are. Their reasons for this interest vary, but the importance of intelligence for success in school and in adult life and the positive reflection of bright children on the intelligence of their parents are central to the rationale. In addition to the parents' and children's personal satisfaction, mental development is of importance to society. Children who are classified as mentally retarded frequently place a financial demand on social institutions, for the high cost of special care for the severely retarded often exceeds the resources of families.

Mental development is a very complex aspect of children. Physical development, genetic contribution, and environmental

101

impact all contribute to the intelligence quotient of an individual. Research with appropriate controls to verify theories on the role of nutrition in human mental development is not conscionable. Instead, observations of the results of unavoidable famine, mild hunger, and diet under normal circumstances are being made to add to the knowledge of nutrition's role. Obviously, this is a slow and scientifically difficult way to learn about nutrition's influence on intelligence.

Maturity and size at birth influence mental capacity; a higher incidence of mental retardation is found among infants weighing under 4 1/2 lb at birth than those of normal weight. Of the approximately three percent of Americans who never achieve the intellectual development of a 12-year-old child, many were either premature or small-for-date babies.

Nutrition is but one of the possible factors influencing the outcome of pregnancy. However, eating an adequate diet during pregnancy is one factor most women can control in this country. A pregnant woman must pay careful attention to an adequate diet, but some assistance from others may be required when the family is not able to provide the necessary food. The Federal Women's, Infants' and Children's program (WIC) provides both nutrition education and food assistance to women economically qualified to participate. WIC has been directed toward the economic segment of society at greatest risk of delivering low birth weight babies.

WIC
Women's, Infants', and Children's Program, a Federal nutrition program directed toward enhancing the health and well-being of qualified partici-pants through the provision of food assis-tance and nutrition education.

Concern regarding nutrition and reproduction includes the time when the mother herself was in her growing years, for height and pelvic dimensions are related to reproductive perfor-mance. Weight at the time of conception is another factor in predicting the quality of a pregnancy. These factors are largely determined by the quality of nutrition over a period of many years prior to pregnancy.

Concern for mental development of the child includes the period of rapid growth from the sixth month of gestation to the time when the child is about one year old. At birth, division of the neuronal cells of the brain has essentially stopped. In animals receiving inadequate protein during gestation, the number of brain cells has been shown to be reduced, and that deficit cannot be altered after birth. A premature birth reduces the length of time avilable in the womb for new brain cells to form. Autopsies of malnourished infants who died before the age of two (Winick, et al, 1970) revealed a reduced number of brain cells. From this finding, it may be inferred that adequate nutrition to permit normal cellular division is required during the period when cells are forming if the brain is to have its normal complement of cells.

Not all portions of the brain develop at exactly the same rate. The cerebellum is most impacted in infants classified as small-for-date newborns. Both weight and number of cells in the cerebellum are especially small in comparison with the rest of the brain (Chase, et al, 1970). Limited formation of myelin lipids is also observed.

In experiments with rats, pups born from rats receiving inadequate protein during pregnancy had only 85 percent of the number of brain cells normally found in rats (Winick, et al, 1972). In these rat brains, the number of cells in the cerebellum was reduced appreciably more than in the cerebrum. When these rats were raised in litters of normal size, the number of brain cells remained correspondingly low, yet they were receiving the level of nutrition ordinarily considered adequate. Increasing nutrient intake during the nursing period by raising these fetally-protein-deprived pups in litters of only three to the time of weaning resulted in an increase in the number of brain cells to nearly normal levels. The serious consequences of protein deficiency during pregnancy and inadequate nutrition during the nursing period were demonstrated by placing some of these rats in litters of 18 until weaning. These rats showed only 80 percent the normal number of brain cells when measured at weaning.

Unfortunately, similar findings have been observed in human infants autopsied after death from malnutrition during the first year. When infants weighed 4.4 lb or less at birth and died of extreme malnutrition during the first year, their brains contained only about 40 percent the normal number of cells. This finding paralleled the rats that had been doubly deprived of protein (during gestation and nursing). In contrast, infants who weighed at least 5.5 lb at birth and died of malnutrition during the first year were found to have a 15 to 20 percent reduction in the number of brain cells (Winick, et al, 1970).

TERATOGENIC
Tending to cause fetal abnormalities.

Undoubtedly, protein is not the only nutrient of significance in brain development. Although human evidence is not conclusive, the results of animal studies strongly suggest that teratogenic abnormalities may be due to inadequacies of certain nutrients during gestation. In rats, an inadequate intake of vitamin A during pregnancy reduced the number of cells in the placenta (Takahashi and Smith, 1973). Inadequate intakes of folate and vitamin B_6 during pregnancy or in the neonatal period caused abnormal electroencephalograms. Evidence that inadequate levels of folate in pregnant women may be associated with renal tube defects in their offspring resulted in the mandatory enrichment of cereals and cereal products with folate (140 μg/100 g flour) in 1998.

INTELLECTUAL GROWTH

One key aspect of a child is intellectual development. Intelligence and intellectual achievement can be measured by a variety of tests, but the factors influencing an individual child's achievements are so varied that they are virtually impossible to isolate. Therefore, it is not possible to state emphatically that malnutrition inhibits the growth of intelligence.

Ordinarily, children who are low in birth weight and/or malnourished in infancy and early childhood are from families of low socioeconomic status. These children's environment is significantly different from that of youngsters in higher socioeconomic groups. Differences in sanitation, food patterns, health care, and educational achievements of family members all contribute to the intellectual development of children at various levels of society. No totally satisfactory techniques for determining the importance of nutrition on intellectual development in early life have been found.

Although it is important to recognize that studies measuring intellectual development in relation to nutrition have limitations because of difficulties in establishing adequate controls, some relationship is nonetheless often inferred. Indonesian children who had been malnourished according to earlier classification were compared (Wechsler Intelligence and Goodenough tests) with their socioeconomic (but not malnourished) counterparts from ages 12 to 15 (Liang, et al, 1967). The researchers found that a poor nutritional state was associated with a lower intelligence quotient than was found in the taller, better-nourished control group.

In India, Bhatia (1958) reported that mental retardation was still evident between 8 and 11 years of age (the ages at which IQs were taken) in children who had been treated for kwashiorkor in earlier years. The greatest handicap was noted in perceptual and abstracting ability, but memory and verbal ability were also impaired. The difference between the former kwashiorkor patients and the control group was greater for those ages 8 to 9 than in the older subjects.

ELECTROENCEPHA-LOGRAM
Tracing of brain waves using an electroencephalograph.

PPM
Parts per million; one part of a specified substance in a million parts of a carrier, which is usually water.

A Jamaican study (Hertizig, et al, 1972) compared males between the ages of 6 and 11 to determine the influence of severe malnutrition prior to the age of 2 on intellectual development. The control subjects were classmates; their achievement level in various areas of intellectual development was measured against similar tests for males formerly hospitalized for malnutrition and against siblings of the hospitalized group; the highest achievement was in the control group, followed by the siblings. The formerly hospitalized males showed the lowest level of intellectual development when measured from 4 and 10 years after hospitalization. The fact that the siblings were found to be below the level of intellectual development measured in classmates from a comparable socioeconomic background suggested the presence of inadequate nutrition in all the children in the "at risk" families.

In families where limited income results in inadequate nutrition for children, there is generally a correlation between the child's height and the intelligence measure. In other words, tall children have a higher IQ than short children when nutrient intake is poor (Cravioto, et al, 1966). This finding does not carry over to more affluent families; the height of children whose nutrition is adequate to approach their genetic growth potential does not appear to correlate with intelligence measurements.

Severe malnutrition before the age of two, particularly within the first six months of life, has a profound influence on intellectual development. A partial recovery can result over time with appropriate nutritional and social intervention. The importance of a stimulating home environment in compensating for early nutritional and environmental influences on intellectual development should not be ignored.

In a summary of the results of several studies on the effects of malnutrition on intelligence, Klein (1975, p. 74–75) formulated the following generalizations:

1. Among the areas of behavioral development typically explored by developmental scales, that of language development is reported to be more severely retarded in subjects who suffered from malnutrition (Cravioto and Robles, 1965; Monckeberg, 1968; Barrerra-Moncada, 1963; Chase and Martin, 1970).

2. A second generalization is that children who are severely malnourished earlier in life (less than 6 months of age) seem to show greater decrements in test performance than do those who become

malnourished later in life (Cravioto and Robles, 1965; Monckeberg, 1968; Chase and Martin, 1970; Pollitt and Granoff, 1967). This distinction between earlier and later malnutrition corresponds roughly with the clinical differentiation between marasmus and kwashiorkor, respectively.

3. Finally, the data tentatively suggest that these differences in performance may be enduring ones (Monckeberg, 1968; Barrerra-Moncada, 1963). Specifically, early onset of malnutrition is associated with more severe decrements in performance in later life.

RESEARCH INSIGHTS

Wauben, I.P.M. and P.E. Wainwright. Influence of neonatal nutrition on behavioral development: a critical appraisal. *Nutr. Rev. 57(2):* 35. 1999.

Eskes, T.K.A.B., Open or closed? A world of difference: history of homocysteine research. *Nutr. Rev. 56(8):* 236. 1998.

Occurrence of spina bifida or anencephaly is the result of a defect between days 21 and 27 of a pregnancy (Eskes, 1998). A problem at the cranial end of the neural tube between 22 and 26 days leads to anencephalus, characterized by lack of development of the central brain and failure to close the neural tube. Between days 23 and 26, spina bifida can result when a defect prevents closure of the caudal part of the tube, thus failing to protect the spinal cord. Researchers traced the possibility of a nutritional cause back to a uniquely high incidence of spina bifida in male births in the Netherlands in the last 2 months of 1945; conception of these males occurred in February and March of that year, a time of severe famine in the country. Eventually, interest focused on folic acid and its possible role in methylating homocyteine to form methionine or conversely demethylating methionine to produce homocysteine. Hyperhomocysteinemia and low methionine were found in almost 1 in every 4 women delivering infants with neural tube defects (NTD). Supplementation with 0.5–1.0 mg folic acid daily allowed normal metabolism of homocysteine. Folate provides methyl groups needed to make methionine and leading ultimately to formation of DNA and RNA during the early stage of pregnancy, a time when demand is very high due to rapid cell division.

Vitamin B_{12} also participates in the methylation of homocysteine to methionine. Practical application of these findings calls for daily supplementation of folic acid 4 weeks prior to conception and continuing through the first 2 months of pregnancy to help prevent neural tube defects in pregnancy. Research is continuing to explore the benefits that folic acid supplementation during pregnancy may have in preventing such congenital problems as heart defects and limb deformities. In adults, the relationship between homocysteine levels and vascular disease is another area of much research activity in which folic acid may play a significant role.

Neurotransmitters may perform such critical roles as regulating neurogenesis, synaptogenesis, and neural migration in the developing central nervous system in the prenatal period. Postnatal developments encompass formation of and changes in synaptic connections, migration of neurons, and myelination of axons. The effects of specific nutrient deficiencies and also general malnutrition on optimal neurologic development and behavior have been explored in animals, but far less information is available for humans.

Wauben and Wainwright (1999) reviewed literature on a wide range of nutrients to draw together current information and identify possibly fruitful directions for future research into the realm of mental and nervous system development. They suggested that the fact that vitamin A stimulates proliferation of stem cells which respond to epidermal growth factor may justify research to see if inadequate vitamin A may alter brain cell growth and differentiation. The effects of serotonin concentration in the brain on neuronal development provide questions for research on possible differences in brain development and behavior in subsequent years. The need by infants for arachidonic acid (20:4 ω-6) and docosahexaenoic acid (22:6 ω-3) in human milk versus the possibility of supplying their precursors linoleic (18:2 ω-6) and linolenic acids (18:3 ω-3), respectively, requires more study in light of the importance of these fatty acids for development of the central nervous system. Animal studies have demonstrated behavioral changes, reduced learning and memory, as well as limited activity when zinc is deficient either during gestation or following birth. Iron performs numerous roles in the central nervous system, for it is involved in myelin formation and maintenance, dopamine metabolism, and is a part of enzymes in amine neurotransmitter systems. Much remains to be learned about these and other nutrients in relation to central nervous system and mental development.

Nutritional intake may have subtle influences on mental development because of the impact specific deficiences may have on the ability of the child to interact with the environment. For example, iron-deficiency anemia is a problem that may occur even when the child is being reared in a family of comfortable means. Children with iron-deficiency anemia are more irritable, less motivated to explore their surroundings, and become tired more quickly than children with adequate iron. As a consequence, their interactions with their environment may be reduced, and their interpersonal relationships with parents and others may be curtailed or reduced in educational value. In short, children with iron-deficiency anemia may have considerably less stimulation toward mental development than other children, but the iron deficiency appears to have no significant influence on the growth of the brain.

Low intakes of nutrients, particularly of vitamins A and C, tend to limit resistance to infections. Sick children have reduced interaction to stimulate mental development in comparison with healthy, active children. The likelihood of having an adequate diet is reduced somewhat in families of low socioeconomic status; these are also the families most likely to have reduced quality of health care and sanitation. Such families may provide minimal mental stimulation to growing children, resulting from the parents' lack of knowledge. This cycle tends to be self-perpetuating.

DEFICIENCY CONDITIONS IN EARLY CHILDHOOD

In developing countries, the combination of very difficult living conditions, limited incomes, and lack of education may trigger life-threatening health problems for newborns and infants. Even when these problems are treated early, the risk of mental retardation persists because of the factors that created the original condition. The three key health problems of a nutritional origin in these children are kwashiorkor, marasmus, and protein-calorie malnutrition.

KWASHIORKOR

Kwashiorkor is the protein-deficiency condition resulting from inadequate intake of protein over a period of time and occurring most commonly in children between the ages of one and four after weaning. Children with kwashiorkor fail to grow normally, and collagen synthesis (important for formation of connective tissue, skin, and bones) is reduced significantly. Obvious changes in the hair occur early in the condition; these

KWASHIORKOR
Protein–deficiency condition occurring in some children between the ages of one and four; symptoms include poor growth impaired collagen synthesis, changes in the hair, moon face, and edema.

include a flag-like or striped appearance when portions of the hair lose pigmentation. Thinning hair is also seen. Development of a "moon face," a very round face due to edema and some added subcutaneous fat, is characteristic of kwashiorkor. Edema, starting in the legs and progressing upward, is another symptom seen as the case develops. Winick (1976, pages 7–12) enumerated additional clinical signs of kwashiorkor.

Poor socioeconomic conditions often accompany the occurrence of kwashiorkor; children living in crowded, unsanitary homes with limited income for food are likely to contract many illnesses. Commonly, the onset of kwashiorkor is traced to an accompanying illness. The combination of a continuing protein deficiency and the challenge to the body presented by a case of the flu or some childhood disease can push the child over into a frank case of kwashiorkor that becomes evident after the triggering problem has been cured. While infants are nursing on their mothers' milk, a marginally adequate amount of protein is being provided. It is when weaning has occurred and an accompanying illness strikes that kwashiorkor can be contracted.

MARASMUS

Marasmus is chronic starvation. It differs from kwashiorkor in that the whole diet is totally inadequate. Children with marasmus are terribly emaciated, causing their heads to look greatly out of proportion to the rest of the body. The arms and legs look like bones with skin stretched over them, although the knees tend to swell. The most likely causes of marasmus are failure to breast-feed in a circumstance where adequate formula feeding is not practical and early cessation of breast feeding.

The symptoms of marasmus are many, and the actual extent of these symptoms is directly related to the severity and duration of the nutritional deficiency. Stunted growth, extreme irritability, lethargy, and very limited interaction with the environment characterize these grossly undernourished children. With proper dietary treatment, many symptoms of marasmus can be alleviated or eliminated; but growth sometimes does not reach its potential.

PROTEIN-CALORIE MALNUTRITION

A related problem, in which both protein intake and calories are inadequate in the diet, is a life-threatening reality to children in families with very limited resources. Protein-calorie malnutrition (PCM) may be viewed as a nutritional problem that

---

MOONFACE
Very round face characteristic of kwashiorkor; caused by a combination of edema and added subcutaneous fatty deposits in the face.

EDEMA
Accumulation of fluid, giving a bloated appearance to the body.

MARASMUS
Nutritional deficiency condition seen in children who have an inadequate intake of many nutrients.

PROTEIN-CALORIE MALNUTRITION
Nutritional deficiency condition resulting from a deficiency of protein and calories in children after weaning; symptoms tend to be intermediate between those of kwashiorkor and marasmus.

PCM
Abbreviation for protein-calorie malnutrition.

ASCITES
Accumulation of fluid in the abdomen, a symptom found in PCM and sometimes in kwashiorkor.

combines the protein-deficiency problems of kwashiorkor with the alarmingly low caloric intake of marasmus. Another term for this condition is protein-energy malnutrition (PEM). Children with protein-calorie malnutrition typically have very low levels of calories and protein-rich foods in their diets. Symptoms include lethargy, increased susceptibility to illnesses, ascites (accumulation of fluid in the abdomen), and decreased interaction with the environment; mental activity in these children is usually greatly reduced.

The individual role of malnutrition in influencing mental development of children with marasmus, kwashiorkor, or protein-calorie malnutrition is impossible to determine. The fact that many children suffering from these conditions are hospitalized results in changes in the stimuli that may influence learning. Of course, the nutritional circumstance is also modified by hospitalization. Even so, the impact of physical problems caused by a slowly developing nutritional deficiency condition certainly has long-lasting effects on the developing child.

SUMMARY

Brain growth is dramatic and important, particularly in the period from about the third month of gestation until the end of the first year of life. Children who are under 4 1/2 lb at birth have an increased risk of being mentally retarded and of having fewer than normal brain cells. Following birth, significant increase in size of brain cells occurs in normal circumstances, but inadequate diets, particularly those low in protein and calories, may result in reduced brain growth. The WIC Program has focused its efforts toward providing supplemental food and nutrition education to women who qualify on the basis of socio-economic need as a means of reducing the likelihood of producing low birth weight babies.

Mental development is a combination of brain growth and learning that results from a child's interactions with the environment. Poorly nourished children are generally apathetic and irritable, making contact with other people more stressful and less educational than is the case for happy, outgoing children who are well fed. The delay in language development that may accompany malnutrition further restricts interchange with others. In addition to mental retardation stemming from protein and calorie deficiencies, an inadequate intake of such nutrients as iron and vitamins A and C may cause considerable interference with normal levels of interaction with other people as a result of illness or lethargy.

Kwashiorkor (protein-deficiency condition), marasmus (virtual starvation), and protein-calorie malnutrition (protein and calorie deficiency) are nutritional problems of great concern in developing nations where sanitation, economic, and educational difficulties make the adequate feeding of newly-weaned children particularly hard to accomplish. Decreased resistance resulting from poor nutrition is often the health threat that triggers these three problems.

BIBLIOGRAPHY

BARRERA-MONCADA, G. *Estudios Sobre Alteraciones del Crecimiento y del Desarrollo Psicologico del Sindrome Pluricarencial (Kwashiorkor)*, Caracas. Editoria Grafos. 1963.

BEARD, J.L., ET AL Iron in the brain. *Nutr. Rev. 51:* 157. 1993.

BHATIA, C.M. *Cited in Performance Tests of Intelligence.* Oxford University Press. London. 1958.

BIRCH, H.G. Malnutrition, learning, and intelligence. *Amer. J. Publ. Health 62:* 773. 1972.

BIRCH, H.G. AND J.D. GUSSOW. *Disadvantaged Children: Health, Nutrition, and School Failure.* Harcourt, Brace, & Jovanovich. New York. 1970.

Chase, H.P. and H. P. Martin. Undernutrition and child development. *New Eng. J. Med. 282:* 933. 1970.

CHEEK, D.B. *Human Growth: Body Composition, Growth, Energy, and Intelligence.* Lea & Febiger. Philadelphia. 1968.

CRAVIOTO, J., ET AL Nutrition, growth and neurointegrative development. *Pediat. 38:* 319. 1966.

CRAVIOTO, J. AND B. ROBLES. Evolution of adaptive and motor behavior during rehabilitation from kwashiorkor. *Amer. J. Orthopsychiat. 35:* 449. 1965.

CARVIOTO, J. AND E.R. DELICARDIE. Mental performance in school age children, findings after recovery from early severe malnutrition. *Am. J. Dis. Children 120:* 404. 1970.

DOBBING, J. Infant nutrition and later achievement. *Nutr. Rev. 41:* 1. 1983.

GIFFT, H.H., ET AL *Nutrition, Behavior, and Change.* Prentice-Hall. Englewood Cliffs, NJ. 1972.

GOYER, R.A. Nutrition and metal toxicity. *Am. J. Clin. Nutr. 61(suppl) 646S.* 1995.

GRANTHAM-MCGREGOR, S. Chronic undernutrition and cognitive abilities. *Human Nutr.: Clin. Nutr. 38C:* 83. 1984.

HERBERT, V. Folate and neural tube defects. *Nutr. Today 27(6):* 30. 1992.

HERTZIG, M.E., ET AL Intellectual levels of school children severely malnourished during the first two years of life. *Pediat. 49:* 814. 1972.

HINE, R.J. What practitioners need to know about folic acid. *J. Amer. Dietet. Assoc. 96(6):* 451. 1996.

HOLST, M. Devlopmental and behavioral effects of iron deficiency anemia in infants based on the 1997 Avanelle Kirskey Lecture Presented at Purdue University. *Nutr. Today 33(1):* 27. 1998.

KLEIN, R.E. AND A.A. ADINOLFI. *Measurement of behavioral correlates of malnutrition. In Brain Function and Malnutrition.* Ed. Prescott, J.W., et al Wiley. New York. 1975. p. 73.

LLOYD-STILL, J.D., ET AL Intellectual development after severe malnutrition in infancy, *Pediat. 54:* 306. 1974.

LIANG, P.H., ET AL Evaluation of mental development in relation to early malnutrition. *Am. J. Clin. Nutr. 20:* 1290. 1967.

LOZOFF, B., ET AL Long-term developmental outcome of infants with iron deficiency. *N. Eng. J. Med. 325:* 1992.

McLAREN, D.X., ED. *Textbook of Paediatric Nutrition.* Livingstone. New York. 1982.

MONCKEBERG, F. *Effect of early marasmic malnutrition on subsequent physical and physiological development. In Malnutrition, Learning, and Behavior.* ed. Scrimshaw, N.S. and J.E. Gordon, M.I.T. Press. Cambridge, MA. 1968.

MONCKEBERG, F. *Effect of malnutrition on physical growth and brain development. In Brain Function and Malnutrition.* ed. Prescott, J.W., et al, Wiley, New York. 1975. p. 15.

POLLITT, E. AND D. GRANOFF Mental and motor development of Peruvian children treated for severe malnutrition. *Revista Interamericana de Psicologia 1:* 93, 1967.

POLLITT, E. AND R.L. LEIBEL. *Iron Deficiency: Brain Biochemistry and Behavior.* Raven Press. New York. 1982.

POMERANCE, H.H. AND J.M. KRALL. Relationship of birth size to rate of growth in infancy and childhood. *Am. J. Clin. Nutr. 39:* 95. 1984.

PRESCOTT, J.W., ET AL *Brain Function and Malnutrition.* Wiley, New York. 1975.

RITCHEY, S.J. AND L.J. TAPER. *Maternal and Child Nutrition.* Harper & Row. New York. 1983.

SHEARD, N.F. Iron deficiency and infant development. *Nutr. Rev. 52:* 137. 1994.

TUCKER, D.M., ET AL Iron status and brain function: serum ferritin levels associated with asymmetries of cortical electrophysiology and cognitive performance. *Am. J. Clin. Nutr. 39:* 105. 1984.

WINICK, M. Nutrition and mental development. *Med. Cl. No. Amer. 54:* 1413. 1970.

WINICK, M. *Nutrition and Development.* Wiley, New York. 1972.

WINICK, M. *Malnutrition and Brain Development.* Oxford University Press. New York. 1976.

WURTMAN, M.D. AND J.J. WURTMAND, ED. *Nutrition and the Brain. 6. Physiological and Behavioral Effects of Food Constitutents.* Raven Press. New York. 1983.

SECTION TWO

Beginnings

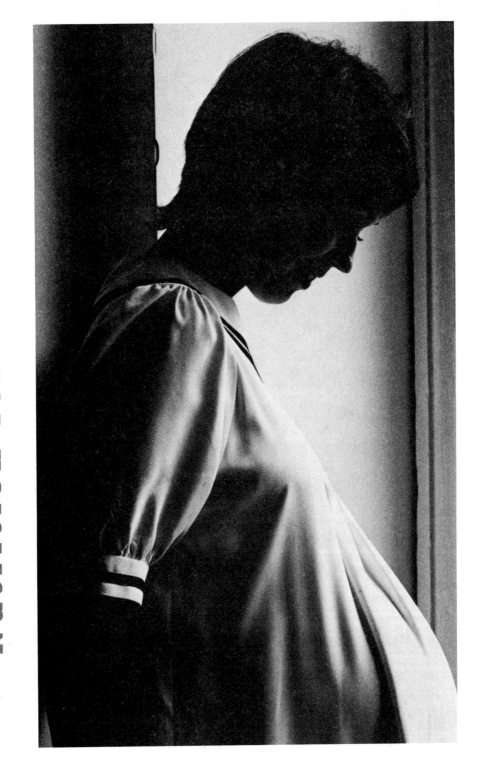

CHAPTER FOUR
Nutrition for the Mother

OVERVIEW

Even with the tremendous amount of research that has been done in the field of nutrition in the last 80 years, myths still predominate in determining the dietary practices of many pregnant women around the world. The awesome responsibility of "eating for two" motivates all kinds of presumably helpful suggestions for pregnant women from mothers, grandmothers, and well-meaning friends who are anxious to help at this exciting time. Some suggestions based on folklore may be helpful to innocuous; others can be harmful, even when given with the best of intentions.

Although there are still gaps in knowledge regarding nutritional needs and appropriate practices during pregnancy,

117

a functional picture is emerging that can provide the basis for good nutrition for pregnant women.

PRE-CONCEPTION — TIME FOR NUTRITIONAL PLANNING

STATUS AT CONCEPTION

Adults are walking case histories of their nutritional habits over the years. Inadequate diets during the growing years result in failure to reach potential height. Ideally, women contemplating pregnancy will have eaten well enough in their early years to be the optimal height for their genetic heritage. The likelihood of bearing a premature or small-for-date baby is minimized in women who have grown well themselves. Once adulthood has been reached, of course, nothing can be done about this problem, but it is reassuring to know that good eating habits that promoted growth in childhood are now an asset in terms of the outcome of pregnancy.

Weight is one indication of nutritional status. Fortunately, with sufficient long-range planning and action, this is a factor that can be altered before pregnancy, when pregnancy is intended. If a woman is normally underweight or overweight, she would be wise to modify her diet either to gain or lose the weight necessary to reach her recommended weight (Table 4.1) before becoming pregnant.

You can easily determine which frame size to use by following these two steps and then comparing the resulting measurement with the figures in Table 4.2.

1. Extend your arm and then bend the forearm upward at a 90° angle, keeping the fingers straight and turning the inside of the wrist toward the body.

2. Place your thumb and index finger from the other hand on the two prominent bones on either side of the elbow. Measure the space between your fingers against a ruler and compare with the figures in Table 4.2.

Even when weight is within the recommended range, some changes in diet may be necessary to provide adequate amounts of all the nutrients. A good way to check on the appropriateness of present habits is to keep a record of all foods

TABLE 4.1   Recommended Weight Ranges for Women of Various Heights and Frames During the Reproductive Years[a]

Height[b]		Recommended Weight (in pounds) by Frame Size[c]		
Feet	Inches	Small	Medium	Large
4	10	102–111	109–121	118–131
4	11	103–113	111–123	120–134
5	0	104–115	113–126	122–137
5	1	106–118	115–129	125–140
5	2	108–121	118–132	128–143
5	3	111–124	121–135	131–147
5	4	114–127	124–138	134–151
5	5	117–130	127–141	137–155
5	6	120–133	130–144	140–159
5	7	123–136	133–147	143–163
5	8	126–139	136–150	146–167
5	9	129–142	139–153	149–170
5	10	132–145	142–156	152–173
5	11	135–148	145–159	155–176
6	0	138–151	148–162	158–172

[a]Adapted by permission of the Metropolitan Life Insurance Company. Source of basic data; 1979 Build Study, Society of Actuaries and Association of Life Insurance Medical Directors of America, 1980.
[b]Height is based on wearing a shoe with a 1-inch heel.
[c]Weight includes 3 lb of clothing. The recommended weight range is based on lowest mortality for women between the ages of 25 and 29.

consumed and their amounts. By adding up the servings eaten and checking the day's total against the Food Guide Pyramid, a useful picture of the adequacy of the day's nutrient intake will emerge. This should be done for at least three days so that habits will be apparent. For instance, if a serving of citrus or other vitamin C source is missing each day, plans can be made to include the missing food at one of the day's meals.

The merits of using the Food Guide Pyramid for analyzing food intake include the facts that analysis is quick and the food groups give a wide range of the nutrients essential to good health. Individual food habits differ considerably from one person to another; a woman planning for pregnancy should record her food intake for several days and compare each day's intake with the

TABLE 4.2   Elbow Breadth for Women of Medium Frame and Various Heights[a,b]

Height with 1 inch heels	Elbow Breadth (inches)
4 ft 10 in — 4 ft. 11 in	2 1/4 to 2 1/2
5 ft 0 in — 5 ft 3 in	2 1/4 to 2 1/2
5 ft 4 in — 5 ft 7 in	2 3/8 to 2 5/8
5 ft 8 in — 5 ft 11 in	2 3/8 to 2 5/8
6 ft 0 in	2 1/4 to 2 3/4

[a]Reproduced by permission of the Metropolitan Life Insurance Co.
[b]Measurements smaller than the above figures for a medium frame indicate a small frame; a value greater than the above is interpreted as being a large frame.

Food Guide Pyramid to find the strengths and weaknesses of her diet.

CHANGING PATTERNS

Once the needed dietary improvements have been identified, change can be initiated, but minor modifications that can be achieved should be attempted first. Modifying food habits is a discouraging and even painful task. Success in making minor changes will help set the stage for shifting patterns to the desired goal. In families, it is helpful if both the prospective mother and father work together to make healthful dietary shifts. Even though the father is not responsible for nutrient intake during pregnancy, he will play a significant part as a role model in shaping his children's food patterns. For the mother, establishing good eating patterns before pregnancy is a good way to ensure that adequate nutrients will be available throughout gestation. Her pattern of healthful eating will also be important in establishing good dietary habits later in her child.

Women who are contemplating pregnancy are advised to be sure that they are ingesting the recommended intake of 400 μg of folate well in advance of pregnancy so that their levels of this key B vitamin will be adequate at the onset of pregnancy. Recognition of the importance of adequate folate prior to and during early pregnancy to reduce risk of neural tube birth defects (particularly anencephaly and spina bifida) has led the Food and Drug Administration to require enrichment of such grain products as flour, breads, cornmeal, and rice with folate (effective

ANENCEPHALY
Birth defect in which a baby is born with no brain and dies before or shortly after birth.

SPINA BIFIDA
Birth defect of spinal cord of varying severity, but that can cause problems with walking, mental retardation, or other dysfunction.

TABLE 4.3　　　Some Suggested Sources of Folate[a]

Food	Serving Size	Folate (μg)
Chicken liver	3.5 oz	770
Breakfast cereals	1/2–1 1/2 cup	100–400
Beef liver	3.5 oz	217
Lentils, cooked	1/2 cup	180
Asparagus	1/2 cup	132
Spinach, cooked	1/2 cup	131
Black beans	1/2 cup	128
Bread	1 slice	38

[a]Bowes, A.D., *Bowes and Church's Food Values of Portions Commonly Used.*
16th ed. Lippincott. Philadelphia. 1994.

in January, 1998). The recommended level of folate intake during pregnancy is 800 μg. However, it is important to recognize that intakes above this level are not recommended and that 1,000 μg is the maximum safe daily level of folate. Food can provide adequate levels of folate (see Table 4.3), but a vitamin supplement may be needed if dietary intake is likely to be low.

If definite changes in weight are needed to prepare for pregnancy, time and some professional help probably are in order. If the goal involves gaining or losing more than five pounds, monitoring by a physician and dietary guidance by a Registered Dietitian are wise adjuncts to the plan. During a weight control program, a diet planned on the Food Guide Pyramid works well to achieve the desired weight while retraining food habits and ensuring that a broad range of nutrients is provided. Appropriate serving sizes are an important part in meeting weight control goals, too.

This period of nutritional concern before pregnancy can be viewed as a training period for both prospective parents to improve their dietary habits. Ideally, the dietary pattern that evolves will be well balanced and in a quantity that maintains a desirable weight and provides adequate levels of nutrients. Breakfast, as well as lunch and dinner, should be part of this pattern. Also, acceptance and appreciation of a wide range of foods and a commitment to eating for good health will evolve as permanent benefits of this program for change.

Advice about establishing good dietary patterns before becoming pregnant will be followed by many people deciding to have children in their late 20s or 30s, because they have the maturity and the time to give serious thought to all the decisions involving pregnancy. However, many adolescents or older women may suddenly find that they are pregnant. Such a discovery does not allow the luxury of preparing for pregnancy by improving food habits before pregnancy. Good dietary management, however, can be the goal throughout pregnancy; this can be quite effective in having a healthy pregnancy.

It should also be mentioned that nutritional preparation for pregnancy applies to any woman, whether she is approaching her first or her fifth pregnancy. Certainly, replenishment of body stores of nutrients before undertaking a subsequent pregnancy is important for her well-being, as well as that of her next child. Family planning, combined with adequate nutrition, can provide the time necessary for recuperation and replenishment. Good dietary practices during this period are recommended to control weight and maintain adequate nutrition.

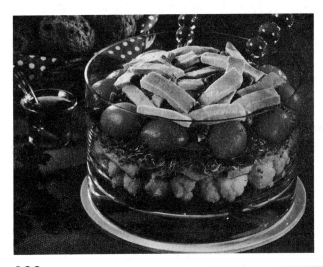

Attractive salads with the dressing served on the side can be made with an array of comparatively low-calorie foods to provide fiber, protein, and many vitamins, and minerals. When combined with a whole-grain bread and a glass of milk, the pregnant woman will be able to enjoy eating well for herself and her fetus.

PHYSIOLOGICAL CHANGES IN PREGNANCY

WEIGHT

The physiological changes occurring during pregnancy dictate the nutritional requirements for this crucial period of life. One of the changes that is most obvious to a pregnant woman is a change in weight, accompanied by a change in balance in the later months, as the rapidly growing fetus shifts her center of gravity. Although some women experience nausea and vomiting, causing some measurable weight loss early in pregnancy, the overall pattern recommended by the Committee on Nutrition of the American College of Obstetricians and Gynecologists (1974) is a linear gain, beginning with the thirteenth week of pregnancy and continuing until delivery. This recommendation continues to be the standard (Committee on Nutritional Status and Weight Gain During Pregnancy Subcommittee on Dietary Intake and Nutrient Supplements During Pregnancy, 1990). The total weight gain suggested falls within the range of 20 to 25 pounds (or even up to 35 pounds was proposed in 1990) for most women, a range that has been viewed as the standard since 1970 (National Research Council, 1970). This recommendation translates into a steady gain of approximately 14 ounces each week, beginning with the thirteenth week. A weight gain of less than 2.2 pounds per month during this period is considered to be inadequate, whereas a gain of 6.6 pounds per month definitely is excessive during the last six months of pregnancy.

Although the above comments focus on the last six months (the second and third trimesters), some attention to weight is appropriate during the first trimester, too. Usually only about three pounds are gained during the first trimester, with this gain beginning very slowly in the second month. Although considerable changes are occurring during this crucial period of differentiation, the actual mass accompanying these changes is quite small. Good dietary habits are important to provide the nutrients needed, but weight gain is not an objective at this time. Beginning with the thirteenth week, the fetal growth and associated changes translate into the weight gain recommendations noted above.

COMPONENTS OF WEIGHT GAIN

Weight gain in pregnancy represents a combination of weight from the products of pregnancy and changes in the mother's body. The weight of the fetus, placenta, and amniotic fluid together represent the products of pregnancy which will be eliminated at birth. Collectively, these ordinarily represent slightly more than 10 pounds of the maternal weight gain noted during pregnancy (Table 4.4). The remaining gain of about 14 pounds is due to some increase in fatty deposits in the mother's body. These contributions are depicted in Fig. 4.1.

AMNIOTIC FLUID
The water-like fluid surrounding the fetus in utero.

CHANGES IN THE BLOOD

Striking changes occur in blood volume and composition during pregnancy. The volume of plasma is constant until about the 12th week, when the volume begins to increase to more than a liter above non-pregnant levels by the 34th week. A small drop

PLASMA
Fluid portion of blood.

TABLE 4.4 **Approximate Weights of the Components of Pregnancy[a]**

Component	Approximate Normal Weight (pounds)
Products of Pregnancy —	
Fetus	7.7
Placenta	1.4
Amniotic fluid	1.8
Total	*10.9*
Maternal Changes —	
Increase in uterus	2.0
Increase in breasts	0.9
Increase in interstitial fluid	2.7
Increase in maternal blood volume	4.0
Increase in fatty deposits	4.0
Total	*13.6*
Combined Total Weight Gain (approximate)	***24.5***

[a]Adapted from H.N. Jacobson, "Nutrition and Pregnancy," In *Maternal and Child Health Practices*, H. Wallace, Ed. Charles C. Thomas, Springfield, IL 1973.

in volume occurs during the final weeks of pregnancy. The increased volume is an aid in carrying nutrients to the fetus and in removing waste.

Red blood cell volume also increases, but at a rate distinctly slower than the increase in plasma volume. The net result is that the concentration of red blood cells and hemoglobin is reduced, a condition referred to as the physiological anemia of pregnancy. This is a normal occurrence in pregnancy; hemo-globin value usually ranges between 11 and 12 per 100 ml late in pregnancy (compared with average values of about 13.5 gm per 100 ml or more for nonpregnant women).

FUNCTIONAL CHANGES

Basal metabolic rate is increased during pregnancy, the result of increased production of thyroxin. Various other endo-crine glands also produce greater amounts of their hormones; these include growth hormone from the pituitary gland,

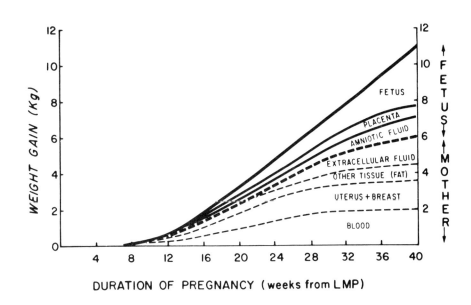

Fig. 4.1   Pattern and components of average maternal weight gain during pregnancy. (Reprinted from Pitkin, R.M. Nutritional support in obstetrics and gynecology. *Clin. Obstet. Gynecol.* 19: 489. 1976.)

parathormone from the parathyroid, and aldosterone from the adrenals.

During the first half of pregnancy; there is an increase in cardiac output of about 1 1/2 liters, from a normal value of about 5 liters for nonpregnant females to an output close to 6 1/2 liters during pregnancy. The heart rate increases, and the stroke volume is larger than before pregnancy. Arterial blood pressure throughout the body and venous blood pressure in the upper part of the body are essentially unchanged by pregnancy, but the legs may experience an increase in venous blood pressure; this contributes to edema and increased discomfort from pressure in the legs. The heart undergoes some enlargement and a slight upward and forward shift as pregnancy causes increased crowding. There is increased blood flow, particularly in the placental region, as well as in the skin and kidneys.

Even breathing is altered by pregnancy. The respiratory rate changes very little, but oxygen consumption increases at least 15 percent as tidal volume increases from appreciable collapse of the lungs at the end of each breathing cycle.

One of the changes noted by many pregnant women is increased salivation in the early phase of pregnancy. Hydrochloric acid secretion is diminished a little in the stomach; but some pregnant women complain of heartburn because the cardiac sphincter relaxes, permitting some backing up of stomach contents into the esophagus. The gallbladder may empty a bit more slowly than normal, causing the bile to become concentrated. In addition, the somewhat relaxed condition of the intestinal walls causes decreased motility and may result in constipation, particularly in the latter stages of pregnancy.

The renal tract dilates by the tenth week of pregnancy and becomes more dilated on the right side than on the left in late pregnancy. This dilation results in an increased urinary capacity and promotes a tendency to develop infections in the region. Urine composition changes, too; amino acids, iodide, sugar, and folate levels are noticeably high in the urine of pregnant women. Two possible consequences of these losses are the megaloblastic anemia associated with inadequate folate levels and an enlarged thyroid gland due to loss of iodide. Urinary volume may be very high early in pregnancy, causing unusual thirst in women at this time.

NUTRITION DURING PREGNANCY

CHANGED NEEDS

The demands for nutrients by the growing fetus and the mother's body during pregnancy are recognized in the Recommended Dietary Allowances and Adequate Intakes (Tables 4.5 and 4.6). Also, the 1989 edition of the Recommended Dietary Allowances indicated a need for 300 additional calories daily during pregnancy.

In the 1998 recommendations, the levels of calcium, phophorus, vitamin D, and fluoride remain the same during pregnancy as prior to becoming pregnant. However, it is important to recognize that many pregnant women may not have been eating adequate levels of all the nutrients previously. This is particularly significant in the case of calcium, phosphorus, and vitamin D because of the likelihood that they may not have formed the habit of including milk at adequate levels in their diets. If this is true for a pregnant woman, she needs to make a special effort to change her dietary habits to include at least 2 glasses of milk daily and preferably more. Continuation of this change after pregnancy will be an aid in protecting against osteoporosis in later life.

Significant increases in the B vitamins (thiamin, riboflavin, niacin, vitamin B_6, folate, vitamin B_{12}, pantothenic acid, biotin, and choline are indicated for pregnancy. Of particular concern is adequate (but not excessive) intake of folate because of its highly significant influence on neural development and role in helping to prevent some birth defects. In fact, attention to adequate folate intake is stressed for all women of child-bearing age who might conceivably become pregnant because adequate folate is important even before a woman knows she is pregnant.

Other nutrients also are needed in significantly larger amounts during pregnancy. In addition to increases in protein, vitamins A, E, K, and C also require a greater intake during pregnancy. The minerals needing to be increased are iron (requirement is double), zinc, iodine, and selenium.

With so much attention being directed to the increased nutritional requirements of pregnancy, it is easy to become too zealous in providing these nutrients through megadoses of supplements. This is a dangerous practice and must be avoided to prevent unnecessary complications. Table 4.7 identifies nutrients that need to be watched carefully to be sure that poten-

TABLE 4.5   RDA and AI for Non-pregnant, Pregnant and Lactating Women[a,b]

Life stage group	Calcium (mg/d)	Phosphorus (mg/d)	Magnesium (mg/d)	Vitamin D (µg/d)[c]	Fluoride (mg/d)	Thiamin (mg/d)	Riboflavin (mg/d)	Niacin (mg/d)
8 to ≤ 18								
Non-pregnant	1300	**1250**	**360**	5	3	**1.0**	**1.0**	**14**
Pregnant	1300	**1250**	**400**	5	3	**1.4**	**1.4**	**18**
Lactating	1300	**1250**	**360**	5	3	**1.4**	**1.6**	**17**
19 to 30								
Non-pregnant	1000	**700**	**310**	5	3	**1.1**	**1.1**	**14**
Pregnant	1000	**700**	**350**	5	3	**1.4**	**1.4**	**18**
Lactating	1000	**700**	**310**	5	3	**1.4**	**1.6**	**17**
31 to 50								
Non-pregnant	1000	**700**	**320**	5	3	**1.1**	**1.1**	**14**
Pregnant	1000	**700**	**360**	5	3	**1.4**	**1.4**	**18**
Lactating	1000	**700**	**320**	5	3	**1.5**	**1.6**	**17**

[a]Adapted from Food and Nutrition Board, Institute of Medicine — National Academy of Sciences Dietary Reference Intakes: Recommended Intakes for Individuals. Washington, D.C. 2000.
[b]Adequate Intakes (AI).   Bold values are RDA.
[c]As cholecalciferol.   1 µg = 40 IU Vitamin D.

Life stage group	Vitamin B$_6$ (mg/d)	Folate (µg/d)	Vitamin B$_{12}$ (µg/d)	Pantothenic (mg/d)	Biotin (µg/d)	Choline (mg/d)
8 to ≤ 18						
Non-pregnant	1.2	400	2.4	5	25	400
Pregnant	1.9	600	2.6	6	30	450
Lactating	2.0	500	2.8	7	35	550
19 to 30						
Non-pregnant	1.3	400	2.4	5	30	425
Pregnant	1.9	600	2.6	6	30	450
Lactating	2.0	500	2.8	7	35	550
31 to 50						
Non-pregnant	1.3	400	2.4	5	30	425
Pregnant	1.9	600	2.6	6	30	450
Lactating	2.0	500	2.8	7	35	550

UL
Maximum level of daily nutrient intake that is likely to pose no risk of adverse effects.

tially harmful levels are not reached. The nutrients highlighted in this listing are calcium, phosphorus, magnesium, vitamin D, fluoride, niacin, vitamin B$_6$, synthetic folate, and choline. The harmful levels will not be reached if a supplement provides 100% of the RDA for the broad spectrum of nutrients. The problems arise with supplements for either single nutrients or multiple nutrients at levels above 100%. Dietary intakes will not reach the ULs.

The rationale for increasing the energy recommendation during pregnancy is based on several factors. The slow, steady rise in basal metabolic rate increases the need for energy for basal metabolism gradually throughout the pregnancy. The formation of new tissue and the growth of the fetus all place additional demands for energy. Simply moving around with the added weight in the latter period of pregnancy requires additional energy, but the tendency to move around less offsets this factor to some degree. The wide diversity in the amount of activity undertaken by pregnant women means that the recommendation for energy needs may be inadequate for physically active pregnant women and too high for those who are quite sedentary. The rate of weight gain during pregnancy is a helpful guide in determining if an individual woman is obtaining enough calories

TABLE 4.6   RDA for Non-pregnant, Pregnant and Lactating Women[a,b,c]

Life stage group	Protein (g)	Vitamin A (µg, RE)	Vitamin E (mg α-TE)	Vitamin K (µg)	Vitamin C (mg)	Iron (µg)	Zinc (mg)	Iodine (µg)	Selenium (µg)
8 to ≤18									
Non-pregnant	44	800	15	55	60	15	12	150	55
Pregnant	60	1300	15	65	70	30	15	175	60
Lactating	65	1200	19	65	95	15	19	200	70
19 to 30									
Non-pregnant	46	800	15	60	60	15	12	150	55
Pregnant	60	1300	15	65	70	30	15	175	60
Lactating	65	1200	19	65	95	15	19	200	70
31 to 50									
Non-pregnant	50	800	15	65	60	15	12	150	55
Pregnant	60	1300	19	65	70	30	15	175	60
Lactating	65	1200	19	65	95	15	19	200	70

[a]Adapted from Food and Nutrition Board, Institute of Medicine — National Academy of Sciences Dietary Reference Intakes: Recommended Intakes for Individuals, revised 1998 (abridged). Washington, D.C. 1998.

[b]First 6 months of lactation.

[c]Based on a weight of 55 kg (120 lb) and a height of 163 cm (64 in) for females age 18 or less and 164 cm (65 in) for females 19 to 24, and 63 kg (138 lb) and 163 cm (64 in) for females ages 25 to 50.

[d]Retinol equivalents. 1 retinol equivalent = 1 µg retinol or 6 µg β-carotene.

[e]α-tocopherol equivalents. 1 mg d-α-tocopherol = 1 α-TE.

TABLE 4.7 Dietary Reference Intakes: Tolerable Upper Intake Levels for Pregnant and Lactating Women[a,b]

Life stage group	Calcium (mg/d)	Phosphorus (mg/d)	Magnesium (mg/d)	Vitamin D (μg/d)	Fluoride (mg/d)	Niacin (mg/d)	Vitamin B$_6$ (mg/d)	Synthetic Folic Acid (μg/d)	Choline (mg/d)
8 to ≤18									
Pregnant	2500	3500	350	50	10	30	80	800	3000
Lactating	2500	4000	350	50	10	30	80	800	3000
19 to 50									
Pregnant	2500	3500	350	50	10	35	100	1000	3500
Lactating	2500	4000	350	50	10	35	100	1000	3500

[a]Adapted from Dietary Reference intakes: Tolerable upper Intake Levels (UL) for Certain Nutrients and Food Components. Food and Nutrition Board, Institute of Medicine — National Academy of Sciences. Washington, D.C. 1998.

[b]UL = the maximum level of daily nutrient intake that is likely to pose no risk of adverse effects. Unless otherwise specified, the UL represents total intake from food, water, and supplements. Due to lack of suitable data, ULs could not be established for thiamin, riboflavin, vitamin B$_{12}$, pantothenic acid, or biotin. In the absence of ULs, extra caution may be warranted in consuming levels above recommended intakes.

[c]The UL for magnesium represents intake from a pharmacological agent only and does not include intake from food and water.

[d]The ULs for niacin and synthetic folic acid apply to forms obtained from supplements, fortified foods, or a combination of the two.

in relation to need. Most pregnant women require about 18 cal/ lb; intake should never drop below 16 cal/lb. Actually, much of the increased energy requirement in the second trimester is due to maternal changes resulting from pregnancy, whereas the fetus is the primary factor influencing increased need in the last trimester.

The increase in protein is not surprising in view of the impressive amount of new tissue that must be formed during pregnancy. When protein is inadequate in the diet, the fetus may fail to reach its genetic potential for length. The recommended intake for protein is made under the assumption that energy available from the diet will be adequate. If this is not the case, some of the protein will have to be used for energy needs and will not be available for building tissue and other protein functions. The problems of premature birth, low birth weights, increased infant mortality, and mental retardation stemming from grossly inadequate intakes of protein and calories were discussed in Chapter 3. Although many people in this country eat far more protein than recommended and are often counseled to reduce their intake of meats, this advice should not be heeded by most pregnant women; the amount recommended in pregnancy is probably quite close to the quantity of protein they have been eating, unless they are vegetarians.

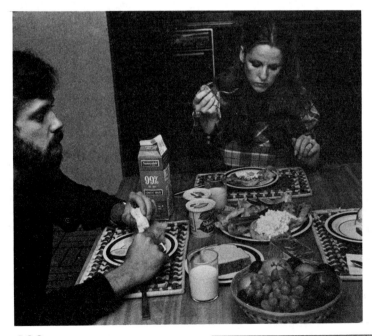

Pregnancy is an important time for the mother and father to examine their dietary patterns and make changes which may be needed in the future when they serve as role models in shaping their children's food habits.

Protein intake needs to be considered very carefully when a pregnant woman is a vegetarian. The combination of low protein intake from some vegetarian diets and reduced utilization of protein from plant sources makes it difficult to provide adequate protein to the body during pregnancy. Increased emphasis on eggs, milk, and cheese can be a practical and realistic way of avoiding difficulties associated with too little protein. An appropriate blend of amino acids can be made available throughout the day if care is taken to include a cereal in combination with a legume at meals. If this is done, the limiting amino acids of these two important plant protein sources will be complemented for optimal utilization.

Clearly, folate is recognized as an extremely important vitamin during pregnancy. Synthesis of DNA and maturation of red blood cells are dependent on adequate levels of folate, and these two processes are vital aspects of pregnancy. Megaloblastic anemia develops when folate intake is inadequate. Pregnant women who are taking supplemental vitamins should be sure that their intake of folate is 400 µg, but is not as high as 800 µg. This upper limit is important to avoid masking of possible low levels of vitamin B_{12}.

Calcium, phosphorus, and vitamin D intakes are recommended at high levels to help promote the availability of calcium and phosphorus to meet the needs of the developing fetal skeletal and dental structures without depleting maternal stores. An inadequate intake of these nutrients will cause some of the necessary calcium and phosphorus to be removed from the mother's bones and transferred to the fetus. There is a wide range of ability to absorb these two minerals from the intestine, but the recommendation has been set high enough to accommodate the variation.

The high recommendation for iron is based on the need for increased erythrocyte formation as a result of the increased volume of blood in the mother. In addition, there will be about 750 to 800 mg of iron incorporated into the fetus. The diet, even when selected very carefully, will not contain nearly the level of iron recommended to insure adequate levels for both the fetus and the mother. When iron intake is inadequate, the fetus appears to have priority over the mother and will draw upon her stores. Actual absorption of iron is highly variable, depending on the need and the form in which the iron is supplied. A supplement of 150 mg of ferrous sulfate (providing 30 mg of elemental iron) is recommended to augment the iron provided in

the diet from meats and other sources. The goal of iron supplementation is to avoid iron-deficiency anemia in the mother so
that she will maintain her optimal energy level and general good
health throughout pregnancy.

Iodine is important for the formation of thyroxine, but an
adequate amount is not difficult to obtain. Use of iodized salt is
sufficient to avoid any possible problem from lack of this mineral.
If iodine is severely restricted during pregnancy, cretinism or
mental retardation may be a consequence. However, the mother
will show evidence of goiter before her fetus is severely affected.

Contrary to previous practice, sodium intake is not
usually restricted today. Actually, sodium needs are increased
during pregnancy as a result of the increase in extracellular
fluids. Diuretics are definitely not recommended during pregnancy because of the increased loss of sodium they trigger.
Normal use of salt in food preparation will be sufficient to meet
sodium needs. The main goal is to maintain a normal pattern,
rather than limiting salt intake sharply. Salt substitutes ordinarily are not recommended because of their lack of sodium.

The benefit of fluoridated water for pregnant women is not
clear because of the limited development of tooth enamel *in utero*.
There is some evidence that there may be some benefit in using
fluoridated water during pregnancy. In view of this possible
benefit, as well as the definite benefit to the nursing infant
following birth, there may be merit in drinking fluoridated water
during pregnancy. The fluoride level should not exceed 1 mg/
liter.

Magnesium, zinc, and manganese have been found to be
potentially harmful at high levels in the diets of some experimental animals. However, these minerals are important at the
levels they ordinarily occur in food. Zinc is of particular importance during cell division. The usual pattern is for the blood level
of zinc to drop somewhat in pregnancy, apparently as a result of
hemodilution (increase in blood volume due to increased fluid
without increased solids). A zinc supplement is not considered
necessary or wise. However, an excessive supplementation of
iron needs to be avoided because iron increases zinc
requirements.

HEMODILUTION
*Increase in blood
volume due to
increased fluid without
a corresponding
increase in solids.*

Vitamin C needs to be increased in pregnancy to provide
for increased collagen formation that is occurring. This vitamin
also aids in the absorption of calcium and phosphorus, both of
which are very important during pregnancy.

The need for more thiamin, riboflavin, and niacin is a direct reflection of the need to process more carbohydrate, fat, and protein during pregnancy. Vitamin B_6 is increased greatly because of protein synthesis occurring throughout pregnancy. Also, the metabolism of tryptophan is modified by pregnancy, but adequate vitamin B_6 counterbalances the problem.

Vitamin E is of particular interest in pregnancy because of its antioxidant action. It has been studied as a possible means of helping to reduce the likelihood of a miscarriage, but results do not support the use of vitamin E therapy for this problem. Another of the fat-soluble vitamins, vitamin K, is important in preventing hemorrhaging in the mother and infant at the time of birth. The routine practice of giving the mother a high dose of menadione (synthetic vitamin K) during or prior to labor was found to cause hyperbilirubinemia (abnormally high bile levels) in a small portion of newborns, especially if they were premature. This practice has been modified to reduce the dosage to the level necessary to prevent hemorrhaging. Another approach is to give natural vitamin K to the mother and the infant.

MENADIONE
Synthetic form of vitamin K; high doses have caused hyperbilirubinemia in some premature infants.

HYPERBILIRUBINEMIA
Abnormally high levels of bilirubin; seen in some premature infants whose mothers received high dosages of menadione in late pregnancy.

"EATING FOR TWO"

Changes are needed in eating habits during pregnancy. That can be easily seen by taking a look at Tables 4.5 and 4.6. The point that stands out is the discrepancy between the recommended intake of various nutrients in comparison with the small increase in calories. If it were not for this inconsistency, a pregnant woman could simply increase the amount of each of the foods she was eating before becoming pregnant. No changes in the pattern would be necessary. However, that is not the case.

Let's consider how appropriate changes can be made by starting with experiences in early pregnancy. Early physiological changes can result in feelings of nausea and, sometimes, vomiting. Severity varies greatly from one woman to another. If the condition is mild, nausea is limited to a short period of the day, usually the early morning hours. This causes little disruption of regular eating patterns. However, a few women experience more severe vomiting problems the rest of the day or even most of the time. Nausea and vomiting, often referred to as "morning sickness" because of the time they occur, will usually diminish and disappear by the end of the first trimester.

MORNING SICKNESS
Nausea and/or vomiting associated with the physiological changes of early pregnancy, but usually stopping by the end of the first trimester.

Nausea is certainly uncomfortable, but it influences nutrition only in its effect on appetite when it occurs. The problem of persistent vomiting does affect nutrition, because an electrolyte imbalance may develop and also some food may fail to reach the small intestine for adequate digestion and absorption. This is not usually a significant problem, but some women may lose weight during this early, crucial phase of pregnancy. For them, attention can be given to providing a nourishing diet and a vitamin and mineral supplement that includes much of the recommended daily amounts at a time of day when they are most likely to be retained.

Some women are helped during this period by eating soda crackers or other plain foods before they get out of bed in the morning. A small amount of a food that is low in fat can have a calming effect. Frequent, small meals are another effective way to reduce feelings of nausea. If these measures are limited in their effectiveness, pregnant women can gain comfort from the encouraging fact that the embryo can obtain necessary quantities of the various nutrients from her body; nausea ordinarily passes before the period when fetal demands become high.

By the beginning of the second trimester, tissue growth begins to increase appreciably, as shown in Fig. 4.1. Fortunately, this is a period when appetite usually is good — if not *too* good. By this time, pregnant women definitely need to eat a diet that provides all the nutrients at recommended levels. Wise selection of a varied diet emphasizing milk, fruits, and vegetables and minimizing fat is important throughout the remainder of pregnancy. Most of the necessary nutrients will be available from food when good choices are made. The nutrient recommended for supplementation is iron, because food levels do not provide optimal amounts. The recommended level of iron supplementation is 30 mg. Women carrying more than one fetus may also need supplementation of folate and vitamin B_6.

One important dietary change in pregnancy is increasing the amount of milk consumed by two glasses to provide additional calcium. Adult women should have as their goal an intake of four glasses daily, and pregnant teenagers are advised to drink at least five glasses daily, preferably six. The milk in most instances should be nonfat milk fortified with vitamins A and D. This represents an increase of 180 cal when two additional glasses are drunk, whereas whole milk would add 320 cal for the two glasses — a figure already 20 cal over the additional 300 cal recommended for pregnancy. When nonfat milk is fortified with vitamins A and D, it is nutritionally an even better choice than whole milk for pregnant women unless they need to gain more weight than is normal during pregnancy. Because appetites tend to exceed need during the second and third trimesters, the calories saved by drinking nonfat milk make it possible to select foods from other groups during this period. Occasional choices of cheese and ice cream can be made to add to the nutrient intake from the milk and dairy products food group, but their calorie burden must be considered when using them. Women who are very active during pregnancy will not have to be so concerned about the possible extra calories from this food group.

Protein intake is important during pregnancy and is recommended at the following levels per kilogram: 1.3 g/day in the first trimester, 6.1 g/day in the second, and 10.7 g/day in the third trimester. The inclusion of a quart of milk a day provides 36 g toward the total of at least 60 g of protein needed daily during pregnancy. Two servings of meat will bring the diet to the recommended protein intake. An egg a day, preferably in the morning at breakfast to help spread the protein intake throughout the day, is also recommended.

Although protein intake is not difficult to maintain at adequate levels when meats can be included, financial constraints or vegetarian food patterns can cause pregnant women difficulty in getting enough protein. Frequent use of poultry and fish, rather than eating only red meats, can be an effective way of getting sufficient high-quality protein at a moderate cost in both calories and money. The animal protein sources, whether red meats or milk, cheese, poultry, and fish, are important as sources of vitamin B_{12}, too. Inclusion of some legumes can be useful in adding variety, as well as protein, to the diet.

Vegetarians should be careful to eat a cereal like rice with legumes to improve the efficiency with which they can use the protein at a meal. Unfortunately, plant sources of protein do not provide vitamin B_{12}, a serious shortcoming for pregnant vegetarians. Inclusion of the recommended intake of milk and eggs is an important way to provide vitamin B_{12}, as well as protein and other nutrients.

Protein content in plant foods is distinctly lower than in animal sources. For instance, a cup of baked beans provides 16 g of protein (and 310 cal), compared with 23 g and (and 245 cal) from a 3-oz serving of braised pot roast. A cup of cooked rice contains only 4 g of protein and (about 185 cal). A tablespoon of roasted peanuts can be used to add 2 gm of protein, but at a cost of 55 cal. Pecans and cashews are similar to peanuts in protein and calories. From these examples, it is clear that the quantities of beans, cereals, or nuts needed to provide necessary protein intake are large and comparatively high in calories.

In the vegetable and fruit group, pregnant women are advised to include a generous serving of a fruit high in vitamin C every day. Special attention should be given to eating a dark green, leafy or yellow vegetable (spinach, carrots, or winter squash, for example) frequently to provide the necessary vitamin A. Serving sizes can be more than 1/2 c, if desired. Actually, fruit and vegetable intake can be significantly increased beyond the recommended minimum of five half-cup servings daily. Not only are they important sources of a wide and useful variety of minerals and vitamins, but they are also key sources of fiber. Their bulk is helpful in satisfying appetites without adding very many calories, and their fiber promotes elimination. Because constipation is a common problem, especially in the last trimester of pregnancy, the stimulation fruits and vegetables provide to intestinal motility is very useful.

Breads and cereals should be included in the pregnant woman's diet at the level of at least six servings daily. However,

RESEARCH INSIGHTS

Hickey, C.A., Sociocultural and behavioral influences on weight gain during pregnancy. *Am. J. Clin. Nutr. 71(suppl):* 1364S. 2000.

Hickey examines factors influencing women to gain less than the amount identified as promoting favorable birth outcomes by the Institute of Medicine in 1990 [lowest weight gain for women with a BMI (body mass index) of 19.8 was 11.5 kg and for those with a BMI between 19.8 and 26.0 was 12.5 kg]. A maternal weight gain within the recommended range was associated with birth of fewer low-birth and high-birth weight infants, large-for-gestational-age infants, and fewer preterm and cesarean deliveries.

U.S. birth certificate information in 1995 indicated that 10.4% of women delivering between 37 and 39 weeks and that 9.3% completing 40 or more weeks gained less than 7.3 kg. Non-Hispanic black women had the highest incidence of low weight gain in pregnancy, followed by Hispanic, and then non-Hispanic white women. Data for maternal weight gain (ignoring length of pregnancy) revealed that American Indians were only slightly less likely to have too low a weight gain than black women; Pacific Islanders were somewhat less likely than Hispanics. Asians were similar to non-Hispanic whites, although Chinese were least likely to be too low in weight gain.

Other factors also appear to influence maternal weight gain during pregnancy. Women in their first pregnancy are more likely to gain the recommended amount of weight than are multiparas. Women who are not married or who are older than 30 years are somewhat less likely to gain enough weight to meet recommendations. Women with more than a high school education are more likely than those with less than an elementary school education to gain the recommended weight during pregnancy. Smokers are more likely to gain too little weight than are non-smokers.

Clearly, pregnant women improve the likelihood of a successful outcome of pregnancy if they gain enough weight to meet the range recommended by the Institute of Medicine (from Subcommittee on nutritional status and weight gain during pregnancy. Institute of Medicine. *Nutrition during Pregnancy*. National Academy Press. Washinton, D.C. 1990). Additional research regarding cultural and psychological influences on weight gain during pregnancy is needed to aid health professionals who are working with women during their pregnancies to help improve outcomes.

if weight gain becomes difficult to control, she should restrict her use of butter and jam on breads and sugar on cereals. The contribution of thiamin, riboflavin, niacin, and iron from breads and cereals is important. The choice of whole grain products to meet the need in this category is very wise during pregnancy, because they are slightly higher in other vitamins and minerals than refined products; they are also excellent sources of fiber, supplementing the fiber in fruits and vegetables.

MEAL PATTERNS

Many eating patterns are found in the United States today, and there are many acceptable ways of meeting nutritional requirements. However, pregnant women need to eat several times a day, following an overall plan to ensure that adequate foods are eaten daily. In particular, protein sources should be distributed throughout the day. Some women will find that four or even more small meals during the day satisfy their needs, whereas others may prefer to eat the traditional three meals and perhaps have one or two appropriate snacks. A single meal a day is definitely not advisable, and even two meals daily will probably not provide appropriate intake.

One pattern that can be suggested to satisfy the nutritional demands of pregnancy is based on eating three meals and an evening snack. This frequency of eating allows good distribution of protein and fits the work schedules that must be considered by many pregnant women. Table 4.8 describes one nutritionally adequate pattern appropriate for pregnancy.

Although the suggested pattern may seem Spartan, it is typical of the type of diet appropriate to the nutritional needs of pregnancy. The nutrient density (the relative concentration of nutrients compared to the proportion of calories) of the foods eaten needs to be comparatively high during pregnancy to ensure that the various nutrients are being provided at the levels required by the body. Milk is an example of a food with high nutrient density, whereas candy and many rich, sweet desserts are very low in nutrient density. As a general dietary rule, desserts of low nutrient density should be avoided during pregnancy.

NUTRIENT DENSITY Comparison of the proportion of various nutrients to calories in a food.

WEIGHT CONTROL

SIGNIFICANCE IN PREGNANCY With today's tremendous emphasis on being thin, there is a need for pregnant women to realize that they should be gaining weight at an appropriate rate during their pregnancies. Too little weight gain presents an unnecessary risk. On the other hand, this word of warning should not be translated into permission to eat everything that may be desired. Excessive weight is likely to result in an increase in maternal fat stores that may remain long after delivery. In addition, weight gain beyond the level recommended by the Food and Nutrition Board (20 to 25 pounds) or the more generous 35 pounds recommended by the Subcommittee on Nutritional Status and Weight Gain During Pregnancy (1990) does not appear to have any particular benefit for the fetus either.

The prospective mother's pre-pregnancy weight influences the amount of weight that is appropriate for her to gain during her pregnancy. In Table 4.9, the recommendations are based on an assessment of body mass index (BMI). This index is calculated by dividing prepregnancy weight by the square of the height (in meters). Note that underweight women are encouraged to gain significantly more weight than obese women, but obese women also need to gain some weight for optimal outcomes of pregnancy.

BODY MASS INDEX (BMI) Ratio of weight/ height^2 in meters.

TABLE 4.8   Suggested Menu Pattern for a Pregnant Woman

Meal	Food	Serving Size
Breakfast	Egg	1
	Whole-wheat toast	1 slice
	Orange juice	6 oz
	Nonfat milk	8 oz
Lunch	Chicken sandwich (w/ whole-grain bread)	3 oz chicken (2 slices)
	Broccoli, steamed	3/4 c
	Nonfat milk	8 oz
Dinner	Spaghetti w/ meatballs in tomato sauce	1 c cooked spaghetti, 3 oz cooked beef
	Mixed green salad, (w/ Italian dressing)	1 c 1 tbs
	Fruit cup	3/4 c
	Nonfat milk	8 oz
Snack	Nonfat milk	8 oz

[a]Adapted from H.N. Jacobson, "Nutrition and Pregnancy," In *Maternal and Child Health Practices*, H. Wallace, Ed. Charles C. Thomas, Springfield, IL 1973.

Adolescents who give birth less than two years after beginning menstruation tend to produce babies that are somewhat lighter than those born of more mature women. Black babies, on the average, are lighter than white babies. Because of these tendencies, very young adolescents and black women are advised to set their weight gain goal during pregnancy toward the upper end of the ranges indicated in Table 4.9. This recommendation, based on the correlation between weight gain during pregnancy and the weight of the newborn, will help to produce infants that are large enough to be at minimal risk.

Short women (62 inches or less in height) probably should attempt to gain about the amount of weight indicated at the lower end of the appropriate range for their BMI. These

TABLE 4.9 Recommended Weight Gain During Pregnancy Based on Pregnancy Body Mass Index[a]

BMI (prepregnancy)	Recommended weight gain (pounds)
<19.8 (underweight)	28–40
19.8–26.0 (normal weight)	25–35
>26.0–29.0 (overweight)	15–25
>29.0 (obese)	At least 15

[a]Adapted from Subcommittee on Nutritional Status and Weight Gain During Pregnancy, *Food and Nutrition Board. Nutrition During Pregnancy*, National Academy Press. Washington, D.C., 1990, p. 5–10.

women are particularly likely to bear infants of high birth weight when their weight gain is excessive. Consequently, birth presents an increased likelihood of complications for both mothers and infants. Even taller women increase their likelihood of bearing infants of high birth weights when they gain an excessive amount of weight during pregnancy.

Too little weight gain during pregnancy is undesirable, too. The principal problem associated with the very limited weight gain is an increased likelihood of prematurity and increased risk for the tiny infant.

The incidence of low birth weight infants has been noted in several parts of the world where pregnant women receive a limited diet as the result of difficult socioeconomic conditions. The least expensive source of calories is usually foods that are rich in carbohydrate, so supplementation of these women's diets with inexpensive carbohydrate foods makes economic sense if it improves the birth weight of their infants. The appropriateness of this supplementation was studied in 1975 by Lechtig, et al, in Guatemala. These workers provided pregnant women in isolated villages with ad libitum supplements, one supplement being sugar and the other a combination of protein and sugar. Surprisingly, even the supplement based only on sugar was effective in achieving a higher birth weight. The protein and sugar supplement also resulted in an increased birth weight, but was more costly than the sugar supplement. This study demonstrated the importance of having sufficient calories in the diet to spare protein for its vital functions, instead of being used for energy. Since most women in the United States have diets that are adequate for good reproductive performance, there is clearly no reason to add sugar. Calories should come from nutrient-dense foods whenever possible for all women who are able to buy the food they need.

Inadequate caloric intake to meet energy needs during pregnancy alters metabolic reactions in the body, because body stores of fat are used to meet the energy deficit. This means that more fat than normal is being metabolized. Because there probably will not be enough carbohydrate to complete the breakdown of the fats, ketcone bodies will start to accumulate; these bodies, as they pass through the placenta, can cause neurological problems in the fetus.

TOXEMIAS OF PREGNANCY AND WEIGHT CONTROL Abnormal patterns of too little or too much weight gain are a potential hazard for the unborn fetus as well as for the mother because of the increased likelihood of abnormal conditions, like preeclampsia, eclampsia, and toxemia. Preeclampsia, eclampsia, and toxemia are collectively known as the toxemias of pregnancy; the degree of symptoms is somewhat milder in preeclampsia than in the other conditions. The symptoms noted in the toxemias include proteinuria (protein in the urine), edema, and hypertension. These problems are seen most frequently in pregnant teenagers, women over 30, very underweight women who fail to gain well in pregnancy, and in women who gain excessively during pregnancy.

Diagnosis of toxemia of pregnancy is based on the presence of all three symptoms. The cause of protein in the urine (proteinuria) in pregnancy is not known, but it is definitely an indication of the possible development of toxemia during pregnancy. Hypertension associated with toxemia is indicated by an elevation in the systolic pressure of 20 to 30 mm mercury above the person's normal value or a rise of 10 to 15 mm mercury in diastolic pressure. This clarifies the point that women who normally have hypertension when not pregnant do not automatically develop toxemia; proteinuria and edema are evident if they develop toxemia.

Edema alone is not an indication of toxemia; swelling of the feet and legs is noted in many women in late pregnancy, particularly when the weather is very warm. Usually, salt restriction and use of diuretics are not appropriate measures to counteract edema.

The problems associated with toxemias vary in severity with the duration and timing of the condition. The liver is vulnerable to negative changes, particularly to hemorrhages. Hemorrhaging may be found in the brain, areas of the heart, the lungs, and the adrenals in extremely severe cases. Infants born of toxemic mothers may be retarded in both mental and physical growth. Some are hypoglycemic following birth, which presents a problem in providing the glucose needed by the brain during this crucial period. Women particularly at risk of developing toxemia are those from poor socioeconomic backgrounds, because their diets may be inadequate during pregnancy.

HYPERTENSION High blood pressure defined in pregnancy as a systolic pressure of 144 mm mercury or a diastolic pressure of 90 mm mercury or both.

ALCOHOL, DRUGS, AND TOBACCO

Foods are not the only substances that have the potential for providing compounds that will influence fetal development. The consumption of alcohol is certainly not an appropriate means of providing nutrients during pregnancy. In fact, the question is whether or not alcohol should be consumed at all during the period of gestation. One thing is perfectly clear: avoiding all alcohol during pregnancy will avoid any possible hazard from this source. The American Council on Science and Health recommends caution in the use of alcohol, with an absolute maximum of two drinks in any day. This recommendation translates into no more than 24 oz of beer, 8 oz of wine, or 3 oz of 80-proof liquor. "Binge" drinking, in which larger amounts of alcohol are drunk on a single occasion, can cause birth defects if consumed at times when critical cell division and differentiation are occurring. In contrast to the recommendation of the American Council on Science and Health, some government groups (the Surgeon General and the Bureau of Alcohol, Tobacco, and Firearms) advocate total abstention during pregnancy, because individual variation and threshold effects of alcohol are not clearly understood at the present time.

FETAL ALCOHOL SYNDROME Serious defects in infants whose mothers drank sufficient quantities of alcohol during pregnancy to harm the fetus; includes changes in the central nervous system, growth deficiencies, facial abnormalities, and organs and structural defects.

Fetal alcohol syndrome is the term applied to the condition of some infants whose mothers were categorized as chronic alcoholics during pregnancy. Abnormalities observed in these children include central nervous system disorders, growth deficiencies, facial abnormalities, and organ and structural defects. These children often have small eye openings, a broad nose with a flattened bridge, and underdeveloped mouth and jaws. Short length and low weight at birth extend to "failure to thrive" in the postnatal period. Mental retardation is present, ranging from mild to severe; coordination is poor, and personality characteristics include irritability and hyperactivity. Cleft palate, defects in blood vessels, extra fingers and toes, abnormal breastbone or spine, or a short neck are other teratogenic effects that excessive alcohol during pregnancy may impose on the infant born with fetal alcohol syndrome.

The effects of drugs on the developing embryo or fetus may be quite different from the effects on the mother. Unfortunately, drug effects may even be lethal to the embryo during the very early phase of pregnancy before a woman is aware that she is pregnant. Effects may range from essentially none to a wide variety of changes seen in the infant after birth. Various hormones may cause some masculinization of females. Anticoagulants can result in hemorrhaging or even fetal death. Even aspirin near the time of delivery can interfere with the appropriate clotting mechanism in the fetus. Other medications may also be transmitted to the fetus, causing a variety of symptoms. Various compounds that are subject to "substance abuse" have been found to cause severe health problems in newborns. Infants of low birth weight are born far more frequently to mothers using the various addictive drugs, including crack cocaine, heroin, LSD, designer-drugs, and amphetamines. Some infants are even born with an addiction. Steps for detoxification are taken after birth. Many babies are irreparably damaged for life by their mother's ingestion of drugs during gestation. Also, life expectancy in these babies is significantly less than babies born to mothers without addictive-drug abuse. Because of possible risks associated with the ingestion of many medications and the use of addicitve drugs, these substances should be eliminated unless prescribed by a licensed physician who is aware of the mother's pregnancy.

The effect of smoking is of significance in pregnancy. The risk of an infant being stillborn or dying in the first few days of life is significantly increased when the mother smokes heavily. Fortunately, there can be some benefit to the infants of smokers if the mothers quit smoking even as late as the fourth month of pregnancy. Growth is depressed when a mother smokes; this effect is apparently due to decreased oxygen availability to the fetus and/or to the consumption of a less adequate diet by women who do smoke. For those who refuse to quit smoking for their baby's health, moderation is the key here.

In summary, the birth defects caused from the mother ingesting alcohol, using addictive drugs, and/or smoking or being exposed to secondary smoke are entirely preventable. No child need suffer the effects caused by these behaviors. It is entirely within the mother's control to prevent the effects of alcohol, drugs, and smoke on her child during pregnancy.

CAFFEINE

Several studies using large numbers of human subjects have not demonstrated a statistically significant relationship between caffeine and birth defects. However, it is known that caffeine crosses the placenta and enters the fetus. In animal studies testing much higher levels of caffeine than would be obtained in routine drinking of coffee, tea, and cola beverages, some congenital malformations, increased spontaneous abortions, and premature deliveries were found. Although similar effects have not been noted in humans, some people feel that decreased caffeine consumption during pregnancy may be prudent.

SUPPLEMENTS

Despite the fact that a good diet provides all the nutrients needed (with the exception of iron), women may still worry about whether they should take massive doses of vitamin supplements as insurance against any possible deficiency. In their enthusiasm for being well nourished, they may fall into the trap of taking megadoses of some of the vitamins — a practice which is likely to be detrimental. Actual cases of vitamin C overdoses during pregnancy have occurred, with the result that the infants develop scurvy after birth because they are no longer receiving the very high dosages available to them *in utero*. To avoid this problem and other possible overdoses, any vitamin supplementation should be limited to no more than the RDA for the various nutrients included in the supplement. The exceptions to this recommendation are iron and folate.

PICA

In some regions, pregnant women exhibit unusual eating behavior in which they ingest large amounts of starch and/or sometimes clay. This craving for such substances is referred to as pica. When clay is eaten, the pica is classified as geophagia; amylophagia is the term for eating starch (Horner, et al, 1991). Research efforts to explain this behavior on the basis of some missing nutrient have been totally unsuccessful. Starch can provide calories, but essentially nothing else; clay does not have the potential for providing energy, but it sometimes contains some minerals (Johns and Duquette, 1991). In cases where this

PICA
Another name for the practice of eating such unusual substances as clay and starch.

GEOPHAGIA
Eating of earthy or clay-like substances.

AMYLOPHAGIA
Eating of starch.

behavior is seen, there is merit in discouraging the intake of substances which may be harmful and seeking food and/or financial aid for needy pregnant women.

THE PREGNANT ADOLESCENT AND NUTRITION

Pregnant adolescents have some unique concerns related to nutrition. The fact that they are still growing themselves places even more importance on nutrition for them than their older counterparts. They are confronted by a dual stress situation, nutritionally speaking. Although the nutrients needed for growth and pregnancy can be easily provided in theory, actual practice may fall far short. First, a pregnancy may be the last thing a young expectant mother wants. A tremendous range of emotions may surge through her as she attempts to adjust to the situation. Relationships with family members and friends may be strained. She is suddenly thrust into the adult world, whether she wants to be or not. The adjustments of pregnancy are great enough for any woman without these added burdens.

According to Story and Alton (1995), about 10 percent of American teenagers become pregnant annually, and just over half of these pregnancies result in births. Perhaps because of the publicity regarding use of condoms to reduce risk of HIV, the pregnancy rate among sexually-active teens has dropped. However, the higher incidence of intercourse among this age group actually has resulted in a higher rate of pregnancies. Added to this picture is the fact that more than 80 percent of teenagers giving birth are from low-income backgrounds; furthermore, about one in five of the first-time mothers ages 15–19 will have a second child in 2 years or less.

Pregnancies in adolescents are complicated by many factors, prominent among which are inadequate prenatal medical care, lack of financial resources, and physical demands for growth of their own bodies (as well as those of the fetus). Prematurity and low birth weight are common results of adolescent pregnancies. Preeclampsia (pregnancy-induced hypertension) and anemia are familiar problems in teen pregnancies.

Teenagers are noted for their independent and sometimes poor food habits. Excesses and deficiencies of nutrients are possibilities as a result of these habits. When a teenage girl becomes pregnant, there is no guarantee that she was well nourished at the time of conception; nor is it certain that she will practice good nutrition patterns during her pregnancy.

These are only a few of the possible reasons a pregnant adolescent will probably need a considerable amount of support, including guidance about her nutrition. Preaching will certainly be received with resistance. Careful exploration of her feelings, ideas, and concerns will help identify some ways in which she can be helped with her diet to enhance the likelihood of a successful pregnancy and to improve her own nutritional status.

Actual dietary plans for individual pregnant teenagers need to be developed based on reported eating patterns. Among the key nutrients is iron, which should be considered in relation to the iron level in the body. Ordinarily, a 30 mg supplement of elemental iron is adequate, but as much as 60 to 120 mg/day may be needed in cases of iron-deficiency anemia. With such high supplementation of iron, a supplement of 15 mg of zinc and 2 mg of copper is wise to overcome the limited absorption of these minerals that results when iron supplementation is very high. Calcium needs can be met by drinking 5 glasses of milk (nonfat is fine) or by taking a 600-mg supplement of elemental calcium (1.5 g calcium carbonate or other source).

LACTATION

The lactation period is often a time of real eating pleasure, because milk production requires an increase in the number of calories that should be included in the diet. In fact, the recommendation is 500 kcal above the nonpregnancy recommendation and even 200 above the level for pregnancy. A few special treats can be worked in occasionally, if desired. Virtually all nutrients are needed at levels at least as high as in pregnancy; a notable exception is folate, which still is recommended at a level well above the amount suggested for the nonpregnant woman. Very minor reductions in a few nutrients are suggested during the second six months of lactation.

Daily milk production itself is estimated to require about 750 kcal. This estimate is based on a woman who produces a little over 3 1/2 c of milk each day. This amount of energy is expected to be available by increasing calories in the diet by 500 (as recommended in the 1989 RDA), and the remaining 250 kcal or so are made available from stores of fat deposited during pregnancy.

Protein need is increased slightly during lactation in comparison with pregnancy, and so is the need for vitamins E, K,

B_6, pantothenic acid, biotin, and choline. Vitamins A and C are increased in the RDA for lactation because of their importance in producing milk with useful amounts of these two vitamins. Thiamin and riboflavin are recommended at increased levels to aid in the utilization of increased amounts of food needed during lactation.

The dietary pattern should include at least a quart of milk. If nonfat milk is used, it should be fortified with vitamins A and D. Two servings from the meat and meat substitutes group will provide the additional protein recommended in the RDA.

Care should be taken to include an adequate amount of iron to replenish iron stores in the mother that may have been reduced during pregnancy and delivery. This will help to build her stores and will add a very small amount of iron to her milk.

Generous use of fruits, vegetables, breads, and cereals will provide necessary quantities of the various vitamins and other minerals. In addition, plenty of liquid is needed. Usually, about three quarts of liquid will be the amount of fluid dictated by thirst to avoid dehydration. The loss of a little less than a quart of fluid daily in the secreted milk accounts for the importance of a generous fluid intake during lactation.

Many ingested substances are incorporated into human milk. This underlines the importance of being careful to avoid drugs as much as possible while nursing an infant. For the same reason, large doses of garlic and other strong-flavored or spicy foods are not recommended. They might cause intestinal distress in the infant.

Diet for lactation is actually quite uncomplicated. An adequate amount of fairly simple foods from the Food Guide Pyramid is the central point of planning. In particular, inclusion of a quart of milk and avoidance of strongly-spiced foods and drugs are the chief points to watch.

SUMMARY

Consideration of nutritional needs during pregnancy should begin well in advance of conception, because nutritional adequacy throughout the mother's growing years influences the outcome of pregnancy. When possible, a woman's diet should be evaluated for adequacy before pregnancy and modified accordingly. Also, weight should be brought into the recommended range.

During pregnancy, total recommended weight gain is approximately 20 to 35 lb, representing the sum of the mother's physical changes, the products of pregnancy, and a small fat reservoir for the mother. Because increased need for nutrients must be provided by foods that contain a combined total of about 300 cal daily during pregnancy, very careful food selections are essential. The appropriate diet pattern includes a quart of milk (usually nonfat fortified with vitamins A and D), two 3-oz portions of meat or meat substitute, generous servings of fruits and vegetables, six servings of whole-grain breads and cereals, plus an iron supplement of 30 mg and 400 μg folate.

Abnormal patterns of weight gain, either too little or too much, may trigger toxemias of pregnancy. Other factors to be restricted during pregnancy to avoid possible harm to the fetus include the consumption of alcoholic beverages, various drugs, and smoking. Although proof of caffeine as a teratogen is lacking, some caution in consuming coffee, tea, and cola beverages is suggested. Massive doses of vitamins or other supplements should be avoided.

Lactation places a special demand upon a woman's body, and nutrient needs are modified somewhat from those of pregnancy. In particular, there is an increase in required calories because of the energy represented in the production of milk. A well-balanced diet with an iron supplement and plenty of liquid are the means of providing the nutritional support for successful lactation.

BIBLIOGRAPHY

ALLEN, C.D. AND C.P. RIES Smoking, alcohol, and dietary practices during pregnancy: comparison before and after prenatal education. *J. Am. Diet. Assoc. 85:* 605. 1985.

ANDERSON, A.S. AND SHEPHERD R. Beliefs and attitudes toward "healthier eating" among women attending maternity hospital. *J. Nutr. Ed. 21:* 208. 1990.

ANONYMOUS Nutritional adequacy of breast feeding. NUTR. REV. 38: 145. 1980.

ARMSTRONG. J.E. AND WEIJOHN, T.T. Dietary quality and concerns about weight of low-income pregnant women. *J. Am. Diet. Assoc. 91(10):* 1280. 1991.

BADART-SMOOK, A., ET AL Fetal growth is associated positively with maternal intake of linoleic acid. *J. Am. Diet. Assoc. 97(8):* 867. 1997.

BINKIN, N.J., ET AL Reducing black neonatal mortality. Will improvement in birth weight be enough? *J. Am. Med. Assoc. 253:* 372. 1985.

BLACKBURN, M.L. AND D.J. CALLOWAY Energy expenditure of pregnant adolescents. *J. Amer. Dietet. Assoc. 64:* 24. 1974.

CANFIELD, L.M., J.M. HOPKINSON, A.D. Lima, B. Silva, and C. Garza. Vitamin K in colostrum and mature human milk over the lactation period. *Am. J. Clin. Nutr. 53:* 730. 1991.

CARROL, P. Safe ingestion of aspartame during pregnancy. *Topics Clin. Nutr. 5:* 1. 1990.

CARRUTH, B.R. AND J.E. SKINNER Pregnant adolescents report infrequent use of sugar substitute. *J. Am. Diet. Assoc. 91(5):* 608. 1991.

CLARREN, S.K. AND D.W. SMITH Fetal alcohol syndrome. *New Eng. J. Med. 298:* 1063. 1978.

COMMITTEE ON DRUGS, AMERICAN ACADEMY OF PEDIATRICS Transfer of drugs and other chemicals into human milk. *Pediatrics 84:* 924. 1989.

COMMITTEE ON MATERNAL NUTRITION *Maternal Nutrition and the Course of Pregnancy.* Food and Nutrition Board, National Research Council. National Academy of Scineces. Washington, D.C. 1970.

COMMITTEE ON MATERNAL NUTRITION *Nutritional Supplementation and Outcome of Pregnancy.* Food and Nutrition Board. National Research Council. National Academy of Sciences. Washington, D.C. 1973.

DUBOIS, S., ET AL Ability of the Higgins Nutrition Intervention Program to improve adolescent pregnancy outcome. *J. Am. Diet. Assoc. 97(8):* 871. 1997.

DUHRING, J.L. Nutrition in Pregnancy. In *Present Knowledge in Nutrition.* Ed. Olson, R.E., et al Nutrition Foundation. Washington, D.C. 5th ed. 1984. p. 636.

ERSHOW, A.G., L.M. BROWN, AND K.P. CANTOR Intake of tapwater and total water by pregnant and lactating women. *Am. J. Pub. Health 81:* 328. 1991.

FIELDING, J. AND A. YANKOUER Pregnant drinker. *Am. J. Pub. Health 68:* 836. 1978.

FINLEY, D., ET AL Food choices of vegetarians and nonvegetarians during pregnancy and lactation. *J. Am. Diet. Assoc. 85:* 678. 1985.

FOOD AND NUTRITION BOARD *Fetal and Infant Nutrition and Susceptibility to Obesity.* National Research Council, National Academy of Sciences. Washington, D.C. 1978.

FOX, H.E., ET AL Maternal ethanol ingestion and occurrence of human fetal breathing movement. *Am. J. Obs. Gyn. 132:* 354. 1978.

FRISANCHO, A.R., ET AL Maternal nutritional status and adolescent pregnancy outcome. *Amer. J. Clin. Nutr. 38:* 739. 1983.

FRISANCHO, A.R., ET AL Influence of growth status and placental function on birth weight of infants born to young still-growing teenagers. *Am. J. Clin. Nutr. 40:* 801. 1984.

GUTCHER, G.R., ET AL Evaluation of vitamin E. status in premature infants. *Am. J. Clin. Nutr. 40:* 1078. 1984.

HABICHT, J.P., ET AL Relation of maternal supplementary feeding during pregnancy to birth weight and other sociobiological factors. *Nutrition and Fetal Development.* Ed. M. Winick. Wiley-Interscience. New York. 1974.

HANSON, J.W., ET AL Effects of moderate alcohol consumption during pregnancy on fetal growth and morphogenesis. *J. Pediat. 92:* 457. 1978.

HEDIGER, M.L., T.O. SCHOLL, J.G. ANCES, D.H., BELSKY, AND R.W. SALMON Rate and amount of weight gain during adolescent pregnancy: Associations with maternal weight-for-height and birth-weight. *Am. J. Clin. Nutr. 52:* 793. 1990.

HERBERT, V. Folate and neural tube defects. *Nutr. Today 27(6):* 30. 1992.

HOOK, E.B. Dietary cravings and aversions during pregnancy. *Am. J. Clin. Nutr. 31:* 1355. 1978.

HORNER, R.D., C.J. LACKEY, K. KOLASA, AND K. WARREN Pica practices of pregnant women. *J. Am. Diet. Assoc. 91(1):* 34. 1991.

JOHNS, T. AND M. DUQUETTE Detoxification and mineral supplementation as functions of geophagy. *Am. J. Clin. Nutr. 53:* 448. 1991.

JOHNSTON, C.S., F.S. CHRISTOPHER, AND L.A. KANDELL pregnancy weight gain in adolescents and young adults. *J. Am. College Nutr. 10:* 185. 1991.

KURPPA K., ET AL Coffee consumption during pregnancy. *New Eng. J. Med. 306:* 1548. 1982.

KRUSE, J. Alcohol use during pregnancy. *Amer. Fam. Physician 29:* 199. 1984.

KURTZWEIL, P. How folate can help prevent birth defects. *FDA Cons. 30(7):* 7. 1996.

LAMMI-KEEFE, C.J. AND R.G. JENSEN Fat-soluble vitamins in human milk. *Nutr. Rev. 42:* 365. 1984.

LECHTIG, A., ET AL Maternal nutrition and fetal growth in developing countries. *Am. J. Dis. Child. 129:* 553. 1975.

LINN, S., ET AL No association between coffee consumption and adverse outcomes of pregnancy. *New Eng. J. Med. 306:* 141. 1982.

LITTLE, R.E. Moderate alcohol use during pregnancy and decreased infant birth weight. *Am. J. Pub. Health 67:* 1154. 1977.

MASON, J.O. Message to Health Professionals about fluorosis. *J. Am. Med. Assoc. 265:* 2939. 1991.

MERCHANT, K., R. MARTORELL, AND H.D. HAAS Consequences for maternal nutrition of reproductive stress across consecutive pregnancies. *Am. J. Clin. Nutr. 52:* 616. 1990.

MILLER, K.A. AND C.S. FIELD Adolescent pregnancy: combined obstetric and pediatric management approach. *Mayo Clinic Proc. 59:* 311. 1984.

MOTIL, K.J., C.M. MONTANDON, AND C. GARZA Basal and postprandial metabolic rates in lactating and nonlactating women. *Am. J. Clin. Nutr. 52:* 610. 1990.

NELSON, M. Vitamin A, liver consumption, and risk of birth-defects. *Brit. Med. J. 301:* 1176. 1990.

NICHOLS, B.L. AND V.N. NICHOLS Nutrition in pregnancy and lactation. *Nutr. Abst. Rev. 53:* 259. 1983.

OUELLETTE, E.M., ET AL Adverse effects on offspring of maternal alcohol abuse during pregnancy. *New Eng. J. Med. 297:* 528. 1977.

PERKIN, J.E. Maternal influences on development of food allergy in infant. *Topics Clin. Nutr. 5:* 6. 1990.

Prentice, A.M., et al Metabolic consequences of fasting during Ramadan in pregnant and lactating women. *Hum. Nutr. Clin. Nutr. 37:* 283. 1983.

RICHMOND, V.L. Thirty years of fluoridation: a review. *Am. J. Clin. Nutr. 41:* 129. 1985.

RINKE, C.M. Infant mortality and the low-birth weight infant. *J. Am. Med. Assoc. 253:* 826. 1985.

RIORDAN, J. AND M. RIORDAN Drugs in breast milk. *Am. J. Nursing 84:* 328.1984.

SALMENPERA, L. Vitamin C nutrition during prolonged lactation. *Am. J. Clin. Nutr. 40:* 1050. 1984.

SERDULA, M., D.F. WILLIAMSON, J.S. KENDRICK, R.F. ANDA, AND T. BYERS Trends in alcohol consumption by pregnant women: 1985 through 1988. *J. Am. Med. Assoc. 265:* 876. 1991.

SEXTON, M. AND J.R. HEBEL Clinical trial of change in maternal smoking and its effect on birth weight. *J. Am. Med. Assoc. 251:* 911. 1984.

SKINNER, J.D. AND B.R. CARRUTH Dietary quality of pregnant and nonpregnant adolescents. *J. Am. Diet. Assoc. 91(6):* 718. 1991.

STEVENS-SIMON, C., K.J. ROGHMANN, AND E.F. MCANARNEY Relationship of self-reported prepregnant weight and weight gain during pregnancy in maternal body habitus and age. *J. Am. Diet. Assoc. 92(1):* 85. 1992.

SUBCOMMITTEE ON NUTRITIONAL STATUS AND WEIGHT GAIN DURING PREGNANCY Food and Nutrition Board *Nutrition During Pregnancy.* National Academy Press. Washington, D.C. 1990.

SUBCOMMITTEE ON NUTRITION DURING LACTATION Food and Nutrition Board. *Nutrition During Lactation.* National Academy Press. Washington, D.C. 1991.

SUBCOMMITTEE ON THE TENTH EDITION OF THE RDAS Food and Nutrition Board. *Recommended Dietary Allowances.* National Academy Press. Washington, D.C. 1989.

* SUSSER, M. Maternal weight gain, infant birth weight, and diet: Causal sequences. *Am. J. Clin. Nutr. 53:* 1397. 1991.

TATE, W.H., R. SNYDER, E.H. MONTGOMERY, AND J.T. CHAN Impact of source of drinking water on fluoride supplementation. *J. Pediatr. 177:* 419. 1990.

VAN RAAIJ, J.M.A., C.M. SCHONK, S.H. VERMAAT-MIEDEMA, M.E.M. PEEK, AND J.G.A.J. HAUTVAST Energy cost of lactation and energy balance of well-nourished Dutch lactating women. *Am. J. Clin. Nutr. 53:* 612. 1991.

WILLIAMS, R. Decreasing the chance of birth defects. *FDA Consumer 30(9):* 12. 1996.

CHAPTER FIVE

Milk for the Infant

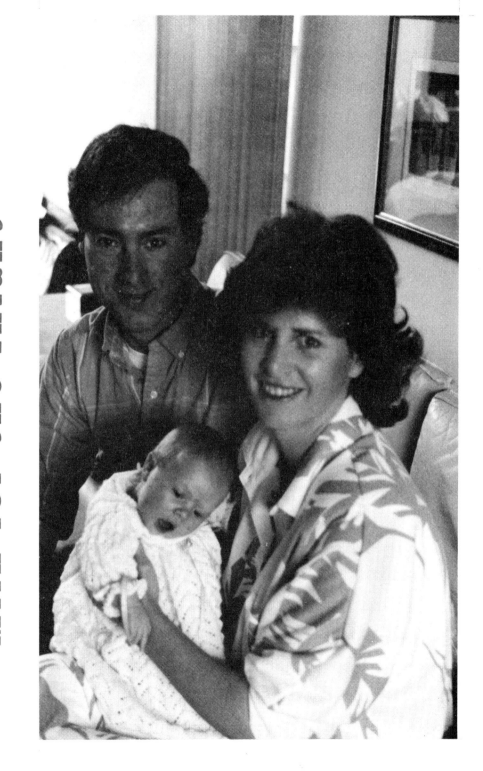

OVERVIEW

Today's new parents include many who are deciding to join the ranks of parents after a decade of getting careers started and sorting out personal priorities! Yes, people in their late twenties and even into their forties, following careful thought, are taking that big step and planning for parenthood. Planning involves making many conscious decisions about the practical aspects of parenthood, as well as the paramount decision to become parents. Parenthood is no longer only for innocent adolescents and eager couples in their twenties. Decisions revolve around such pragmatic questions as whether the mother will continue in her career, who will help with the care of the newborn, and what will be the best way to feed the new baby? These are important questions, particularly for older parents who are making rapid changes from a financially comfortable and independent lifestyle to one in which a constant responsibility in the form of the newborn assumes center stage.

Whatever the ages and lifestyles of prospective parents, they will need to proceed with the care of their newborns immediately after birth. A key aspect of this care is feeding. Fortunately, there is really only one decision regarding this responsibility — whether to breast-feed or bottle-feed. For many parents in this country, this is not an easy decision. Some factors to be considered in making the decision are discussed in this chapter.

WHAT ARE THE ALTERNATIVES?

For most babies, the alternatives are whether to give them human milk by breast-feeding or to bottle-feed with a formula (usually based on modified cow's milk). Although they are both milk, human milk and cow's milk vary considerably in their composition. Proponents of the practice of breast-feeding loudly praise the merits of human milk while deriding cow's milk to be as good for infants as human milk. Others champion the parents who opt for bottle-feeding. In the past few years, we have gone from a nation that blushed and shied away from any talk of breast-feeding to one where parents may be openly criticized unless their children are raised at the breast. Emotions have run amazingly high and people have been remarkably vocal in shoving their opinions on infant feeding practices at any prospective parent within earshot.

Why has the banner of breast-feeding been raised so high and waved so vigorously? No doubt there are as many reasons as there are proponents of breast-feeding, but considerable credit for its resurgence as an important and appropriate means of feeding infants certainly goes to the La Leche League and its enthusiastic members. The renewed interest across the nation in "natural" ways of living, which was essentially a backlash against the impersonalization of technology, provided just the right framework in which to launch a concerted drive toward returning to the natural act of breast-feeding.

The strong interest in breast-feeding that developed in the 1980s has continued, particularly among well-educated, higher income women. In 1995, almost 60 percent of new mothers nursed their infants during the very early days of life. However, the figure dropped to about 23 percent after 6 months. For the past several years, the WIC (Women's, Infants, and Children's) federal program in the U.S. Department of Agriculture has promoted lactation among its participants. Since this program reaches many women from families with low incomes, some progress has been made toward expanding breast-feeding in this population, too.

Because feeding is done primarily to provide the body with the nutrients needed for life and growth, a look at the composition of human and cow's milk will help clarify the facts behind the two feeding alternatives. Human milk starts out as a fluid called colostrum for the first few days of the infant's life. The mother's secretion then changes gradually into mature human milk. The composition of her milk, however, will vary during a feeding; it is much lower in fat at the beginning of the feeding than later in the feeding. Nevertheless, some reasonable comparisons can be made between the secretions of the human mother and the milk available from dairy cows.

COLOSTRUM

COLOSTRUM
Thin, yellowish fluid secreted by new mothers in the first days after delivery; good source of antibodies.

The mother's body undergoes some crucial changes after delivery, for she is making the transition from providing for her infant via the placenta to secreting the necessary nutrients as a result of lactation. Mammary glands in the breasts are able to accommodate this transition quite rapidly; the quantity of flow increases gradually during the first few days, stimulated by the nursing efforts of the infant. During the transition period, colostrum is normally produced during the first three to six days following delivery. Initially colostrum is a thin, yellowish fluid and then it gradually evolves into mature milk by the end of the first week. Although the composition of colostrum comsumed by the newborn varies a bit initially depending upon the elapsed time from birth, energy value, lactose, and fat levels are lower than in mature milk. Protein content, however, is higher. Of particular importance is the antibody content of colostrum, for this is the means of transferring additional health protection to the infant after birth. Even if breast feeding is practiced for only a few days, the transfer of these antibodies will provide important protection for newborns. The nutrient content of colostrum is particularly well-suited to newborns and is somewhat different from either human or cow's milk (Table 5.1).

HUMAN MILK

The increased energy value in mature human milk as compared to colostrum is the result of a dramatic increase in carbohydrate to a level almost twice as high as that of colostrum. Fat content also increases, but only by about one-third. Surprisingly, the protein level in mature milk drops to only about 40 percent of the amount in colostrum.

Human milk generally is considered the best choice for feeding the newborn. Usually, this is a very practical and nutritionally sound decision. In many countries with difficult living conditions, limited educational opportunities, and incomes below the poverty level, mothers may have to nurse their infants if their babies are to have any chance of survival. Many mothers in the United States do have options in deciding how to feed their babies, for both breast and bottle-feeding can be successful under the right conditions.

The mother's diet will influence the nutrient composition of her milk because the vitamin C and iron in her milk correspond to the adequacy of these nutrients in her diet. On the other hand, protein, carbohydrate, and fat content are essentially constant, regardless of the mother's nutritional status. Recommendations for nutritional intake during lactation are intended to ensure adequate nutrients to meet the mother's needs.

COW'S MILK AND COW'S MILK FORMULAS

As can be seen from Table 5.1, there are significant differences in human and cow's milk. For human infants to thrive, modifications must be made if cow's milk is used in feeding. In

TABLE 5.1   Composition of Colostrum, Human, Milk, Cow's Milk, Cow's Milk-Based Formula, and Soy-Based Formula per 100 ml

	Cal-ories	Pro-tein (g)	Fat (g)	Vit. A (IU)	Vit. D (IU)	Vit. E (IU)	Vit. C (mg)	Thia-min (mg)	Ribo-flavin (mg)	Nia-cin (mg)	Pyri-doxine (μg)	Fol-ate (μg)	Vit. B$_{12}$ (μg)	Cal-cium (mg)	Phos-phorus (mg)	Mag-nesium (mg)	Iron (mg)	Zinc (mg)	Cop-per (mg)	Io-dine (μg)
Milk																				
Colostrum[a]	58	2.7	2.9	296	—	1.5–2	4.4	0.015	0.29	0.075	—	—	—	31	14	—	0.09	0.57	0.05	12.2
Human	77	1.1	4.0	240	22	2	5	0.01	0.04	0.2	10	5.2	0.3	33	14	2.3	0.1	4–5	0.024	3.0
Cow's	65	3.5	3.5	140	42.4[d]	0.4	1	0.03	0.17	0.1	64	5.5	4	118	93	1.2	Trace	3–5	0.06	4.7
Formula[c]																				
Milk-Based	67	1.5–1.6	3.8	212	42.4	2	5.5	0.05–0.07	0.06–0.11	0.74–0.95	40	5–10	0.1–0.2	46–54	32–41	4.1–5.2	0.15	0.36–0.5	0.04–0.07	10
Soy-Based	67	1.9	3.9	212	42.4	2	5.5	0.04	0.06	0.95	40	5–10	0.2–0.3	74	53	5–7.8	1.27	0.3–0.5	0.04–0.06	10

[a]Data from Food and Nutrition Academy of Science, *Composition of Milks*, National Research Council Publication No. 254, National Research Council, Washington, D.C., 1953. Dash represents no data available.

[b]Data from *Composition of Foods, Dairy and Egg Products*, *Ag. Handbook 8-1*, Agricultural Research Service, U.S. Department of Agriculture, Washington, D.C. Rev. 1976; Picciano, M.F. and H.A. Guthrie, Copper, iron and zinc contents of mature human milk, *Am. J. Clin. Nutr. 29*: 242, 1976; and *Trace Elements in Human Nutrition*, World Health Organization Technical Report Series No. 532, Geneva, 1973.

[c]Data from product labels; iron-fortified Enfamil, Similac, and Isomil.

[d]Vitamin D-fortified.

the past, diluted canned evaporated milk was combined with corn syrup or dextrimaltose and sterilized for infant feeding. This may still be used as an inexpensive method of feeding, as long as a vitamin C supplement is given.

Many infants who are not breast-fed receive modified cow's milk formulas, with varying modifications according to the manufacturer. These formulas are usually based on the use of nonfat milk, with fat being provided by any of several different vegetable oils. Lactose or some other form of carbohydrate is also added. The addition of various vitamins and minerals brings these formulas to levels comparable to human milk. They are available with or without an iron supplement.

Formulas are marketed in ready-to-feed form requiring merely the addition of a nipple for feeding. This form already contains the appropriate amount of water. Another option is the concentrated formula to which an equal amount of boiled water is added to dilute the product to the correct concentration before feeding. Sterile feeding bottles and nipples, as well as sterile water, are required for safe use of this type of formula. The total cost, however, is usually slightly less than that of the ready-to-feed formulas. A powdered formula that must be reconstituted with sterile water and poured into feeding bottles is also available. Sometimes the granules may fail to dissolve, however, resulting in clogged nipples during feeding. This inconvenience is counterbalanced by the ease of storing the powder for a reasonable time and the savings that may result from its low cost.

NUTRIENT COMPARISONS

FAT

The amount of fat in human milk and in milk-based formulas is quite similar. Cow's milk without modification is half a percent lower in fat than human milk. Regardless of the type of milk being fed, milk fat is an important source of energy for the infant. Milk's level of almost four percent fat is sufficient to spare protein for its unique functions in the body instead of being used immediately for energy. Because infants have a limited stomach capacity, this level of fat helps provide sufficient energy in a form concentrated enough to be held comfortably at one feeding. The ability to provide sufficient caloric intake without excess volume by adding fat is of particular importance in premature infants, whose capacity is even more limited. In the normal, full-term infant, it is not necessary to increase the amount of fat above the four percent level.

The fats in milk perform additional functions besides providing energy: they are carriers of the fat-soluble vitamins A and D, and linoleic acid the essential fatty acid, is supplied by the lipid in milk. With an inadequate intake of linoleic acid, infants will develop a somewhat dry and scaly skin; growth may eventually be stunted.

DHA (docosahexanoic acid) is a polyunsaturated fatty acid that is of particular importance in the brain tissue. Since brain growth is occurring rapidly during early life, dietary intake of DHA may be of special interest in the diet of newborns. Related to DHA intake also is the inclusion of the essential fatty acids (linoleic and linolenic) from which DHA can be synthesized. In Europe, infant formulas are fortified with DHA and arachidonic acid, another polyunsaturated fatty acid involved in brain tissue development. However, fortification of infant formulas with these fatty acids is not done in the United States at the present time despite the fact that the World Health Organization recommends fortification with DHA at the level of 40 mg DHA/kg of infant body weight.

DHA
Docosahexanoic acid; polyunsaturated fatty acid important in the development of brain tissue and intellectual performance.

The level of DHA in human milk is dependent on the diet of the woman. American women tend to eat diets low in fish, which may account for the fact that their milk has low levels of DHA compared with breast milk in other populations around the world. The significance of the comparatively low levels of DHA in human milk in the U.S. is still not known in terms of the impact on the IQ of breast-fed American infants. There may be merit in encouraging pregnant and lactating women to consume an abundance of fish in their diets.

Lipids in human milk appear to be well utilized in the form in which they occur. The comparatively high proportion of saturated fatty acids in cow's milk is not considered as valuable to infants as the higher level of polyunsaturated fatty acids provided in vegetable oils. Therefore, vegetable oils are added to nonfat milk in making infant formulas. These oils are valued not only for their linoleic acid content, but also for their fluid nature. Fats need to be emulsified in the small intestine for optimal enzyme action, digestion, and absorption. Fluid oils can be readily emulsified in the body to promote digestion.

If evaporated milk formulas are being used, the original fat contained in whole milk will be present. This fat is lower in linoleic acid than vegetable oils that are added to formulas, which is a slight disadvantage nutritionally. Homogenization of the milk being evaporated changes the fat into small fat globules that can remain suspended in the milk. Homogenized milk can thus be emulsified and digested for absorption more readily than plain cow's milk. Even with improved emulsification resulting from homogenization, formulas using whole cow's milk still have the disadvantage of containing a comparatively high level of saturated fatty acids.

Modification of the type of fats in formulas may be of significance because of the fat's influence on cholesterol levels in infants. Formulas containing coconut, corn, soybean, or safflower oil promote lower serum cholesterol levels in infants than products containing butterfat. The relationship of this fat in infants to the possible development of atherosclerosis in adulthood is not fully understood. Fomon (1974) suggested possible hazards of a low serum cholesterol level in infancy; normal cholesterol levels may be important to challenge development of the enzyme systems of metabolism needed to degrade cholesterol in the body. Moreover, myelination of the brain may require dietary cholesterol if the process is to continue at the normal rate. On the basis of these arguments, the necessity of feeding infants to achieve a low serum cholesterol value in the very early years is certainly open to question at the present time.

PROTEIN

Protein is essential for growth and development of infants. The vital need for amino acids from proteins to synthesize the proteins needed for tissue growth can be met admirably by breast-feeding. This may seem surprising when the protein content of human milk (1.1 percent) is compared to that of cow's milk (3.5 percent). On the basis of quantity, one would surely predict that infants would grow more rapidly on cow's milk than on human milk, yet this is not the case. In fact, cow's milk has to be diluted to reduce its protein level for improved utilization.

Part of the reason for the difference in digestibility between human milk and cow's milk lies in the characteristics of curd formation resulting from both types. The chief difficulty infants encounter when digesting cow's milk protein is the hardness of the protein curd that forms in the stomach. In technical literature, curd toughness is called curd tension. Milk that is consumed by the infant passes into the stomach, where a dramatic change takes place in the physical state of the milk. Rather than remaining in a smooth, fluid form, the proteins in

HOMOGENIZATION

Forcing of milk through very tiny apertures to split fat globules into smaller particles to prevent the fat from floating to the top.

CURD

Mass formed when protein is denatured, a process ordinarily the result of heating or the addition of acid.

CURD TENSION

Hardness or firmness of a protein curd; a soft curd is digested more readily than a hard curd.

the milk coagulate, forming curds similar to those formed in making cottage cheese. These curds must make intimate contact with proteolytic enzymes in the small intestine so that the protein molecules can be split into their component amino acids in preparation for absorption through the intestinal wall.

If the curd formed by the protein is a very soft, almost fluid mass, it is a comparatively simple matter for the enzymes to make close contact for efficient digestion of protein to the individual amino acids in preparation for absorption. Enzyme action is much less effective on hard, tight curds. The protein curd from human milk which forms in the infant's stomach is soft enough to be digested easily, whereas the curd from cow's milk is much harder. This difference in curd tension is a likely explanation why infants grow almost as well on the lower protein content of human milk as they do on cow's milk.

Digestion of cow's milk protein is aided by two processes: homogenization and pasteurization. Both these procedures modify protein by denaturing some of its molecules. However, pasteurization is not done solely to improve digestibility. The primary reason for pasteurizing milk is to make it safe by killing potentially harmful microorganisms through controlled use of heat. Raw milk (unpasteurized milk) can be the source of microorganisms causing tuberculosis, undulant fever, and salmonellosis, as well as other illnesses. Any microorganisms that happen to find their way into raw milk will still be viable when consumed. These organisms can also be present in pasteurized milk, but the heat reatment involved in pasteurization will kill them.

A comparison of the total amount of protein in human and cow's milk provides only part of the picture. Levels of the various essential amino acids in the two types of milk are also of interest; they are not exactly the same despite the fact that they are both complete proteins. Table 5.2 includes amino acid analysis of these two types of milk and the levels considered to be necessary for infants and children. All the essential amino acids are present in amounts that are adequate or somewhat greater than needed in both types of milk. From the standpoint of protein content, either type of milk can be used quite satisfactorily in infant feeding.

CARBOHYDRATE

The carbohydrate in milk is necessary for the energy it contributes and the role it plays in metabolizing fatty acids. Human milk is almost twice as high in carbohydrate as cow's

TABLE 5.2 Comparison of the Amino Acid Requirements of Infants and Children with the Amino Acid Content of Human and Cow's Milk (g/16g N)[a]

	Human Milk	Cow's Milk	Infant[b]	Infant[c]	Children[d]
Arginine[e]	4.1	3.7	—	—	—
Histidine	2.2	2.7	2.4	—	—
Lysine	6.6	7.9	7.7	7.5	10.7
Leucine	9.1	10.0	10.9	10.9	8.0
Isoleucine	5.5	6.5	6.6	9.2	5.3
Methionine	2.3	2.5	4.8	3.3	—
Cystine[e]	2.0	0.9	—	—	—
Total sulfur amino acids[g]	4.3	3.4	6.2[f]	—	4.8[f]
Phenylalanine	4.4	4.9	6.6	6.5	4.8
Tyrosine	5.5	5.1	—	—	—
Total aromatic amino acids[h]	9.9	10.0	—	—	—
Threonine	4.5	4.7	4.4	6.3	6.1
Tryptophan	1.6	1.4	1.6	1.6	1.6
Valine	6.3	7.0	6.7	7.6	5.9

[a]From *Evaluation of Protein Quality*, Publ. 1100, National Research Council of National Academy of Sciences, Washington, D.C., 1963.
[b]Recalculated from the data given in *Evaluation of Protein Nutrition*, Publ. 711, National Research Council of National Academy of Sciences, Washington, D.C.
[c]Realculated from L.E. Holt, Jr., P. Gyorgi, E.L. Pratt, S.E. Snyderman, and W.M. Wallace, *Protein and Amino Acid Requirements in Early Life*, New York Univ. Press, New York, 1960.
[d]Recalculated from the data of I. Nakawa, T. Takahashi, and T. Suziki, *J. Nutr., 73:* 186 and *74:* 401, 1961.
[e]Nonessential amino acids.
[f]Methionine requirements in absence of cystine.
[g]Includes cysteine, cystine, and methionine.
[h]Includes phenylalanine and tyrosine.

milk. Lactose is the principal carbohydrate in both types of milk. To compensate for the low carbohydrate content of cow's milk, formulas are prepared with added carbohydrate to approximate the level found in human milk. Sometimes lactose is added as the carbohydrate, but corn syrup or sucrose are other popular and less costly forms.

Human milk also contains a large number of different oligosaccharides representing a wide variety of sugars, including lactose. These carbohydrate compounds, which are a bit larger than lactose, are of recognized importance in helping to protect the health of neonates even though they are present in small

OLIGOSACCHARIDES Carbohydrates containing between 3 and 10 units of simple sugar joined into a molecule.

amounts. The oligosaccharides in human milk are often found as glycolipids (joined with lipids) and as glycoproteins (attached to a protein). Various milk oligosaccharide compounds appear to aid in blocking such infectious agents as *E. coli, Campylobacter, C. jejuni,* and *Streptococcus pneumoniae* and also toxins produced by *E. coli, V. cholerae, C. jejuni,* and *S. dysenteriae.*

Other nitrogen-containing oligosaccharides in human milk aid in the production of acetic acid in the intestines of infants by promoting the growth of *Bifidobacterium bifidum var. Pennsylvanicus* (previously designated as *Lactobacillus bifidus*). The acidic condition promoted by *B. bifidum* helps block multiplication of harmful microorganisms, thus providing some protection against diseases. Cow's milk is less effective than human milk in protecting against microbial infections.

Honey should never be added to infant formulas. This admonition is given because spores of *Clostridium botulinum* occasionally make their way into honey. The toxin resulting from the presence of this microorganism is lethal to infants, even in extremely tiny amounts. Other sugars are utilized equally well by infants and do not represent any risk to them. Therefore, there is absolutely no reason to risk the possibility of infants developing botulism through the use of honey as the carbohydrate addition in formulas.

MINERALS

Calcium and phosphorus levels are dramatically different in human and cow's milk. Undiluted cow's milk has more than three times the amount of calcium and six times the amount of phosphorus contained in human milk. Because these minerals are so involved in growth, cow's milk might be expected to promote growth much better than human milk. However, this does not prove to be the case. At the end of the first three months, there is no signficant difference in height or weight as a result of the type of milk fed; formula-fed infants are larger at one year.

Iron needs to be provided by the time an infant is six months old; stores of iron established during the fetal period will be sufficient to meet demands until then if the mother has had adequate iron during pregnancy. By six months, the infant needs iron in the diet. Human milk does not provide enough iron, nor does cow's milk. Cow's milk-based formulas are available with iron added, but breast-fed infants will need to get their iron from iron-enriched cereals or a supplement until cereals are added to the diet.

Fluoride is an important mineral in infant development because of its role in reducing the incidence of dental caries. However, this mineral is inadequate when infants are breast-fed unless a supplement is given. Cow's milk is also quite low in fluoride. Only ready-to-feed formulas with added fluoride in them meet the recommended intake of 0.5 mg per day. Fluoridated water used in diluting concentrated formulas is one means of getting the necessary fluoride. Breast-fed infants can be given a supplement of 0.5 mg daily to compensate for the lack of fluoride in human milk.

VITAMINS

Both human and cow's milk contain adequate amounts of vitamin A and the B vitamins to meet infant needs. The vitamin notably low in cow's milk is vitamin C. Milk from adequately nourished mothers will contain enough vitamin C for infants. The inadequacy of cow's milk can be met by inclusion of sufficient vitamin C in formulas made from cow's milk. In the rare case when an infant is being fed a formula prepared at home from evaporated milk, vitamin C can be provided by feeding 2 oz of orange juice daily.

Vitamin D is not naturally present in sufficient quantities in either type of milk to meet the infant's needs. Cow's milk and cow's milk formulas ordinarily will be fortified with vitamin D at the level of 400 IU (10 µg) per quart. Human milk contains only a little vitamin D, making a vitamin D supplement appropriate for breast-fed infants. This supplement is particularly important for dark-skinned babies because of their limited formation of vitamin D from exposure to sunlight.

Vitamin K is present in higher amounts in cow's milk than in human milk, but both types are adequate once lactation is well established. Parenteral administration of a single dose of vitamin K_1 at a level of 0.5 to 1.0 mg is sufficient to prevent potential problems of hemorrhaging when given at birth. Consequently, the small difference in vitamin K between the two types of milk is not important.

Premature infants are given a vitamin E supplement of 17 mg daily to compensate for their inadequate levels of vitamin E at birth. Breast-fed infants receive more vitamin E in human milk than those given cow's milk, but the level of this fat-soluble vitamin in both types of milk appears to be adequate to meet the need for vitamin E.

OTHER FACTORS IN THE DECISION

The previous discussion regarding the specific nutrient differences between the two types of milk made it clear that either human milk, a cow's milk formula, or a combination of the two is an appropriate choice when viewed from the perspective of nutrition. Consequently, other factors may determine whether a baby should be breast-fed or bottle-fed. Most parents facing this decision in the United States truly have a choice. This is one of those enviable decisions where there really is no wrong choice; either of these choices results in satisfactory growth. The correct decision is the one that will give both the baby and the parents a good start together.

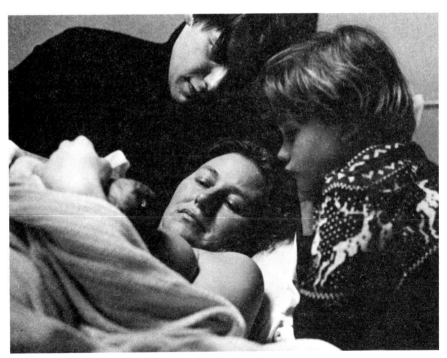

The decision to breast or bottle feed the newborn is one involving dynamics of the entire family.

SAFETY

In areas where refrigeration may be nonexistent and living conditions are far from sanitary, there is no question as to the appropriate type of feeding. Nursing reduces the likelihood of illness from a contaminated milk supply (at the same time providing antibodies against infection) and may well make the difference between survival and death for newborns. Most American homes have good refrigeration, safe water, and are clean and convenient for sanitary bottle-feeding preparation. With literate parents who have some instruction in the necessary sanitary precautions to assure a safe formula in a clean container, the safety of bottle feeding is not a problem. Nevertheless, there is considerably more room for human error leading to unsafe milk being given by bottle than in breast-feeding. The fact that breast-fed infants have fewer respiratory problems than infants fed by bottle supports the greater safety and antibody protection of human milk.

Families who like to travel or who enjoy outdoor activities may find it a problem to keep bottles and formula ready for a hungry infant. The need for refrigeration and bottle preparation disappears when the infant is breast-fed. An adequate and safe milk supply is available as needed wherever the family may be if the mother is breast-feeding. This argument for breast-feeding is counterbalanced in part by the fact that ready-to-feed formula does not require refrigeration until the container is opened. If the amount in a container is intended for a single feeding, refrigeration is not necessarily a problem when a baby needs to be fed away from home. An additional convenience is that ready-to-feed formulas do not require a source of sterile water for dilution, as is true for concentrated products.

Producers of baby formulas are rigidly monitored to ensure that the conditions under which the formula is prepared are sanitary. The actual heat processing of the formula is also under constant scrutiny to ensure a safe and sterile product for babies. Until these containers are opened, the formula remains sterile. Any opened containers must be refrigerated to retard spoilage from growth of potentially harmful microorganisms. Because milk is such a good medium for the growth of microorganisms, opened containers should be stored no more than two days before being used, preferably no more than a day. Nipples, bottle covers, and people's hands all need to be thoroughly washed and absolutely clean before handling the formula container and feeding the baby. When these precautions are observed, bottle-feeding is safe and nourishing for infants.

Usually, human milk is perfectly safe for babies. The milk is sterile as it moves directly from the mother's breast into the infant's mouth. There is no opportunity for contamination as long as the mother cleanses her nipples before nursing and washes her hands thoroughly.

DDT
Dicholoro–diphenyldi-chloroethane; water-insoluble insecticide observed to have toxic effects on some verte-brates.

PCB
Polychlorinated biphenyl; environ-mental pollutant found in industrial waste and used as insecticide.

PBB
Polybrominated biphenyl; environ-mental pollutant in industrial waste.

Some thought must be given to what the mother consumes when she is lactating. Many substances find their way directly into the milk supply, and not all of these are of benefit to the nursing infant. For instance, there is the distinct possibility that traces of many medications will make their way into the mother's milk and ultimately reach the baby. Such medication as birth control pills, diuretics, atropine, steroids, reserpine, hallucinogens, anticoagulants, morphine and its derivatives, bromides, antithyroid drugs, anthaquinones, dihydrotachysterol, and antimetabolites are incorporated into the lactating woman's milk (Arena, 1970). Environmental pollutants such as DDT, PCB, and PBB may be in human milk if the mother lives in an area where contamination is occurring. The full impact of these various substances on infants is not known, but the small size of the infant makes these contaminants a potentially greater problem to babies than to mothers. Nicotine is transmitted in the milk of mothers who smoke cigarettes or marijuana. Ten cigarettes or more smoked by mothers daily are sufficient to transmit harmful levels of nicotine to infants. On the other hand, if mothers drink liquor at a level of up to two cocktails daily there is no evidence of growth problems in infants.

PHYSICAL CONSTRAINTS

Sometimes the physical condition of the mother may make breast-feeding undesirable. For instance, mothers with problems like kidney disease have already placed a considerable strain on their bodies during pregnancy and clearly should not undergo the additional physical strain of lactation. If the mother has a communicable health problem, such as tuberculosis or AIDS or ingests drugs, breast-feeding represents a distinct hazard to the infant and is very unwise.

For their own well-being, mothers sometimes require medications to treat physical problems. When this is the case, the effect of this medication on the newborn must be known before making a decision to breast-feed. Secretion of the medication in the mother's milk poses a potential hazard and should certainly be considered if the mother wishes to breast-feed. The ready availability of excellent commercial formulas makes it unnecessary to risk breast-feeding if there is any question regarding the safety of a mother's medication.

Mothers who use drugs, smoke, or drink heavily will transmit these substances to the infant through their milk. From the infants' standpoint, breast-feeding under these circumstances is not nearly as desirable as use of a commercial formula. Good intentions on the part of the mother are not the issue; if she has not altered her substance abuse during pregnancy, bottle-feeding is an appropriate choice.

Prematurity may dictate the need for use of special formulas rather than breast milk. High-calorie formulas (100 cal per 100 ml compared with the usual caloric concentration of about 58 cal per 100 ml of breast milk) efficiently supply necessary energy without overcrowding the infant's small capacity. For these hospitalized infants, careful monitoring of nutrient intake and frequent adjustments by the dietitian-physician team are needed to ensure optimal progress during the very first days of life.

Although this is not ordinarily a problem, a few women may have an inadequate supply of milk for their infants, making it necessary to use a bottle in addition to nursing. The practice can be continued for a short time as a means of gaining the benefits of the antibodies in colostrum and early milk. However, extended use of this dual feeding process is time-consuming and often frustrating to both mother and child. About two to four weeks is as long a time as is sensible to continue this pattern.

Inverted nipples make it difficult for infants to nurse well. Infants born with a cleft palate may experience considerable difficulty in nursing. Other infants may tend to become exhausted from the effort of nursing before they have received enough milk. Although reasons like these seem to contraindicate it, most women and infants are fully capable of successful breast-feeding.

IMMUNITIES

While the infant's immune system is developing the first year, the body's defenses rely on the passive immunity afforded through placental transfer of immunoglobulin G (IgG) and the immunities afforded by human colostrum and milk. Immunoglobulins A and E (IgA and IgE) are abundant in

IMMUNOGLOBULIN A Protein in colostrum and human milk that affords some immunity from respiratory and gastrointestinal tract infections.

IMMUNOGLOBULIN E Protein in colostrum that provides some protection against infections in infancy.

colostrum. Immunoglobulin A, in particular, provides protection for mucous membranes. IgA continues to be secreted in human milk, providing useful protection until the baby's immune system begins to become effective at about six months of age. Human milk also includes antibodies effective against some viruses and bacteria to help avoid infections in the gastrointestinal tract and respiratory system. By stimulating growth of *L. bifidus*, *E. coli* growth, which causes diarrhea, is inhibited.

LACTOBACILLUS BIFIDUS
Microorganism effective in inhibiting infections by slowing growth of Escherichia coli *that result from greater acidity in the bowel.*

Cow's milk formulas do not provide these protections. However, formula-fed infants are usually protected by appropriate attention to good hygiene and sanitation, although they generally have a somewhat higher infection rate than breast-fed infants.

CONVENIENCE

One of the real advantages in breast-feeding is the convenience. No time needs to be set aside for preparing formula. It is not necessary to plan ahead to be sure there is formula available, nor are trips to the store to buy bottle-feeding supplies and formula necessary. The supply is ready and available without conscious planning and effort. However, the mother must be present, or she must make plans if she is going to be absent for the next feeding time. This can certainly be done, but the need to do this offsets the convenience afforded by breast-feeding.

For mothers who have other children besides the newborn, breast-feeding may be a real advantage because she can use the time that would be involved in formula preparation to do other things. Actually, the timesaving feature of breast-feeding may be a greater advantage to the mother with her first born than it is to the mother with other children, for she will already have mastered or at least be expected to cope with the time management problems that are new to the first-time mother.

ALLERGIES

Generally, few allergy problems occur in infants who are breast-fed, whereas there is an increased potential for an allergic response in infants fed cow's milk. This does not mean that most infants who are fed on formula will experience problems of allergies. Consideration of allergic potential when deciding on breast or bottle feeding is usually important only when there is a previous history of allergies in the families of either parent. If there is a likelihood that the newborn will have allergies, breast-feeding is a desirable choice to minimize feeding difficulties.

BONDING

Breast-feeding is a useful part of the process of bonding between mother and infant. The close physical relationship can give mothers a sense of fulfillment and knowledge that they are helping to ensure that their children are adequately nourished. The infant responds well to the warm, close relationship with the mother. Therefore, breast-feeding is often an appropriate method because of its psychological benefits to both mother and child.

The situation just described is idealized, although it does occur often. However, breast-feeding does not automatically effect a close psychological bonding between a mother and her infant. Not every woman is overjoyed at being a mother. Sometimes mothers need to adjust slowly to the concept of motherhood, and the adjustment may be easier if the infant is bottle-fed rather than breast-fed. The somewhat greater freedom accorded to the mother who is bottle-feeding may be crucial to the mother's adjustment to her new role. If that is the case, breast-feeding and its confining schedule would only accentuate the sudden change in her life and would benefit neither mother nor child from a psychological perspective.

A mother with other children in the family may find that breast-feeding, rather than promoting the psychological bond between herself and the new addition, actually causes a feeling of antagonism or resentment in her other children because of the displacement they feel. She may find it difficult to give adequate care to her other children while she is nursing the newborn, particularly if the weather is nice and the other children are playing outdoors at feeding time. This may cause her to feel anxious and tends to interrupt the desired warm relationship of nursing.

Women who have opted to breast-feed their infants usually are enthusiastic about the experience and choose to breast-feed subsequent children. This certainly endorses the pleasurable experience of breast-feeding, which is typical. Clearly, breast-feeding is a good choice when the outcome is such a positive experience.

On the other hand, bottle-feeding need not be a cold and impersonal experience. Excellent bonding can also occur with bottle-feeding if the baby is cuddled and held comfortably during

When infants are fed by bottle, fathers have an excellent opportunity to share in the responsibilities and joys of feeding them.

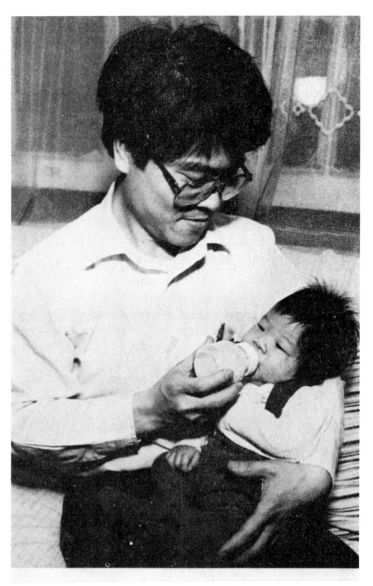

each feeding. Feeding can be a quality time when bottle-feeding is the choice. The important thing is to create a happy and warm relationship by holding and talking to the baby exactly as in breast-feeding.

FEELINGS OF OTHER FAMILY MEMBERS

In view of the fact that either breast or bottle feeding can provide an adequate and appropriate answer to the feeding question, the feelings of other family members should be considered in making the decision. Particularly in the past few years, parenting has become a dual responsibility in many families. Fathers are enjoying the opportunity to become intimately acquainted with their children. Newborns often are such sleepyheads that feeding may be their major activity when they are awake. Fathers can have the pleasure of participating in the feeding responsibility when infants are bottle-fed by either using formula or expressed breast-milk. Sometimes a compromise can be reached in this regard by preparing an occasional bottle, which the father can give. This gives him some opportunity to experience the very pleasant closeness of feeding.

Not all fathers are fascinated with caring for a newborn. Some clearly prefer to have their wives breast-feed and are perfectly willing to forgo this aspect of parenting. They may also

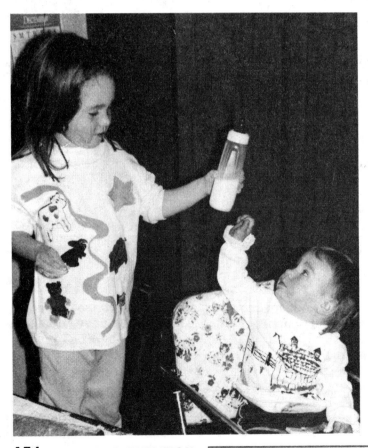

Even while they are still quite young, older children in families can be helped to adjust to the newest member by being a "helper" in bottle-feeding the baby.

be perfectly willing to have their wives make all decisions regarding the mode of feeding.

A new baby represents an adjustment for all members of the family, not just the mother and father. If there are other children, they are going to have a definite response to the baby, whether positive or negative. With bottle-feeding, they can help the mother hold the baby's bottle during feedings when they wish to do so. Responsible older children can even hold the baby and feed the bottle under appropriate supervision. When siblings are able to help in the baby's care, they can get acquainted with the baby and begin to enjoy the new family member.

Children can help with other aspects of the baby's care if breast-feeding is the choice. They do not have to be completely isolated from caring for the infant. They may enjoy sitting close to their mother when the newborn is nursing. This can be a pleasant time for the whole family to be together. The feelings of all family members toward the new baby will influence the merits of breast-feeding and its success.

EMPLOYMENT

The typical family pattern has undergone extensive changes in the past few decades. Between the high cost of living (particularly housing costs) and the priority of women's careers, a growing number of women including new mothers can be found working away from home. Economic need or career demands may dictate a very early return to the job following delivery. It is certainly easier for women to breast-feed their infants if they can stay home for at least a month after birth to become accustomed to the new routine and responsibility and to get their milk flow well established. This adjustment period will make it easier for them to arrange the details of expressing and storing their milk safely for the sitter to feed to their infant while they are at work. Breast milk can be fed to infants when their mothers work outside the home, but planning, with particular attention to adequate refrigeration of expressed milk, is essential to the safety of the human milk supply.

Women who work very few hours each day may be able to nurse their babies just before leaving for work and as soon as they return home. Another alternative for some women who are fortunate enough to live near their work or near their sitters may be to leave work briefly and nurse their infants at the necessary time. Few work places are prepared to have mothers bring their babies to work for nursing, but this is certainly a desirable situation from the perspective of the lactating woman and her infant.

When women need to return to work very soon after delivery, they may find that bottle-feeding is a good solution. Someone else can prepare the formula and do the feeding while she is at work, and the baby will not have to adjust to her work schedule for feedings. If this is the appropriate decision from the parents' point of view, they should feel perfectly comfortable that their decision is sound and will be an excellent way of meeting nutritional needs for growth and development. Certainly, they should not feel at all guilty about choosing to bottle-feed, as long as it is being done under sanitary conditions with warmth and human interaction.

COST

Breast-feeding appears to be virtually without cost, for there is no direct purchase of formula or feeding and sterilizing equipment. This does not represent the total picture. As was noted in Chapter 4, lactating women must increase their total food intake to provide the added energy and nutrients being expended in milk production. Food choices made to meet these demands influence just how costly breast-feeding is, although there is no way to set a specific figure. With prudent choices in the market, breast-feeding can be less costly than bottle-feeding.

Bottle feeding costs vary depending on the specific solution chosen. Ready-to-feed formulas are clearly most costly and somewhat better nutritionally than those prepared with canned evaporated milk. Concentrated and dried infant formulas are comparable in nutritive value to ready-to-feed varieties and may cost slightly less. Purchasing formulas by the case or in quantity at the time of special sales can be a way to help keep the cost of bottle-feeding as low as possible.

Some costs associated with the choice between breast-feeding and bottle-feeding have been examined by researchers in the federally-funded Women, Infants, and Children (WIC) program. The delay in onset of menstruation and subsequent pregnancies resulting from breast-feeding for as long as 6 months was deemed to be an economic benefit; reduced visits to doctors and less need for medicine among breast-fed infants provided further savings (Montgomery and Splett, 1997). These researchers concluded that promotion of breast-feeding by mothers who participated in WIC was justified because of both economic and health benefits.

PERSONAL MOTIVATIONS

For women who have been plagued by the conflict between appetite and excessive weight gain in late pregnancy, the increased caloric budget of lactation may be a real incentive to breast-feed. They will need about 500 cal more during lactation than in the pre-pregnant state (200 cal more than needed during pregnancy). Psychologically, this increase can be a real boost.

On the other side of the coin is the concern some women have about their figures. The breasts become enlarged and somewhat heavy during lactation. Whether lactation causes a permanent change in her figure depends on the woman herself. There will be little permanent stretching of breast tissue if the mother is careful to wear properly fitted brassieres at all times, including when she goes to bed at night. If this is done, there should be little change in her figure once breast-feeding is discontinued.

Breast-feeding is a normal part of the total reproductive cycle and may benefit the mother in two very tangible ways. The nursing process, with its associated hormones, aids in returning the uterus to its normal size more quickly. This role can be noted by the uterine contractions often felt during nursing. In addition, the risk of breast cancer is somewhat lower among women who have nursed infants compared with those who have not. For some women, the delay in subsequent conception as a result of lactation's tendency to deter ovulation is yet another benefit. Breast-feeding is not a guarantee against conception, however, and should not be viewed as an effective contraceptive measure. A study done by Bioiosa in Nigeria in 1955 found that the average time for the subjects' first menstrual period after delivery was 16 months for women who breast-fed as opposed to 55 to 59 days for nonlactating women.

SOCIETAL INFLUENCES

Decision about breast- or bottle-feeding may be influenced by societal attitudes as much as by scientific or practical considerations. Although breast-feeding has been gaining considerably in its acceptability among American women in the upper social classes, there are still women who do not feel that breast-feeding is socially acceptable. Conversely, others feel definite pressure to breast-feed because that is the method with societal approval. In other words, breast-feeding has achieved a high status among the upper classes and the upwardly mobile.

The La Lache League has generated considerable support for breast-feeding. Its work, public support from the medical profession, and social pressure are combining to encourage mothers to breast-feed, whereas they probably would not have opted for this procedure had they been faced with the choice 30 years ago when it was considered prestigious to have enough money to buy formula.

Pressures for American women with limited incomes to return to work conflict with the social pressure to breast-feed. Social pressure can create unnecessary feelings of guilt in women who have elected to bottle-feed their infants. In the United States, such pressure is truly unnecessary, for these women can be expected to have excellent outcomes by bottle-feeding their babies.

THE ACTUAL DECISION

The final decision regarding breast or bottle-feeding is really the domain of the people who will be involved in the actual care of the baby. It is not the business of grandparents, aunts and uncles, or interested neighbors. If the mother has strong feelings in favor of breast-feeding, she should be given the support necessary to help her nurse successfully. She may need encouragement and some guidance on techniques and management of breast-feeding to fit her lifestyle. Conversely, for the mother who really does not wish to breast-feed, support for her decision may also be needed. The important point is that the mother be comfortable with her decision and confident that she is using a feeding method that is appropriate for her and her infant.

Discussions between the mother and father are particularly useful in arriving at the decision. Frequent visits to the doctor during the final weeks of pregnancy afford a convenient way of getting background information the couple may desire. Both the mother and father need to be supportive of the feeding technique chosen. It is very difficult for a mother to breast-feed successfully if her husband prefers the baby to be bottle-fed. Of course, the reverse situation may also be found. When a husband is determined that his baby will be breast-fed and his wife is not pleased with the idea, breast-feeding is not a satisfactory answer. Prospective parents need to share their true feelings about breast versus bottle feeding when they are contemplating which method to use. Since either method can be quite satisfactory in the United States, the psychological aspects of the decision are of great importance. Unless feelings are shared openly, the decision may be made with incorrect information and assumptions.

Parents need have no misgiving about their feeding decision, for either method of feeding can provide a very warm and comfortable relationship between parent and child. The quality of the bonding and the joy in the new relationships are the focal points of the feeding situation. Bottle-fed and breast-fed babies respond beautifully to either form of feeding when the person doing the feeding creates a warm and secure environment.

Sometimes breast-feeding is chosen, but circumstances intervene to make this inadvisable. For instance, there may sometimes be too little milk available. If this is the case, a supplemental bottle can be given as needed to provide sufficient food for the infant. Usually, it is impractical to continue this practice for more than about one month.

BREAST-FEEDING

PHYSIOLOGICAL ASPECTS

Functioning of the mammary glands in lactation is particularly stimulated by prolactin, a hormone from the anterior lobe of the pituitary gland. This hormone is suppressed during pregnancy by comparatively high levels of estrogen and progesterone. At delivery, these female sex hormones are reduced; prolactin increases, an increase which is enhanced by the sucking of the infant.

The infant is able to promote release of colostrum or milk by sucking on the mother's nipple. Sucking is effective in stimulating the hypothalamus to trigger release of oxytocin, a hormone from the posterior pituitary responsible for contracting the myoepithelial cells around the alveoli. This causes the milk to be ejected into the lactiferous ducts (Fig. 5.1), which carry the milk to the lactiferous sinuses. The nursing infant is able to remove the milk from the sinuses. During the early period of a feeding, the infant stimulates the let-down reflex by sucking on the nipple; this makes it easy for the infant to obtain the colostrum or milk in large lactiferous ducts and sinuses.

PROLACTIN
Hormone produced in the anterior lobe of the pituitary that plays an instrumental role in the stimulation of milk.

OXYTOCIN
Hormone produced in the posterior lobe of the pituitary gland, stimulating contraction by the myoepithelial cells, and promoting transport of the milk from the alveoli via the lactiferous ducts to the lactiferous sinuses.

MYOEPITHELIAL CELLS
Cells surrounding the alveoli that contract to force milk into the lactiferous ducts.

ALVEOLI
Honeycomb-like compartments where milk is formed.

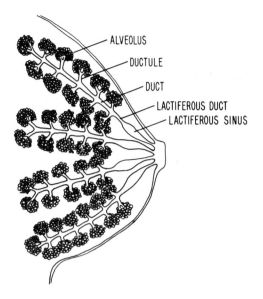

Fig. 5.1   Diagram of breast structures essential to lactation process.

Labels in diagram:
ALVEOLUS
DUCTULE
DUCT
LACTIFEROUS DUCT
LACTIFEROUS SINUS

The early phase of nursing removes the milk that has collected in the lactiferous sinuses and ducts. Meanwhile, the nursing process increases the amount of oxytocin, stimulating the contractions of the myoepithelial cells. Increased oxytocin is the result of increased blood flow to the breasts during nursing. As the process continues, milk is removed from some of the remote or small alveoli that were not involved in the initial part of the feeding. This removal of milk in the second part of nursing is referred to as the draught. The draught reflex aids in getting the remainder of the milk removed from the breast and is important in helping the infant get an adequate amount of milk.

The let-down reflex is important for successful lactation. Favorable conditioning promotes the reflex to such an extent that milk may start to drain from the breast without any sucking action. This can be inconvenient and is not a necessary development for lactation. Response at sucking is quite sufficient. Unfortunately, psychological factors may interfere with the normal let-down reflex. Emotionally-charged situations, like family arguments, can interfere with successful nursing. This may be the result of a burst of adrenaline causing constriction of blood vessels, reducing the input of oxytocin for the stimulation

LACTIFEROUS DUCTS
Passageways for transferring milk from the alveoli to the lactiferous sinuses.

LACTIFEROUS SINUSES
Holding areas for milk received from the lactiferous ducts.

DRAUGHT
Second phase of nursing in which the milk is removed from the distant alveoli, which were not emptied in the first phase.

DRAUGHT REFLEX
Reflex action promoting the emptying of the alveoli distant from the nipple.

LET-DOWN REFLEX
Reflex triggered by the infant's sucking promoting the release of milk from the lactiferous sinuses and ducts at the beginning of feeding.

of milk flow. Alcohol also has a depressing effect on the let-down
The innate action of a reflex.
newborn to extract
colostrum or milk from
the breast. ## ESTABLISHING LACTATION

Successful lactation is aided by appropriate preparation
of the nipples in the last part of pregnancy. Because breasts are
enlarged during lactation, nursing brassieres promote comfort
and convenience during the final stage of pregnancy, as well as
during lactation. By opening the flaps for a while each day, the
nipples can gradually become accustomed to some friction; this
helps reduce their sensitivity. Additional help can be provided by
gently rolling the nipples about 90° between the thumb and index
finger briefly a couple of times daily during the last ten or twelve
weeks of pregnancy.

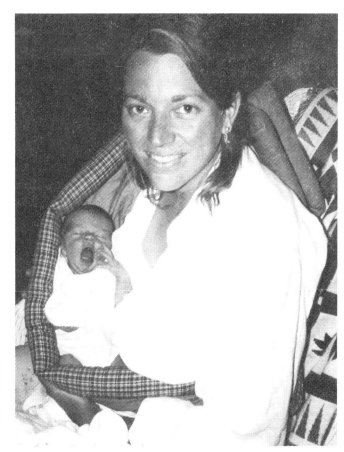

Breast-feeding, with its very close
interaction between mother and
infant, is an effective way of
promoting bonding between the
two while also providing excellent
nutrition for the baby.

RESEARCH INSIGHTS

Ndauti, R., et al., Effect of breastfeeding and formula feeding on transmission of HIV-1: a randomized clinical trial. *J.A.M.A. 282:* 1167. 2000.

This study was conducted in Nairobi, Kenya, to measure the frequency with which infants born of HIV-1-seropositive, antiretroviral motherds became infected with HIV-1 via breastfeeding; mortality rates between breastfeeding and formula feeding were compared. There were 401 mother-infant pairs in the actual study, with 212 mothers being assigned randomly to the group doing breastfeeding and 213 to the formula feeding group. Thorough instruction was given regarding formula feeding preparation and feeding techniques; all women had access to water from the municipal water supply, a situation that often may not be true in rural Kenya and other parts of Africa where HIV-1-infected mothers often are living. Subjects had follow-up visits monthly the first year following delivery and visits every three months the second year to obtain the data, which included samples of maternal milk, infant blood, and physical examinations. Infants were given the regular immunizations regardless of the mode of feeding being used.

Both groups of infants were considered at risk for becoming infected with HIV-1, but the infants being fed breast milk showed a greater frequency (16.2 percent higher) of infection than the formula group. The first 6 months of breastfeeding resulted in transmission of HIV-1 infections at a significantly greater frequency than was measured in the following 18 months of the study. The mortality rates for HIV-1-infected infants in both feeding groups was not signficantly different. However, infants in the formula group who were HIV-1-free at the age of 2 had a significantly higher survival rate than comparable infants in the breastfeeding group. Under the conditions of this study, formula feeding was found to avoid 44% of infections.

On the basis of this study, breastfeeding by HIV-1-infected mothers is not recommended because of the ease of transmission of HIV-1 by this feeding technique, particularly during the early part of life (up to 6 months). However, the risks of unsafe formula preparation, handling, and feeding have to be overcome if infants are to be fed safely using formula rather than breast milk.

The infant's sucking reflex is an important part of establishing successful lactation, and this reflex is particularly strong within about half an hour of birth. Because of this, infants may even be put to the breast in the delivery room. In any event, a brief opportunity for nursing within the first six hours of life is recommended. Although little nourishment may be provided in this early nursing, it does serve to stimulate milk production and to transfer some of the colostrum. Although the sucking reflex diminishes rather quickly, it usually returns within a couple of days at quite an adequate level. A very strong sucking reflex can cause some pain to the mother, whereas an infant with a weak sucking reflex and a limited appetite may fail to stimulate the breasts sufficiently to establish a good milk supply promptly. In this situation, the mother may have to provide some stimulation to evoke the initial milk let-down response. Fortunately, production and delivery processes are usually successful within the first week or less.

ROOTING REFLEX
Natural tendency of an infant to turn the head toward the cheek being stroked.

The sucking reflex is not the only reflex that promotes breast feeding. The rooting reflex causes the infant to turn toward the cheek being stroked. If the mother strokes the baby's cheek closest to the nipple, the infant will automatically turn toward the breast and contact the nipple when properly held. Appropriate use of this reflex simplifies the process of helping the baby begin to nurse.

NURSING

Nipples should be washed with water only in preparation for feeding. For successful nursing, the mother and infant must both be comfortable. Nursing can be done either with the mother lying down or sitting up. There is a possibility of the mother falling asleep and then smothering the baby without realizing it when feeding lying down. Particularly at first, the mother may be

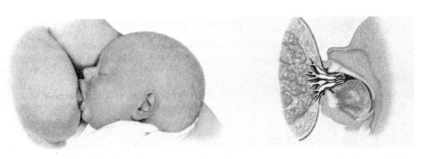

The proper position of the infant's mouth on the breast.

more comfortable if she nurses lying on her bed. To do this, she should find a comfortable position on her side, using a pillow to help her maintain the position if necessary. This will position one breast so that the nipple can be reached comfortably by her infant, who is cradled in her arms in a way that provides easy access to her nipple. The situation is reversed to permit the infant to feed from the other breast. Alternatively, the mother may prefer to sit in a comfortable chair that has an arm on which she can rest. By placing the infant on a pillow, the baby's head can be cradled easily into the appropriate position for nursing without causing the mother to become tired quickly.

To promote successful lactation and avoid painful nipples, it is important that the baby have most of the areola (pigmented portion of the breast) in its mouth. The areola can be flattened a bit between two fingers to help the baby grasp it. Sometimes a full breast makes it a bit difficult for the baby to breathe. This problem is handled very easily if the mother places a finger gently on her breast to create a small cavity for the baby to breathe easily.

When the areola is positioned well into the mouth, good sucking can be done rhythmically by the infant. The first part of nursing will release an abundance of milk, but the draught phase requires more persistence. The mother can facilitate the draught phase a bit by massaging her breast gently in a circular pattern to help move her milk toward the nipple. When the breast has been emptied, the mother can gently push her finger into the corner of the infant's mouth to release the suction without hurting the nipple.

New mothers wonder whether both breasts should be offered at a single feeding. The answer depends on the infant's appetite and the supply of milk. For proper stimulation of milk production, breasts should be emptied of the draught, not just the first portion of the milk supply. Mothers can feel when the draught phase is occurring because of some tingling in the breasts. A simple way of handling this question is to allow an infant to nurse from five to ten minutes on each breast at each feeding for the first few days. This stimulation is helpful in establishing the desired balance between supply and demand. Gradually, the time on each breast is lengthened to a maximum of 15 minutes. About ten minutes is sufficient for babies who are nursing rather vigorously. The first breast offered should be alternated each feeding.

BREAST MILK IN A BOTTLE

Mothers who have to be away from their babies at feeding time for part of the day, but who still wish to breast-feed, need to express their milk into sterile bottles and freeze it for subsequent feedings. This process is easiest if an electric breast pump is available, although manual pumps or simple manipulation of the breasts is possible, if sometimes a bit difficult. For manual removal, a gentle motion is used. The thumb is placed above the nipple, and the index finger is opposite the thumb on the other side of the nipple. Gentle pressure is applied, moving from near the ribs toward the nipple to help move the milk through the ducts to the lactiferous sinuses for excretion. This pressing motion is repeated lightly all around each breast so that breasts are emptied sufficiently.

Human milk, just like cow's milk, unfortunately is a good medium for the growth of microorganisms. This means that great care must be taken to collect the milk in sterile form in sterile bottles. Careful washing of hands with soap and water and gentle washing of the nipples with clear water should be done in preparation for expressing human milk. The collected milk should be frozen immediately and kept frozen until just before it is fed. Cold temperatures are essential to slowing the growth of microorganisms that may have found their way into the milk during its collection.

WEANING

The duration of lactation varies considerably, depending on circumstances. When possible, breast-feeding is probably advantageous for the first five to seven months of life. Sometimes breast-feeding needs to be stopped sooner. By the time solid foods become part of the infant's diet, there may be some convenience in gradually shifting the baby to a bottle or cup after six months of age. Some mothers choose to continue breast-feeding beyond this time, but there seems to be limited benefit to the child from prolonged breast-feeding.

Ideally, the weaning process should be gradual. The breast can be withheld at one of the day's feedings when other food or some milk is given in a cup or bottle. This will start the process of diminishing the mother's milk supply and training the infant to accept a new form of feeding. After three or four days, another nursing period can be deleted by substituting the supplemental feeding. This process is continued until the infant is nursing at only one feeding on alternate days. Then, finally, nursing is omitted altogether. This slow transition makes the "drying up" process quite simple.

FORMULA FEEDING

SELECTION

If infants are to be fed by bottle, a cow's milk formula is usually a satisfactory choice. Excellent formulas are available, their specific ingredients and proportions having been carefully chosen to approximate the nutritional composition of human milk (see Table 5.1). Among these formulas, parents must choose not only a brand, but also the form to be used. The greatest convenience is afforded by read-to-feed products, but liquid concentrates and powdered forms are easy to use if a sterile water supply is convenient. Pediatricians or dietitians can work with parents to help them in their selection of an appropriate product.

Infants with an allergic response to cow's milk will need a different type of formula. Sometimes a goat's milk formula can be used. In other instances, a soybean milk formula is the choice. The soybean formula is made with added methionine to improve the amino acid profile and enhance protein utilization. Special formulas for children with a variety of health problems can be discussed with a dietetian or physician.

Regardless of specific formula consideration, infants should be receiving a formula in which the calories from protein, fats, and carbohydrates are distributed in the ranges indicated below:

Protein	7–10% of total calories
Fats	30–55% of total calories
Carbohydrates	35–50% (the remainder) of total calories

Commercial formulas based on these guidelines are often made with nonfat milk as the base. This is done to permit the replacement of butterfat with oils like soybean, corn, or coconut, for infants absorb them better. Their different fatty acid composition provides a better source of linoleic acid and reduces the sour smell if babies spit up.

The comparatively high level of fat (usually about 3.8 percent) in formulas is needed to provide an adequate amount of energy in the volume of food an infant can be expected to eat. Formulas are designed to provide 67 cal/100 ml of formulas (20 cal/fl oz). An infant will normally drink about 3 tablespoons of formula per pound of body weight every day. Undesirable weight gain often occurs when infants over four months regularly eat more than 45 cal/lb each day.

Despite the concern some people feel about having such high levels of fat in formulas, evidence is lacking to support their theory that this practice will predispose these babies toward heart disease later in life. If infants are fed nonfat milk or even milk with two percent fat, caloric intake is much too low to meet energy needs.

Sometimes the question is raised regarding the use of sweetened condensed milk for preparing formula. This type of milk definitely is not recommended because of the extremely high proportion of carbohydrate due to its added sugar. In fact, the calories from carbohydrate in sweetened condensed milk represent about two-thirds of the total calories. In addition, its total calorie content is about five times greater than a comparable amount of whole milk.

FORMULA PREPARATION

Unless the product chosen is a ready-to-feed formula, preparation will be necessary. This may simply involve sterilizing the various items being used and adding the appropriate amount of boiled and partially cooled water (using fluoridated water where available or adding prescriptive fluoride). The specific formula being used should be one recommended by your physician or dietitian. Usually, infants will drink about 1 qt of milk or formula daily once they are past the neonatal stage. A day's supply can be made all at one time and then refrigerated for use within a 24-hour period. By making formula at a convenient time during the day and being sure to make enough to last for 24 hours, there will be a safe bottle of milk available for a breakfast feeding, as well as during the night. Enough bottles should be prepared to provide a fresh bottle at each feeding. This may mean making as many as eight bottles of formula at first and then reducing the number, but filling them with a larger quantity of milk to meet the changing feeding habits of the growing baby.

EQUIPMENT The equipment necessary for bottle-feeding depends on the type of milk being prepared. Bottles can be made of plastic or glass, or they may be holders designed for use with disposable plastic liner. Any of these will work fine. Glass bottles have the minor disadvantage of being breakable, although they are remarkably sturdy in use unless the baby is in training for Little League pitching. Disposable liners have the advantage of minimizing the amount of air swallowed while the baby is eating, because the liner collapses and does not retain air as the formula is sucked out. There are various nipples to choose from; any type is fine as long as the holes permit the formula to move through at an appropriate rate. The covers that come with the bottles are well suited to their purpose and should be used according to instructions.

STERILIZING METHODS   Careful preparation and sanitary handling of formulas are essential to the well-being of bottle-fed newborns to avoid infections and illnesses transmitted through the food supply. If plastic or glass bottles are used, they must be scrubbed well with a bottle brush as the first step in formula preparation. The covers and nipples also require a thorough scrubbing in hot, soapy water. Nipples should have hot soapy water squeezed through them to insure that the holes are open and clean. Then, they should be thoroughly rinsed in hot running water to remove all traces of detergent. At this point, the remainder of the formula preparation can proceed by either the aseptic or the terminal method (Fig. 5.2–5.4).

TERMINAL METHOD Sterilization of bottles and formula at the same time in a boiling water bath for 20 to 25 minutes.

If water is to be added to a concentrated formula, a word of caution is warranted. Although most tap water is free of lead, this heavy metal can pose a threat to infants if the water used in formula preparation does contain lead. Most of the possible hazard can be eliminated simply by running cold water for about a minute before collecting cold water and using only water from the cold water tap for preparation of formula. This practice will eliminate lead that could have settled in the tap during the night when the water was not being used or lead brought into solution from hot water coming into contact with lead used in the plumbing system. Also, water that is boiled for aseptic formula preparation should be boiled just five minutes. Extended boiling concentrates any lead that may be present in the water. Their small body size makes infants much more vulnerable than older children to the harmful effects of lead.

ASEPTIC METHOD Formula preparation method in which bottles and other equipment are sterilized by processing in boiling water for five minutes and then combined with formula under very sanitary conditions.

Assembly of bottles and formula using the aseptic method is done with extreme care to avoid contamination of the formula and feeding equipment, because no additional heat processing is done after the formula is bottled. This is why the tongs are so important, and why it is imperative that persons preparing the formula be sure to wash their hands thoroughly with hot water and soap before this final stage. The actual assembly of the bottles and formula is quick. The cans of formula are placed in a sink, and boiling water is poured over the tops to cleanse them before the sterilized water is poured to the correct level in the bottles. With the sterilized tongs, a nipple is inverted on the top of each bottle; covers are added and tightened manually. The completed bottles are then stored in the refrigerator for use within 24 hours. If necessary, formula prepared by the aseptic method or the terminal method can be kept a maximum of 48 hours in the refrigerator.

FEEDING TECHNIQUE

Babies are remarkably adaptable to different feeding techniques. Traditionally, formulas have been warmed to approximate the conditions of breast-feeding, but this procedure is not really necessary. Babies will accept cool formula if that is what they are accustomed to drinking, and there appears to be no digestive problem caused by the cool liquid. This can be quite a convenience when bottle-feeding, for it eliminates the problem of trying to get a bottle warmed away from home and avoids a possible delay with a crying baby while waiting for a bottle to warm. The risk of burning the delicate tissues of the baby's mouth with formula that is too hot is also avoided.

The feeding situation and the way the baby is held for a bottle should be essentially the same as for breast-feeding. A quiet and happy atmosphere is ideal, particularly when there is a comfortable chair available for a relaxing and social feeding time with the baby. Some soft music in the background can be a nice way of promoting the pleasant environment desired for establishing good rapport between the baby and the person doing the feeding. The key to successful bottle-feeding is emphasis on a pleasant and comfortable relationship between the two; socialization and feeding are then achieved naturally and simultaneously. Propping the bottle should definitely be avoided; babies need this social exchange, and feeding is one of the very few times when infants are awake enough to have contact with parents and others in their young lives.

A few mechanical aspects of feeding need to be mentioned to avoid frustrations resulting from poor delivery of formula during bottle feeding. The nipple needs to have holes that permit the milk to pass in drops at a regular pace from the inverted bottle, rather than flowing in a stream. A sterile needle can be used to enlarge the holes if the flow is so slow that too much effort

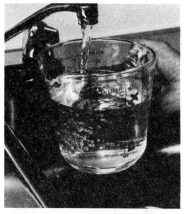
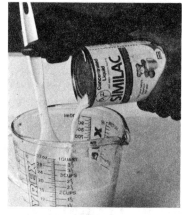
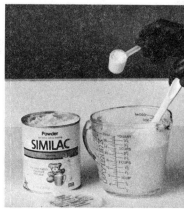
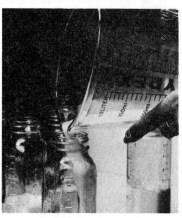
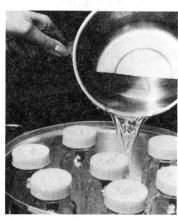
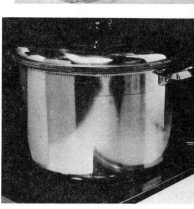

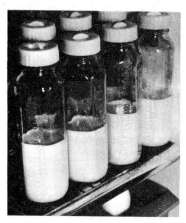

Fig. 5.2 After nipples, bottles, collars, and caps have been scrubbed well with a bottle brush in hot, soapy water and rinsed thoroughly and the formula can has been scrubbed, rinsed, and opened with a clean opener, sterile bottles of formula can be prepared by any of the following methods: *terminal heating*, *aseptic method*, or *single-bottle method*.

Terminal heating method — 1) Measure required amount of water into clean pitcher. 2) Measure the amount of formula needed to follow your physician's orders (usually equal amounts of concentrated fluid formula and water or a level scoop of powdered formula for each two fluid ounce of warm water). 3) Pour enough of the mixed formula into each bottle for a feeding, making enough bottles for the entire day. Fill one bottle with tap water to be sterilized for drinking, if desired. Place the nipples, caps, and collars loosely on the bottles. 4) Place the prepared bottles on a rack in the sterilizer and add three inches of water. 5) After the water comes to a boil, boil for 25 minutes. Leave bottles in the covered sterilizer until cool enough to remove comfortably. 6) Remove bottles, tighten caps, and refrigerate until feeding time. After each feeding, discard any remaining formula and rinse bottles and nipples.

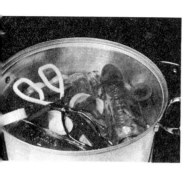
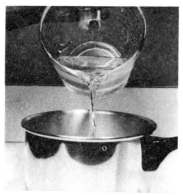
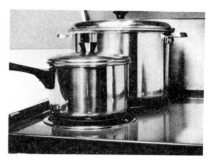
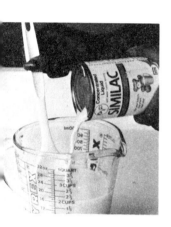
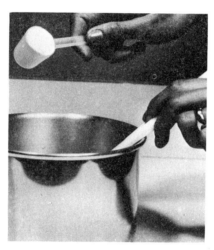
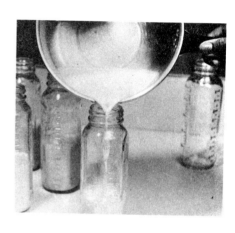
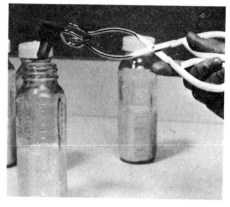

Fig. 5.3 *Aseptic method* — 1) Place bottles, nipples, collars, caps, mixing spoon, can opener, measuring pitcher, and tongs in rack in the sterilizer and cover items with water. Begin to heat the covered sterilizer. 2) pour the amount of water required for the formula preparation into a clean pan, and place the covered pan over the heat. 3) When the water in each container comes to a boil, continue to boil for five minutes. Cool to room temperature while still covered. 4) Measure the correct amount of formula into the sterilized water in the pan (equal amounts of concentrated fluid formula and sterilized water or a level scoop of formula powder for each two fluid ounces of sterilized water at about 100°F). 5) Pour the amount of mixed formula necessary for a single feeding into the bottle, making enough bottles for the entire day. Use tongs to place nipples, collars, and caps on the bottles. Store in refrigerator until feeding time. Discard any formula left in the bottle after a feeding, and rinse the bottles and nipples.

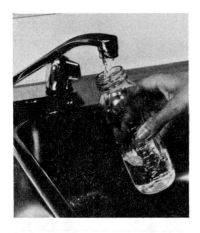
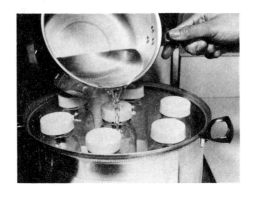
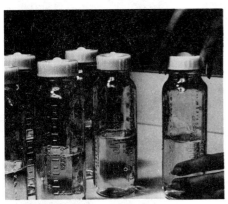
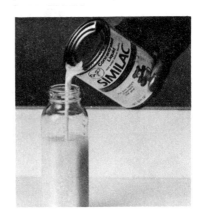
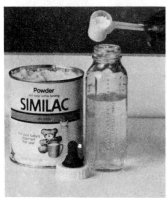

Fig. 5.4   *Single-bottle method* — 1) Add the specified amount of tap water to each bottle needed for a day's feedings. 2) Put nipples and caps loosely on bottles, and place the assembled bottles in a rack in the sterilizer. Add water in the sterilizer to the level of the water in the bottles. Bring the water to a boil in the covered sterilizer and continue to boil 25 minutes. 3) When the covered sterilizer has cooled enough to handle the bottles, remove them and tighten the caps. 4) To feed a bottle, remove the cap and nipple and add the correct amount of formula (equal parts of concentrated fluid formula and water or a scoop of powdered formula for each 2 fluid ounces of water). Replace the nipple and collar, shake the formula, and feed. Discard formula remaining in the bottle after a feeding, and rinse the bottle and nipple.

is required for the infant to get the formula. When nipples get so old that they let the milk run out too rapidly, they should be discarded; the baby should have to suck on the nipple to obtain the formula.

When a bottle feeding is going properly, small air bubbles will be seen passing up the sides of the bottle. If bubbles are not seen, the nipple has probably collapsed, causing a partial vacuum that interferes with the flow of milk. This can be remedied easily by turning the bottle upright and loosening the cap just a bit to let air enter the bottle again.

Throughout the feeding, an occasional check for air bubbles passing into the bottle should be made to be sure that the nipple has not collapsed. If infants are sucking on a collapsed nipple, they will ingest a considerable amount of air, which may make them quite uncomfortable. Well-designed nipples in good condition usually do not collapse, but this problem may develop as they weaken from repeated sterilizations. The problem of ingested gas can be relieved by interrupting the feeding occasionally and holding the baby upright against your shoulder while gently thumping the back of the baby. This technique helps the baby to burp and expel any gas that may be trapped in the stomach. This is a great help in avoiding colicky cries of discomfort after feedings.

Sanitation is a key word when doing bottle-feedings; feeders should be sure to wash their hands thoroughly with hot, soapy water in preparation. The bottle of formula can be warmed, if desired. The nipple should then be placed on the bottle, being sure to avoid handling the part of the nipple that will go into the baby's mouth. Only fresh bottles of formula should be used at feedings. Any remaining formula from a feeding should be discarded, never saved and fed later. The risk of infection is simply too great to permit this small economy.

SPECIAL SITUATIONS

DIARRHEA

Infants are susceptible to minor intestinal disruptions and may develop diarrhea in varying degrees of severity. A physician should be contacted to determine the correct treatment for the condition causing the diarrhea. Usually, some change in feeding is made as a part of the treatment. Sometimes formula or breast milk is withheld for a day, but fluid intake must not be restricted. The fluid might be skim milk diluted with an equal amount of water or a commercial electrolyte solution for babies. An alternative to either of these is carrot soup prepared by diluting strained carrots with an equal amount of boiled water. The object of these various choices is to replace electrolytes that were lost excessively in diarrhea. More importantly, these alternatives provide good sources of the water that is so necessary for the infant without unduly increasing the renal solute load. Use of bouillon is definitely not recommended, because its high levels of sodium and chloride provide a large renal solute load. These substances, which must ultimately be excreted in the urine, place high demands on the kidneys to concentrate liquid and form urine.

RENAL SOLUTE LOAD Solutes (especially electrolytes and protein) that must be excreted by the kidneys.

Fluid intake should be just under 4 tbsp/lb of body weight daily, plus the amount of fluid estimated to have been lost in the feces. However, infants running fevers will need somewhat more fluid than this to compensate for the insensible perspiration losses. Their fluid needs may run as high as 5 tablespoons per pound.

INSENSIBLE PERSPIRATION Water lost through the lungs and skin, exclusive of loss through sweating.

If diarrhea persists four days or longer, a physician may be required to treat the illness. Additional dietary measures are needed to compensate for nutrient losses. Commercial formulations that eliminate lactose and butterfat can be helpful. Soy-based formulas are often appropriate. Infants who are intolerant to various sugars during bouts of diarrhea may be deficient in disaccharidases needed for digestion of disaccharides. Often, glucose can be absorbed effectively by these infants. In instances where diarrhea persists and requires unusual diet controls, careful reading of the labels of commercial formulations will be invaluable in ascertaining the type of carbohydrate being used. A suitable carbohydrate must be included in the diets of infants with diarrhea. Otherwise, they will be unable to metabolize fats normally and will become hypoglycemic.

PREMATURITY

While in the hospital, premature infants (those whose gestational age is 270 days or less or who weigh less than 5 1/2 lb at birth) have special requirements as a consequence of the higher proportion of water in their tissues and their less-developed systems. They will not be able to nurse as vigorously, and their enzyme systems are less prepared to handle food.

Despite these limitations, these infants' nutritional needs are high and must be provided for optimal gain.

Breast-feeding is appropriate for premature infants who weigh at least 4 lb 6 oz and are free of respiratory problems. Infants weighing between 3 lb 5 oz and 4 lb 6 oz can be given 1 to 3 teaspoons of distilled water by bottle about four hours after birth. If this feeding goes well, the baby is given a 10% glucose solution at seven hours and ten hours after delivery, each feeding consisting of 1 to 3 teaspoons of the glucose solution. At thirteen hours, the feeding consists of a formula containing equal parts of 10% glucose solution and a high-calorie milk-based formula (100 cal/100 ml formula). The first day, the feedings will be given at three-hour intervals at a level of 1 to 3 teaspoons of the glucose-formula mixture. Subseqeuent days should provide an increase in the amount of formula very gradually (usually about 1 teaspoon daily). The glucose solution can be replaced very gradually in the formula, but care must be taken to be certain that urine osmolality (ion concentration) is maintained between 300 and 400 mosmol (milliosmoles) per liter.

Formulas providing 100 cal/100 ml formula are usually made with about 11% of the calories coming from protein and about 50% from vegetable oils added to nonfat milk. Corn syrup solids are often added to augment lactose in the milk. Infants consuming this high-calorie formula need enough to provide at least 64 cal/lb of infant weight each day. This quantity is enough to avoid an unduly high renal solute load in these premature infants.

Infants weighing less than 3 lb 5 oz, or larger infants who are unable to suck, will require intravenous feeding to provide 10 g of glucose and 2 meq each of sodium and potassium per 100 ml of liquid. Gavage (tube) feedings are introduced as soon as possible, using a soft tube to deliver food to the stomach at intervals of two to three hours. The intravenous feedings can be eliminated gradually as gavage feeding is established. Protein needs range from 2.8 g/100 cal to 1.6 g/100 cal when weight is up to 6 1/2 lb. The small quantity of formula necessitates vitamin supplementation. This should be started in the third day and should be at the level indicated in the RDA, with iron being added to the supplement when the baby starts to gain weight. Feeding of premature infants is best done in a hospital, where effective monitoring is possible.

SUMMARY

During the first four to six months of life, infants are fed with either breast milk or a formula, usually one based on cow's milk. Breast-feeding definitely is recommended whenever this method is a good choice for both mother and infant. The decision of breast- or bottle-feeding is influenced by many factors; these include safety, convenience, allergies, bonding, feelings of other family members, mother's employment outside the home, physical constraints, cost, personal motivations, health aspects, and social influences. Most American families truly have a choice, for both breast- and formula-feeding are capable of supporting excellent growth and development in most children. Although cow's milk is notably higher in protein, calcium, phosphorus, and some other vitamins and minerals than human milk, modifications in composition are made commercially to produce cow's milk-based formulas that are quite similar to human milk. One important reason for breast-feeding is the merit of breast milk in transferring protective substances to the infant in the early colostrum as well as in mature milk. The reduced possibility of allergic response, the convenience of nursing, and safety are other sound reasons for breast-feeding. Bottle-feeding is a perfectly acceptable solution to feeding infants, provided they are held while being fed. The feeding situation is an important time for infants to develop rapport with those around them, and this can be accomplished with other family members as well as with the mother when bottle-feeding is the choice.

Breast-feeding can be accomplished very satisfactorily by most women who wish to nurse their infants. The let-down reflex promotes the release of milk during the early phase of nursing. The draught reflex aids in moving the milk from the outer alveoli through the lactiferous ducts and sinuses for excretion to the infant during the nursing period. Infants should consume adequate milk if they are allowed to nurse from five to ten minutes on each breast at a feeding.

Careful attention must be paid to ensuring that bottle-fed infants are given formula that is absolutely safe. Enough formula for 24 hours can be prepared at one time in the correct number of bottles to provide a fresh bottle at each feeding. Bottles should be sterilized for at least the first three months of a baby's life. Persons handling formula preparation should be sure to wash their hands thoroughly and to time the sterilization accurately, whether it is being done by the terminal method (formula sterilized in bottles while the bottles are being sterilized) or by the aspetic method (bottles, nipples, and caps sterilized and then filled with sterile formula). Refrigeration of the prepared formula is necessary until feeding time, when it can be given to the infant cool or heated.

Special attention needs to be given in feeding infants who have diarrhea. After a brief period when they receive only water or an electrolyte solution designed for treatment, nonfat milk diluted with an equal amount of water or electrolyte solution can be used until the diarrhea stops. Emphasis needs to be on ensuring that fluid intake is in excess of 4 tablespoons per pound body weight, with the amount increasing to 5 tablespoons in some instances of fever and excessive fluid losses.

Premature infants have high nutritional needs in relation to their body size and should be cared for in a hospital. Intravenous glucose feedings are used until gavage feedings of glucose solution and a high-calorie milk-based formula can be started. Gradually, the formula being used is altered as the infant gains weight. Originally, these infants need as much as 2.8 g of protein per 100 cal of formula, but that requirement drops gradually to about 1.6 g by the time the infant weighs 6 1/2 pounds.

BIBLIOGRAPHY

ABRAMS, C.E., ET AL Hazards of over-concentrated milk formula. *J. Am. Med. Assoc. 232:* 1136. 1975.

AHN, C.H. AND W.C. MACLEAN, JR. Growth of exclusively breast-fed infant. *Am. J. Clin. Nutr. 33:* 183. 1980.

ALLEN, C.D. AND C.P. RIES Smoking, alcohol, and dietary practices during pregnancy: comparison before and after prenatal education. *J. Am. Diet. Assoc. 85:* 605. 1985.

AMERICAN ACADEMY OF PEDIATRICS COMMITTEE ON NUTRITION Nutritional needs of low-birth-weight infants. *Pediat. 60:* 519. 1977.

ANDERSON, S.A., ET AL History and current status of infant formulas. *Am. J. Clin. Nutr. 35:* 381. 1982.

ANONYMOUS Human milk as a source of long-chain polyunsaturated fatty acids for preterm human infant neural tissues. *Nutr. Rev. 42:* 247. 1984.

ANONYMOUS Morbidity in breast fed and artifically fed infants. *Nutr. Rev. 38:* 114. 1980.

ANONYMOUS Nutritional adequacy of breast feeding. *Nutr. Rev. 38(4):* 145. 1980.

ANONYMOUS Introduction of solid foods and total energy intake in exclusively breast-fed infants. *Nutr. Rev. 48:* 280. 1990.

ARENA, J. M. Contamination of the ideal food. *Nutr. Today 5(4):* 2. 1970.

ARON, S.S., ET AL Honey and other environmental risk factors for infant botulism. *J. Pediatr. 94:* 331. 1979.

BEE, D.E., T. BARANOWSKI, D.K. RASSIN, C.J. RICHARDSON, AND W. MIKRUT Breast-feeding initiation in a triethnic population. *Am. J. Dis. Child. 145:* 306. 1991.

BEERENS, H., ET AL Influence of breast-feeding on the bifid flora of the newborn intestine. *Am. J. Clin. Nutr. 33:* 2434. 1980.

BHOWMICK, S.K., K.R. JOHNSON, K.R. RETTIG Rickets caused by vitamin D deficiency in breast-fed infants in southern United States. *Am. J. Dis. Child. 145:* 127. 1991.

BLACK, R.F. Transmission of HIV-1 in the breast-feeding process. *J. Am. Diet. Assoc. 96(3):* 267. 1996.

BLACK, R.F., J.P. BAIR, V.N. JONES, AND R.H. DURANT Infant feeding decisions among pregnant women from a WIC population in Georgia. *J. Am. Diet. ASsoc. 90:* 255. 1990

BROWN, R.D. Breast feeding and family planning: a review of relationships between breast feeding and family planning. *Am. J. Clin. Nutr. 35:* 162. 1982.

BUTTE, N.F., ET AL Effect of maternal diet and body composition on lactational performance. *Am. J. Clin. Nutr. 39:* 296. 1984.

COMMITTEE ON DRUGS, AMERICAN ACADEMY OF PEDIATRICS Transfer of drugs and other chemicals into human milk. *Pediat. 84:* 924. 1989.

COMMITTEE ON NUTRITION, AMERICAN ACADEMY OF PEDIATRICS Commentary on breast feeding and infant formulas, including proposed standards for formula. *Nutr. Rev. 34:* 248. 1976.

COMMITTEE ON NUTRITION, AMERICAN ACADEMY OF PEDIATRICS Relationship between iron status and incidence of infection in infancy. *Pediatr. 62:* 246. 1978.

DALLMAN, P.R., ET AL Iron deficiency in infancy and childhood. *Am. J. Dis. Child. 131:* 463. 1977.

ELLIS, L.A. AND M.F. PICCIANO Milk-borne hormones: regulators of development in neonates. *Nutr. Today 27(5):* 6. 1992.

FOMON, S.J. Human milk and small premature infants. *Am. J. Dis. Child. 131:* 463. 1977.

FOMON, S.J., ET AL Cow milk feeding in infancy: gastrointestinal blood loss and iron nutritional status. *J. Pediatr. 98:* 540. 1981.

FORD, K. AND M. LABBOK Who is breast-feeding? Implications of associated social and biomedical variables for research on consequences of method of infant feeding. *Am. J. Clin. Nutr. 52:* 451. 1990.

FORSYTH, B.W.C. Colic and effect of changing formulas. *J. Pediat. 115:* 521. 1989.

GARCIA, R.E. AND D.X. MOODIE Routine cholesterol surveillance in childhood. *Pediat. 84:* 7541. 1989.

GIOIOSA, R. Incidence of pregnancy during lactation in 500 cases. *J. Obstet. Gynec 70:* 162. 1955.

HOLMAN, S.R. Infant feeding in Roman antiquity. *Nutr. Today 33(3):* 113. 1998.

HOLST, M.C. Developmental and behavioral effects of iron deficiency anemia in infants. *Nutr. Today 33(1):* 27. 1998.

KALLEN, D. Effects of nutrition on maternal-infant interaction: a symposium. *Fed. Proc. 34:* 1571. 1975.

KEMPER, K. B. FORSYTH, AND P. MCCARTHY Jaundice, terminating breast-feeding and vulnerable child. *Pediat. 84:* 773. 1989.

KNOWLES, J.A. Excretion of drugs in milk — a review. *J. Pediatr. 66:* 1068. 1965.

LALECHE LEAGUE INTERNATIONAL *Womanly Art of Breastfeeding.* Franklin Park, Illinois. 1958.

LAMMI-KEEFE, C.J. AND R.G. HENSEN Fat-soluble vitamins in human milk. *Nutr. Rev. 42:* 365. 1984.

LEPAGE, G., ET AL Composition of preterm milk in relation to degree of prematurity. *Am. J. Clin. Nutr. 40:* 1042. 1984.

LEVINE, B.S. . . .about DHA. *Nutr. Today 32(6):* 248. 1997.

LONNERDAL, B. AND E. FORSUM Casein content of human milk. *Am. J. Clin. Nutr. 41:* 113. 1985.

LOZOFF, B., ET AL Mother-newborn relationship: limits of adaptability. *J. Pediatr. 91:* 1. 1977.

LUCAS, A. AND T.J. COLE Breast milk and neonatal necrotising enterocolitis. *Lancet 336:* 1519. 1990.

LUCAS, A., ET AL Latent anaphylactic sensitisation of infants of low birth weight to cows' milk proteins. *Br. Med. J. 289:* 1254. 1984.

MACY, I.G., ET AL *The Composition of Milks.* Publ. 254. National Research Council of National Academy of Sciences, Washington, D.C. 1953.

MCMILLAN, J.A., ET AL Iron absorption from human milk, simulated human milk, and proprietary formulas. *Pediatr.60:* 896. 1977.

MARTINEZ, G.A. AND J.P. NALEZIENSKI 1980 update: recent trend in breast-feeding. *Pediatr. 67:* 260. 1981.

MONTGOMERY, D.L. AND P.L. SPLETT Economic benefit of breast-feeding infants enrolled in WIC *J. Am. Diet. Assoc. 97(4):* 379. 1997.

NATIONAL ACADEMY OF SCIENCES SUBCOMMITTEE ON NUTRITION DURING LACTATION. Who breast-feeds in the United States. In *Nutrition during Lactation.* National Academy Press. 1991. p. 28.

NEWBURG, D.S. AND J.M. STREET Bioactive materials in human milk. *Nutr. Today 32(5):* 191. 1997.

NEWTON, N. Psychologic differences between breast and bottle feeding. *Am. J. Clin. Nutr. 24:* 993. 1971.

NICHOLS, B.L. AND V.N. NICHOLS Nutrition in pregnancy and lactation. *Nutr. Abstr. Rev. 53:* 259. 1983.

NOMMSEN, L.A., C.A. LOVELADY, M.J. HEINIG, B. LONNERDAL, AND K.G. DEWEY Determinants of energy, protein, lipid, and lactose concentrations in human milk during first 12 months of lactation: Darling Study. *Am. J. Clin. Nutr. 53:* 457. 1991.

O'CONNOR, P.A. Failure to thrive with breast feeding. *Clin. Pediatr. 17:* 833. 1978.

O'MALLEY, B.A., A.C. BROWN, M. TATE, A.A. HERTZLER, AND M.H. ROJAS Infant feeding practices of migrant farm laborers in morthern Colorado. *J. Am. Diet. Assoc. 91(9):* 1084. 1991.

OSAKI, F.A. Iron-fortified formulas and gastrointestinal symptoms in infants: a controlled study. *Pediatr. 66:* 168. 1981.

POLITT, E. AND S. WIRTZ Mother-infant feeding interaction and weight gain in first month of life. *J. Am. Diet. Assoc. 78:* 596. 1978.

POSTKITT, E.M.E. Infant feeding: a review. *Human Nutr.: Appli. Nutr. 37C:* 271. 1983.

REEVE, L., ET AL Vitamin D of human milk: identification of biologically active forms. *Am. J. Clin. Nutr. 36:* 122. 1982.

ROCHE, A.F. AND J.H. HIMES Incremental growth charts. *Am. J. Clin. Nutr. 33:* 2041. 1980.

SAMPSON, H.A. Infantile colic and food allergy: Fact or fiction? *J. Pediat. 115:* 583. 1989.

SCHAEFFER, A. AND S. DITCHEK Current social practices leading to water intoxication in infants. *Am. J. Dis. Child. 145:* 27. 1991.

SCIACCA, J.P., ET AL Influences on breast-feeding by lower-income women: an incentive-based, partner-supported educational program. *J. Am. Diet. Assoc. 95(3):* 323. 1995.

SERDULA, M.K., K.A. CAIRNS, D.F. WILLIAMSON, M. FULLER, AND J.E. BROWN Correlates of breast-feeding in a low-income population of whites, blacks, and Southeast Asians. *J. Am. Diet. Assoc. 91(1):* 41. 1991.

SIMONIN, C., ET AL Comparison of fat content and fat globule size distribution of breast milk from mothers delivering term and preterm *Am. J. Clin. Nutr. 40:* 820. 1984.

SONG, W.O., ET AL Effect of pantothenic acid status on content of the vitamin in human milk. *Am. J. Clin. Nutr. 40:* 317. 1984.

STYSLINGER, L. AND A. KIRKSEY Effects of different levels of vitamin B_6 supplementation on vitamin B_6 concentrations in human milk and vitamin B_6 intakes of breastfed infants. *Am. J. Clin. Nutr. 41:* 21. 1985.

TUTTLE, C.R. AND K.G. DEWEY Potential cost savings for Medi-Cal, AFDC, Food Stamps, and WIC programs associated with increasing breast-feeding among low-income Hmong women in California. *J. Am. Diet. Assoc. 96(9):* 885. 1996.

VICTORIA, C.G., ET AL Is prolonged breast-feeding associated with malnutrition? *Am. J. Clin. Nutr. 39:* 307. 1984.

CHAPTER SIX

Nutrition During Infancy

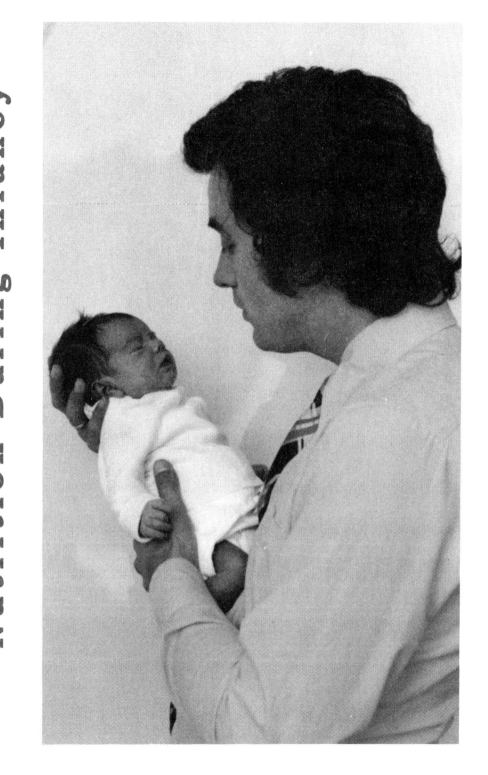

NUTRITIONAL NEEDS

RDA FOR THE FIRST YEAR

The abrupt transition from the fetal period to the neonatal phase creates a sudden need to provide necessary nutrients from external sources. The levels suggested by the Food and Nutrition Board of the National Research Council and the Institute of Medicine — National Academy of Sciences are divided into two age periods during the first year: from birth to six months and from six months to one year. This permits refinements in the recommendations to accommodate dramatic increases in body size during the first year and the resultant modification in needs.

Tables 6.1 and 6.2 present the RDA and the estimated amounts of additional selected vitamins and minerals for which RDA and AI values have not yet been established. When using

205

TABLE 6.1   AI for the First Year of Life[a,b]

Nutrient	0–6 months	6–12 months
Calcium (mg/d)	210	270
Phosphorus (mg/d)	260	275
Magnesium (mg/d)	30	75
Vitamin D[c] (μg/d)	5	5
Fluoride (mg/d)	0.01	0.5
Thiamin (mg/d)	0.2	0.3
Riboflavin (mg/d)	0.3	0.4
Niacin[d] (mg/d)	2	4
Vitamin B_6 (mg/d)	0.1	0.3
Folate (μg/d)	65	80
Vitamin B_{12} (μg/d)	0.4	0.5
Pantothenic acid (mg/d)	1.7	1.8
Biotin (μg/d)	5	6
Choline (μg/d)	125	150

[a]Adapted from Food and Nutrition Board, Institute of Medicine —
National Academy of Sciences Dietary Reference Intakes:
Recommended Intakes for Individuals. Washington, D.C., 2000.
[b]For healthy breastfed infants, the AI is the mean intake.
[c]As cholecalciferol. 1 μg cholecalciferol = 40 IU vitamin D.
[d]As dietary folate equivalents (DFE). 1 DFE = 1 μg food folate = 0.5 μg
of folic acid from fortified food or supplement consumed with food =
0.5 μg of synthetic (supplemental) folic acid taken on an empty stomach.

these figures, it is important to remember that these are not intended to be strictly applied to individual infants. The RDA for an infant up to six months of age are based on a hypothetical infant weighing 13 pounds and measuring 24 inches long. The counterpart in the second six months is assumed to weigh 20 pounds and be 28 inches long. Most infants are not these precise sizes, but recommendations for calories are stated in calories per kilogram as an aid in making appropriate adjustments for variations in body size. Even then, the RDA are not intended to be rigidly interpreted for individual children; they are merely useful guidelines.

TABLE 6.2   Recommended Dietary Allowances for the First Year of Life[a]

Nutrient	0–6 months[b]	6–12 months[c]
Protein (g)	13	14
Vitamin A (μg RE)[d]	375	375
Vitamin E (mg α-TE)[e]	4	6
Vitamin K (μg)	5	10
Vitamin C (mg)	40	50
Iron (mg)	6	10
Zinc (mg)	5	5
Iodine (μg)	40	50
Selenium (μg)	15	20

[a]Adapted from Food and Nutrition Board, Institute of Medicine — National Academy of Sciences Dietary Reference Intakes: Recommended Intakes for Individuals. Washington, D.C., 2000.
[b]Based on weight of 6 kg (13 lb) and height of 60 cm (24 in).
[c]Based on weight of 9 kg (20 lb) and height of 71 cm (28 in).
[d]Retinol equivalents. 1 retinol equivalent = 1 μg retinol or 6 μg β-carotene.
[e]α-Tocopherol equivalents. 1 mg d-α-tocopherol = 1 α-TE.

MILK, FORMULAS, AND THE RDA

A practical means of approaching the study of dietary adequacy during the first year of life is to compare the nutrients provided in a quart (32 fl oz or 944 ml) of human milk or formula with the RDA. Such a comparison is provided in Table 6.3. This amount of milk or formula is used as the basis of comparison because this quantity is generally considered to be the maximum amount of milk appropriate in an infant's diet. Appetite beyond this amount should ordinarily be satisfied with solid foods suited to the developmental capability of the infant. The addition of solid foods is considered later in this chapter.

The energy value of a quart of human milk or formula provides for the needs of most infants until they weigh about 14 pounds, according to the RDA recommendation. However, infants who need a higher caloric intake prior to the initiation of solid foods between the ages of 4 and 6 months can be given additional milk or formula to supply energy needs.

TABLE 6.3   Comparison of the RDA[a] and the Nutrient Content of 1 Qt of Human and Cow's Milk-Based Formula[b]

Nutrient	RDA		Amount/quart	
	0–6 months	6–12 months	Human Milk	Cow's milk-based formula
Energy (cal)	kg x 108	kg x 98	727	632.5
Protein (g)	13	14	10.4	14.2
Vitamin A (µg RE)	375	375	686	606
Vitamin D (µg)	5	5	5	10
Vitamin E (mg)	4	6	2	2
Vitamin K (µg)	5	10	—	—
Vitamin C (mg)	40	50	47	52
Thiamin (mg)	0.2	0.3	0.1	0.5
Riboflavin (mg)	0.3	0.4	0.4	0.6
Niacin (mg equiv.)	2	4	1.9	7.0
Vitamin B_6 (mg)	0.1	0.3	0.09	0.4
Folate (µg)	65	80	49	47
Vitamin B_{12} (µg)	0.4	0.5	2.8	0.9
Calcium (mg)	210	270	312	434–509
Phosphorus (mg)	200	275	132	302–387
Magnesium (mg)	30	75	22	39–49
Iron (mg)	6	10	0.9	12
Zinc (mg)	5	5	4–5	3–5
Iodine (µg)	40	50	28	94
Selenium (µg)	15	20	—	—

[a]*Recommended Dietary Allowances*, Food and Nutrition Board, National Academy of Sciences — National Research Council, Washington, D.C., 10th ed., 1989; Food and Nutrition Board, Institute of Medicine — National Academy of Sciences Dietary Reference Intakes: Recommended Intakes for Individuals. 1998; Food and Nutrition Board, National Academy of Sciences — National Research Council Recommended Dietary Allowances, revised 1989 (abridged). 2000.
[b]Data from *Composition of Foods, Dairy and Egg Products, Ag. Handbook 8–1*, Agricultural Research Service, U.S. Department of Agriculture, Washington, D.C., Rev. 1976; Picciano, M.F. and H.A. Guthrie, Copper, iron, and zinc contents of mature human milk. *Am. J. Clin. Nutr. 29:* 242, 1976; product label — iron-fortified formula.

Human milk is lower in thiamin, niacin, vitamin B_6, and folate than the values stated in the RDA, yet growth is considered excellent for nursing infants without any supplementation of these vitamins. Iron is far below the amount needed once the infant's original body stores have been depleted.

Cow's milk-based formulas are adjusted to approximate the RDA for several nutrients. For example, thiamin, niacin, vitamin B_6, and iron levels in iron-fortified formula are consistent with RDA values. Although cow's milk is diluted to reduce its protein level, protein content of most formulas remains appreciably higher than human milk. This decision reflects the fact that human protein is utilized more efficiently by infants than the protein in cow's milk, even when the cow's milk has been homogenized and heat-processed.

SUPPLEMENTS

PPM
Parts per million; system of indicating how many parts of a substance are contained in a million parts of water.

INFANTS OF NORMAL WEIGHT Supplementation of the milk-based diets for infants of normal weight at birth depends on the milk being fed. However, a parenteral administration of vitamin K (0.5 to 1.0 mg phytylmenaquinone) should be done routinely in the hospital at delivery regardless of the anticipated type of feeding.

Breast milk is quite low in vitamin D; for this reason, vitamin D should be given daily (5 to 7.5 µg each day). Formulas are prepared with sufficient vitamin D to meet infant needs when 1 qt of formula is consumed. Vitamin D supplementation should never provide more than 10 µg (400 IU) daily, and this is provided as soon as 1 qt of cow's milk-based formula is consumed daily.

Infants who are being fed only human milk will receive sufficient vitamin C, but infants receiving a cow's milk formula will need a supplement of this vitamin unless the formula has vitamin C added to it. This means that formulas made at home with evaporated milk will need to be supplemented with vitamin C. This can be accomplished by feeding the infant at least 2 fl oz (4 tablespoons) of orange juice or a vitamin C-fortified fruit juice daily. Commercially-prepared formulas contain sufficient vitamin C.

Folate needs to be supplemented for infants consuming goat's milk or evaporated milk formulas. This supplement is intended to provide the RDA (65–80 µg), thus offsetting the low folate levels in these products.

Iron is stored at very useful levels in infants who are born at term. In fact, the supply of iron deposited during the fetal period is sufficient to meet the needs of these infants for four months or longer. Iron released from red blood cells when they are destroyed after about 70 days is reused to make new erythrocytes, but this source of iron is inadequate for the infant's growing needs after about four months. By this time, a source of iron may be necessary for breast-fed infants. Ordinarily this is most appropriately provided in iron-fortified infant cereals. However, infants who begin these cereals by six months of age do not usually become anemic if they are being breast-fed. Although there is very little iron in human milk, infants' iron absorption appears to be unusually efficient (as high as 49 percent). This far exceeds the 10 percent or less absorption efficiency for the iron in cow's milk. However, commercial formulas fortified with iron at a level sufficient to meet infant needs are available and are the formula of choice for infants after they are four months old. Six tablespoons of iron-fortified infant cereal will provide about 14 mg of iron.

Infants being fed evaporated milk formulas receive an inadequate supply of iron in the formula, as is also the case for commercial formula products with no added iron. These infants will need an iron supplement by about four months of age; iron-fortified infant cereals can be used to meet this need when they become part of the diet by six months of age or a little earlier. However, use of an iron-fortified formula may be a more appropriate choice between the ages of four and six months if economy makes it important to keep an infant on a formula made with evaporated milk as long as possible. If a commercial formula is already being fed, the shift to an iron-fortified formula should be made when the infant is between three and four months old; this will cost no more, and the fortified product eliminates the possibility of the infant becoming iron-deficient.

Fluoride supplementation is recommended at levels that vary according to the fluoride level of the water supply. Supplementation must be done very carefully to avoid the possibility of an intake sufficient to cause mottling of teeth. Table 6.4 presents the levels of supplementation recommended by Fomon (1974, p. 351). The American Academy of Pediatrics Committee on Nutrition recommends that children between the ages of two weeks and two years receive a supplement of 0.25 mg fluoride per day (Barness, 1981).

PREMATURE OR SMALL-FOR-DATE INFANTS   Nutrient needs of premature or small-for-date babies are particularly high in relation to capacity and may require more supplementation than is needed for other infants. Limited ability to absorb fat interferes with the availability of vitamin D in premature infants, which makes it wise to supplement vitamin D up to a level of 10 μg (400 IU) daily, at least until milk intake is about 1 qt each day. A supplement of 17 mg of vitamin E is also recommended for the first three months of a premature baby's life.

Because of their premature births, these infants' iron stores are smaller than normal; in fact they are likely to be exhausted by the time the baby is two months old. These infants should probably be fed an iron-fortified formula at about two months of age, or even earlier, to augment the iron already in the body. However, these infants clearly need a vitamin E supplement at the same time. Iron fortification increases the possibility of developing a vitamin E deficiency, a problem which is compounded by the high levels of polyunsaturated fatty acids normally used in feeding premature infants.

Protein and calcium requirements are elevated for premature infants in their first weeks of life. Protein at the level of 3 to 5 g/kg of body weight promotes the best weight gain in these tiny babies, a level well in excess of the recommendation for infants of normal weight. In fact, this level is about double that

TABLE 6.4   Recommended Fluoride Supplementation During the First Year of Life[a]

Milk or Formula	Level of Supplementation (mg/day) if Water Fluoride Concentration is:			
	0.3 ppm	0.3–0.7 ppm	0.8–1.1 ppm	1.1 ppm
Human milk	0.5	0.5	0.5	0
Cow's milk	0.5	0.5	0.5	0
Commercial formula				
Ready-to-feed	0.5	0.5	0.5	0
Concentrated liquid	0.5	0.25	0	0
Powder	0.5	0	0	0[b]
Evaporated milk formula	0.6	0.25	0	0

[a]From Fomon, S.J., *Infant Nutrition*, Sanders, Philadelphia, 2nd ed. 1974, p. 351. Levels are designed to provide about 0.5 mg fluoride daily.
[b]Water used for reconstituting powdered formula should not provide more than 1.1 ppm (parts per million) of fluoride.

suggested for optimal growth of most infants. This protein intake should provide for good growth, although some infants may benefit from small increases in their intake of four amino acids (histidine, tyrosine, arginine, and taurine). The merits of supplementation of these four amino acids are still under study. premature infants also have greater calcium needs than full term infants. Formulas made with evaporated milk ordinarily have a higher content of calcium in proportion to calories than commercial formulas. Fomon et al (1977) indicated that the content should be about 132 mg calcium in each 100 cal of formula, a level approximately double that provided in commercial formulas with the lowest calcium levels (about 60 mg per 100 cal).

CAUTIONS   Formulas prepared especially for infants do not contain excessive levels of any nutrients, but vitamin supplements can be purchased easily and adminstered at potentially harmful levels by well-meaning parents attempting to ensure that their babies are getting all the nutrients they need. The two vitamins that represent particular risks are vitamins A and D.

Toxic levels of vitamin D for infants may be as low as 25 µg daily, only about five times the recommended intake. The symptoms of hypervitaminosis D (the condition resulting from too high an intake of vitamin D) begin with a loss of appetite, vomiting, and weight loss. Blood calcium levels are high, and deposition of calcium in the blood vessels, lungs, and kidneys can result in death if the overdose is not halted. These symptoms can only be created in this country through the use of a vitamin D supplement; vitamin-D fortified milk and formulas are the only dietary sources of vitamin D for most children. However, cod-liver oil is a rich source of this vitamin and presents a potential problem for infants receiving generous supplements of it.

Vitamin A is provided in generous amounts when a quart of formula or human milk is consumed by infants. There is no need to supplement this vitamin. In fact, high dosages may result in infants developing hypervitaminosis A over an extended period during infancy. Continual administration of vitamin A at levels about eight times above the RDA can create such symptoms as loss of appetite, blurred vision, loss of hair, cracked and dry skin, headaches, nausea, and irritability. These symptoms can be reversed by discontinuing the supplement, but the problem should never occur in the first place. Infants should not be given a vitamin A supplement.

HYPERVITAMINOSIS D Condition characterized by high blood calcium levels and calcium deposits in the blood vessels, lungs, and kidneys, as well as by loss of appetite, nausea, and weight loss as a result of too high an intake of vitamin D.

HYPERVITAMINOSIS A Condition marked by loss of appetite, blurred vision, loss of hair, cracked and dry skin, headaches, nausea, and irritability as a result of too much vitamin A.

FEEDING SCHEDULES

The one truism about infants and their feeding schedules is that schedules were meant to be broken. Just when a parent begins to count on a routine feeding schedule, the baby's appetite changes. Flexibility is an essential of parenting. This situation can be quite frustrating for parents who prefer living by a schedule, yet it may be quite comforting to others to know that some variation in schedule occurs normally.

One very practical question that is usually asked right away is: "How often should a baby be fed?" Two schools of thought exist to answer this question. At one end is the school that believes babies need to eat at regular intervals throughout the day. For parents who are uncertain about caring for their babies, this approach provides a bit of comfort; the clock makes the decision when to feed. The other end of the spectrum is represented by those who feel that babies must be fed whenever they are awake. This pattern, when followed precisely, can prove to be quite exhausting to parents of wakeful babies.

DEMAND FEEDING
Feeding a baby any time the infant insists on being fed.

Each family works out its own feeding routine with varying degrees of success. However, for families just starting to get acquainted with their new babies and their feeding routines, a melding of the two schools of thought may prove to be helpful. The demand feeding system, in which infants are fed on demand, can be combined with the clock-watching technique quite successfully when some flexibility is allowed. After all, it does seem silly to wake up a sleeping baby just because the clock says it's time to eat. A sleeping baby is not going to die of malnutrition even if the time between feedings is fairly long. On the other hand, a crying baby who finished eating an hour ago certainly does not need to be fed to satisfy what new parents may be misinterpreting as a cry to eat versus a cry for attention or diaper changing.

Somewhere between these extremes, a feeding routine can be worked out to keep the parents happy and the baby adequately fed. In general, a fairly routine eating schedule evolves with a little help from parents or caregivers. Infants who are very small when they are born need to be fed much more often than babies who are of normal weight at birth. Premature and small-for-date babies may need to eat every 1 1/2 to 2 hours at first, whereas larger newborns may want to eat at least every 3 hours and sometimes every 2 hours for the first few days.

As infants gain weight, they can be encouraged to a schedule in which they eat about every 4 hours, although breast-fed infants may eat more frequently. This schedule will mean six feedings every day at first, but this frequency is easier to manage than the days when tiny babies need eight or more feedings. Generally, babies who weigh at least 8 lb are comfortable when they eat at intervals of about four hours.

To help babies establish a reasonable time span between feedings there must be adequate intake at each feeding. This usually means a feeding time of 10 to 20 minutes. If babies fall asleep after nursing for only about 5 minutes, they usually have not consumed enough food to enable them to wait another three or four hours before eating again. A soft light and some pleasant conversation by the feeder can help babies stay awake until they have had enough food to satisfy them for at least three hours. This suggestion does not mean that babies should be encouraged to eat as much as possible at each feeding. Babies should not be urged to eat; the idea is to help them stay awake to satisfy their hunger. When they are awake, but no longer eager for food, the feeding should end. Overfeeding is definitely not recommended.

Generally, it is unwise to get in the habit of giving a baby more food soon after a meal. If a well-fed baby rouses after sleeping for an hour or so, a gas pain is much more likely to be the cause than a hunger pang. Burping, and perhaps a change of diaper, may be all that is necessary when a baby demands attention an hour or two after eating. The baby will probably go back to sleep until it is almost time for the next feeding.

Sometimes parents and babies drift into a pattern of frequent feedings, a situation which exhausts them all. If this occurs, parents can gradually extend the time between feedings to about four hours if the baby weighs at least 8 lb. For wakeful babies, this may mean a bit of playtime or simply very slow feeding preparations. Sometimes rocking a baby in a rocking chair or a little conversation to help pass the time can be diversions to extend the time between feedings. This will help parents and infants feel comfortable about simply sharing some time together. After all, eating does not have to be the entire focus of interaction between parents and children, even in the early days of life.

As a baby grows older, efforts can be made to eliminate the middle-of-the-night feeding. A good feeding at about 10 p.m., or whenever convenient just before the parents plan to go to bed, is important. Gradually, babies will be able to sleep for longer stretches when all is quiet and dark at night. Many babies can sleep six to eight hours at night without the middle-of-the-night feeding by the time they are a month to six weeks old. Babies who are small at birth may require two months or a little longer before they can sleep through the middle-of-the-night feeding.

Parents are often motivated to begin solid foods at the last feeding of the evening in an attempt to hasten the time when infants will sleep through the night. Although this is a tempting idea, evidence of this practice's efficacy is lacking. A solid cause-and-effect relationship between feeding solids and sleeping through the night has not been demonstrated to date.

THE FEEDING SCENE

Feeding time for babies should be calm and sociable. For most neonates, this is the primary time available to get

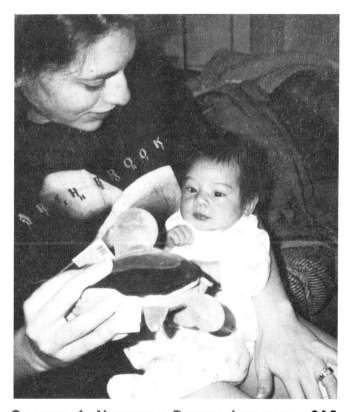

A bit of playtime helps in extending the time between feedings.

acquainted with the world and, specifically, with their parents. Everything is new and different from the protected environment of the womb. Sights, sounds, and smells are new experiences. The act of nursing is unlike the fetal situation. Mealtime is a stimulating, nourishing, and sometimes exhausting time for babies. Parents or others feeding babies can help establish a pattern of pleasant eating by creating a favorable environment.

Feeding should be done in a place that is comfortable for both the baby and the person doing the feeding. The temperature should be comfortable, and the setting should be away from traffic and distractions, so that eating is the primary event. Loud noises can be particularly disruptive. Shouts and banging of doors or pots and pans can startle a baby badly and upset what otherwise would have been a comfortable and pleasant meal. Harsh sounds like the ringing of the telephone can interrupt a baby's enjoyment of eating. On the other hand, soft background music or soothing conversation, even a song by the feeder, can add pleasure.

It is a wise mother who encourages other family members to participate in feeding the baby if they wish. Even when the mother is breast-feeding, she can encourage a sibling to let the baby cling to an eager little finger. Fathers can also share in the feeding by joining in conversation or by preparing a baby for the feeding. When babies are being fed by bottle, fathers and older children can actually participate in the feeding experience directly. One of the nicest aspects of parenting today is the deep involvement of fathers in caring for their children, including helping with the feeding. These shared moments by parent and siblings help bring the new baby into the family circle.

When a feeding is finished, infants need to be changed, burped, and placed on their backs in their beds for a period of quiet sleep. This marks the end of a pleasant social time. It is very important to avoid the habit of putting a baby to bed with a bottle. Although this may seem like a simple way of getting a baby to fall asleep quietly and quickly, it creates risks for the infant. There is a possibility that the baby may choke. A more likely problem is the insidious attack that this practice can mount on baby teeth when they start to erupt. Milk draining slowly into the baby's mouth will create a pool in which bacteria form acid from the sugar in milk; this promotes dental caries in the deciduous teeth. Dental caries in such young children is sometimes referred to as "nursing bottle syndrome." The

NURSING BOTTLE SYNDROME
Decay of baby teeth caused by routinely giving babies a nursing bottle when they are put to bed.

important preventive measure to avoid nursing bottle syndrome is to make it a policy never to put babies to bed with a bottle.

SOLID FOODS

Practices in infant feeding change from time to time. One significant change in the past few years has been the increased emphasis on the delay in feeding solid foods to supplement breast milk or formula. Formerly, cereals were added within the first month or even in the first two weeks of life. Now it is recommended that solid foods be delayed until at least four months, and preferably about six months of age. Recommendations for when beikost (the German word for foods other than milk or formula) should be introduced to infant diets are based on developmental progress in feeding skills, sensory experiences, and nutritional needs.

BEIKOST
Infant foods other than milk and formula.

DEVELOPMENTAL PROGRESS IN FEEDING SKILLS

When infants are very young, they have the reflexes and skills necessary to obtain milk from a nipple and swallow it. For the first few weeks, babies have an extrusion reflex that causes them to push out food placed toward the front of the tongue. This reflex is cited as one reason that babies are not ready for solid foods during the early period of infancy. The extinction of the extrusion reflex by the time the baby is four months old makes feeding of solids an easier process.

EXTRUSION REFLEX
The automatic expulsion of solid food if it is placed on the front part of a baby's tongue in the first few weeks of life.

Lip closure improves slowly so that babies about eight months old have good control of closing their lips. This ability facilitates drinking from a cup, but infants can begin drinking from a cup before they completely master lip closure.

A key ability required for successful beikost feeding is the movement of food from the front of the mouth to the back for swallowing. Of course, babies vary somewhat in their rate of development, but this coordinated movement of food for swallowing can be managed by many infants at about three months or slightly later. Until this can be done easily and the extrusion reflex has been extinguished, the feeding of solid foods can frustrate both baby and feeder.

CRITICAL PERIOD
A particularly important time for developing a developmental skill; usually around six months for chewing.

Chewing is another developmental skill that babies must master in their progress toward eating a regular diet. The ability begins with rotary motions, followed by vertical movement of the jaw, and is usually ready to be put into practice by six months of age. At this critical period, babies should receive beikost every day to permit this practice, which enables them to learn to chew and accept food textures that are different from milk.

Development of feeding skills involves the hand, as well as the tongue and mouth. By six months of age, babies are beginning to grasp objects and even carry them to their mouths with a bit of difficulty. However, they can feed themselves finger foods with reasonable success by seven or eight months. A piece of zweiback or cracker can be mouthed and also passed from one hand to the other.

SENSORY EXPERIENCE

Until solid foods are introduced into the infant's life, feeding acquaints the sense of taste, smell, and touch only with human milk and/or formula, and possibly with orange or other fruit juice. Breast milk may provide somewhat broader flavor

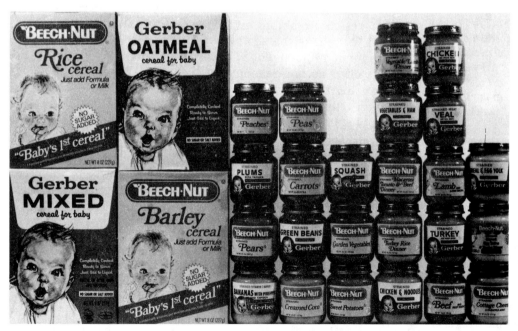

Numerous cereals, fruits, vegetables, meats, egg yolks, and combinations of these basic strained foods are available to add variety to babies who are between four and six months old. These can be made in the home, too.

experiences for babies than formula because of the variety of foods and spices that the mother may be ingesting. However, flavor experiences remain limited until beikost is gradually introduced to extend the breadth of flavors the infant gradually learns to accept. The sweetness of milk is just the beginning of becoming acquainted with flavors. Although there is nothing wrong with the experience to that point, feeding can certainly provide far more exciting textures, aromas, and flavors when the menu is broadened. Despite the limited ability of an infant to chew regular table foods, adventure can be brought in by introducing pureed foods. Even infant cereals diluted with enough milk to make them fluid can introduce new sensory experiences. Babies appear to be mystified and surprised when they first encounter a small spoonful of cereal on the tongue. As variety expands into an array of vegetables and fruits, their acquaintance with the world and its remarkable assortment of foods begins to broaden. Strained meats add still different types of flavors and tactile perceptions in the mouth.

A considerable amount of pleasure in life is afforded through food, with its infinite palate of colors, aromas, flavors, and textures. The foundation for learning to enjoy a broad spectrum of foods is established through early experiences. The gradual introduction of solid foods is an important step in educating babies to experience and enjoy many foods, not simply milk. In particular, infants are ready to chew and swallow pureed foods by around six months of age. This experience is important for them, because they are receptive to changes in food textures and flavors at this time. When solid foods are withheld until very late in the first year, infants may be unwilling to accept the new feeding experience. They may already be set in their attitude toward food and reject the unfamiliar.

NUTRITIONAL ASPECTS

Very early introduction of beikost is not recommended at the present time because infants who receive beikost in the first few weeks of life may be overfed or may replace some of their milk with cereal. Human milk or a balanced commercial formula is an excellent way to provide necessary nutrients in amounts a baby can consume comfortably for at least the first four months of life. At about this age, large babies may begin to show signs of needing more food than they are getting from human milk or formula alone. For them, a quart of either milk will simply not provide sufficient energy for their growing and increasingly active bodies. By six months of age, most babies have reached this stage.

Added nutrients, particularly iron, are first obtained from cereals then from other types of beikost; these foods enhance the vitamins and minerals contained in milk.

The rationale for the timing of starting to feed solid food is the development of feeding behaviors and the physical development needed to move the food to the back of the mouth and swallow it, rather than being pushed out by the undamped extrusion reflex. Since nutritional needs can be met from formula feeding or breast milk, possibly with minor suppplementation, there is no compelling nutritional reason to start solid foods earlier than this.

Considerable controversy has developed regarding the possible relationship between early introduction of solid foods and obesity in later life. A critical period for increasing the number of fat cells is from birth through the first six months of life; considerable increase in fat cells still occurs, but at a somewhat slower rate, in the second half of the first year. This information has raised the question of whether or not the additional calories provided by solid foods might result in overfeeding of infants and development of an excessive number of fat cells, thus setting the stage for a lifetime of battling excess weight. Although this has been a popular theory, research efforts to prove it have not been conclusive to date. Even when the number of fat cells is greater than normal in infancy, research has not shown that this situation is responsible for obesity later.

RESEARCH INSIGHTS

Krebs, N., Dietary zinc and iron sources, physical growth, and cognitive development of breastfed infants. *J. Nutr. 130:* 358S. 2000.

Mennella, J.A. and G.K. Beauchamp, Early flavor experiences: research update. *Nutr. Rev. 56(7):* 205. 1998.

Birch, L.L. and K. Grimm-Thomas, Food acceptance patterns: children learn what they live. *Pediatr. Basics 75:* 2. 1996.

Despite the fact that the iron in human milk is absorbed very efficiently, infants need a supplemental source of iron by about 6 months of age. The usual practice to meet this need is to introduce iron-fortified cereal as gruel sometimes as early as 4 months and certainly by 6 months. Human milk also is quite low in zinc by 3 months postpartum and needs to be supplemented from other food by at least the sixth month. Krebs (2000) tested the effects of adding beef versus iron-fortified cereal as the first food to complement human milk, beginning between the ages of 5 and 7 months and continuing through 1 year. Fruits and vegetables were allowed to be added during the test period, but neither the beef nor the cereal test group could be fed the other test food throughout the test.

Acceptance of meat or cereal as the first complementary food was statistically the same. Absorption of zinc from cereals and from beef was similar, but the greater amount of zinc in beef provided more absorbed zinc in the infants fed beef versus those fed cereal in this experiment at 7 months. Those fed iron-fortified cereal had a higher iron intake than those fed beef. By the age of 9 months, no significant differences in growth, development, and biochemical indices for iron and zinc were noted between the two groups.

Mennella and Beauchamp noted that a fetus contacts glucose, lactic acid, and various other flavorful compounds beginning around the 7th week in utero, which provides experiences on which taste and flavor acceptance can develop after birth. A clear preference for sweet taste in foods can be seen even when an infant begins to nurse. A subsequent demonstration of this liking for a sweet taste is the ready acceptance of fruits when they are added to the diet later in the first year of life. Meat flavors are not sweet like fruit, but Krebs found that acceptance was good when beef was offered as the first solid (pureed) food, i.e., sweet taste was not a requirement for acceptance. This finding was in agreement with the work of Birch and Grimm-Thomas who found that repeated exposure to new foods is important for acceptance, particularly foods lacking a sweet taste.

ADDING CEREALS

Enriched cereals prepared in flaked, dehydrated form for infant feeding are the first type of solid food in most children's experience. Cereal is added between four and six months of age when a quart of formula or breast milk alone no longer seems to satisfy the baby. These infant cereals are manufactured with added thiamin, riboflavin, niacin, vitamin C, and iron to enhance their nutritional value. Iron enrichment is particularly important, for cereals are the primary source of dietary iron during the first year and effectively compensate for the low iron content in a milk diet.

Aside from their nutritional benefits, cereals are valuable for their texture. Textural characteristics of a cereal being fed can be varied gradually, beginning with a very dilute mixture with some noticeable flakes of cereal and continuing until the cereal is thick enough to provide some practice in chewing and passing the thickened paste from one side of the mouth to the other by about nine months of age. The feeder can dilute dry cereal flakes to a consistency suited to the infant's stage of development in coordinating the movement of food in its mouth.

A pleasant feeding experience when cereal is added is determined to a large extent by proper dilution of the cereal. Adults ordinarily expect hot cereals to be quite thick, but this consistency is much too difficult for the young and inexperienced infant to manipulate in the mouth and swallow. Practice can be gained by starting out with a very thin cereal mixture that is only slightly thicker than the liquid that has been fed up to this point. This can easily be placed on the baby's tongue with a demitasse or other small spoon appropriate for the baby's mouth. Some of the cereal may run out of the corners of the mouth at first, but this is not a sign that the cereal is disliked. It merely reflects the baby's inexperience and need for developing coordination of the tongue, jaws, and lips. Coordination will develop with practice and patience.

Problems with keeping cereal in the mouth long enough to be swallowed can be eased by the feeding technique used. When the food is placed toward the back of the tongue, swallowing is fairly easy even for an inexperienced baby. Even then, some cereal is likely to be propelled forward by the tongue and onto the lips and face. The spoon can be used gently to gather the cereal and place it once again on the back of the tongue. Babies will learn to coordinate tongue movements and swallowing rapidly. Parents or caretakers should realize that spilling is part of the process of learning to eat and is not a rejection of the food.

Cereal choices for infants include rice, barley, oatmeal, and mixed grains. A single grain should definitely be fed first, and rice is usually recommended because it is unlikely to cause allergic responses. Usually, infants' digestive tracts are sufficiently mature by the age of four months to digest rice cereal for absorption. If new allergic symptoms like rashes, breathing problems, or sneezing are noted before the next milk feeding, it is wise to switch to a different grain the next time cereal is fed. The offending grain can be tried again in a month or two after the digestive tract has had more time to mature.

Rice or any other cereal being introduced should first be fed in a very small amount, beginning with about 1/4 teaspoon dry cereal mixed with enough milk to make an extremely thin

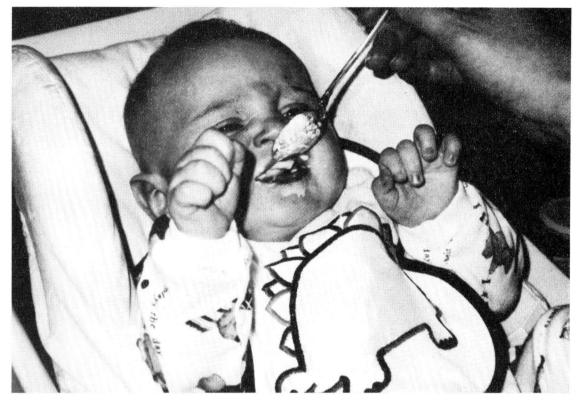

The texture of diluted cereal is a surprise to this baby, but it soon is accepted.

gruel. Nursing mothers may wish to express some breast milk for this dilution or use some ready-to-feed formula. Each time the cereal is fed, the amount can be increased slightly until 1 tablespoon dry cereal is being used at a feeding. The same cereal grain should be fed for at least two weeks before trying a different grain. In this way, any possible allergic response can be related to a specific cereal.

Cereal is ordinarily considered a breakfast food served with sugar. There is, however, no reason to add sugar to a baby's cereal. The added calories in sugar are not appropriate, because they are not accompanied by any nutrients. Furthermore, there is no merit in encouraging babies to develop a preference for sweet foods. Having cereal for breakfast is another tradition that can be ignored when feeding infants. Parents often prefer to feed cereal around 10 p.m., just before going to sleep. However, cereal can be fed at another meal if that fits a family's routine better.

VEGETABLES AND FRUITS

There is no rule as to whether fruits or vegetables should be added after cereals are well established. Some people prefer to add fruits to the diet next, but others think that babies will accept vegetables better if they have not experienced the sweetness of fruits first. Either approach seems to work well. This decision can be made without worry; there really is no bad choice as long as they are added to the diet on a regular basis by six months or slightly later.

Each new pureed fruit or vegetable should be added very gradually, starting with about 1/2 teaspoon the first day. The next day, the portion of the same food can be increased a little. Once a baby has become accustomed to a new fruit or vegetable, the maximum serving size should be about 1 tablespoonful for most infants. The food being fed at a meal should be removed from the jar so the feeding spoon does not contaminate the remainder in the jar.

From the baby's standpoint, it is wise to introduce a variety of vegetables and fruits instead of just one or two. The early period of life is a highly experimental time for the infant, and the variety of experiences that can be provided by an assortment of fruits and vegetables should not be ignored. Babies can develop a sense of adventure with food if they are given different experiences in eating.

Although variety is important, each fruit or vegetable should be started in small amounts to avoid possible allergy problems. However, vegetables and fruits are generally less allergenic than cereals. Pureed single fruits or vegetables are good choices during the early phase of adding foods to the diet, because the food causing an allergic response can be identified if mixtures have not been fed.

MEATS AND EGGS

Meats and egg yolks are usually added soon after fruits and vegetables are being fed regularly. An important reason for adding meats and egg yolks is to provide a dietary source of iron to supplement the iron in cereals. They also add flavors and textures quite different from those of pureed vegetables and fruits.

Strained meats prepared by baby food manufacturers can be a real convenience. The many types available can save considerable labor in preparing strained meats at home. Baby food meat products are well suited to the infant's nutritional needs and eating experience, although they may not be particularly appealing to the feeder. It is important that parents do not convey negative feelings about meats. They should be fed with the same enthusiasm used in feeding fruits. Remember that meats and egg yolks are fine sources of the B vitamins and copper, in addition to iron.

Canned egg yolks are convenient to use and have the distinct advantage of avoiding the problem of left over whites. Egg yolks are usually accepted well and do not trigger allergies; whites may cause allergic responses unless they are withheld until near the end of the first year. On the contrary, it is recommended that meats and yolks be fed very soon after the baby reaches the age of six months.

Occasionally, high meat dinners and cottage cheese may be served as the main course of a meal near the end of the first year. These items add variety and sufficient protein for older, hungry babies, but are not sufficiently concentrated sources of energy for babies with small appetites. In 4 1/2 oz of a high meat dinner, there will be about 8 1/2 g of protein, as contrasted with approximately 19 g from the same quantity of strained meat.

BREADS AND PASTAS

When infants are around nine months old, they enjoy trying to hold foods in their fingers and putting them in their mouths. Zwieback and teething biscuits are examples of bread products that can be useful as babies begin to learn to feed themselves. These foods, when they are made with enriched flour, are useful as sources of the B vitamins and some iron. Hard-textured breads can be useful in easing teething problems, too. Although these are useful foods in the diet, they should be limited so that they do not interfere with appetites at meals. About four teething biscuits or pieces of zwieback should be the maximum each day, with fewer servings for babies with small appetites.

Occasionally, babies enjoy having potatoes or pasta added to meals at eight or nine months. These items can be chewed easily, yet offer pleasing variations in texture. Small servings of these foods are fine, as long as milk consumption is adequate and appropriate amounts of fruits, vegetables, and meats are eaten.

DESSERTS

A baby's nutritional needs to support the impressive rate of growth during the first year are great in proportion to a relatively small capacity. Nutrient-dense foods that provide significant levels of nutrients in relation to calories are wise choices. Desserts should not ordinarily be included. An occasional dessert or fruit or custard can be fed, but such items as cookies, cakes, and candies are best omitted.

COMMERCIAL BABY FOODS

Strained baby foods are a definite convenience, though somewhat costly. A wide selection of strained fruits, vegetables, meats, egg yolks, pasta and meat combinations, high meat dinners, vegetable and meat dinners, and fruit and cereal combinations can be purchased in small screw-top jars. These products have undergone a series of changes consistent with knowledge of infant nutritional needs. In the past they were often flavored with added sugar, monosodium glutamate (MSG), and salt. To help reduce the ratio of solids to liquids and reduce the renal solute load, MSG (a flavor enhancer) has been eliminated from strained baby foods, and salt levels have been markedly reduced. Sugar has also been eliminated as an additive in some strained baby foods or has been reduced in quantity. The raitonale for reducing sugar in the diet is based on the 1) the infant's need for nutrient-dense foods, 2) the wisdom in not establishing a strong bias for sweet foods, and 3) concern for the cariogenic effects of sugar in children's diets.

MSG
Monosodium glutamate; flavor enhancer formerly used in strained baby foods, but now voluntarily eliminated by companies producing strained baby foods.

The first strained commercially-prepared baby foods designed for infants are marketed in 2.5-oz jars, consistent with the limited capacities of babies 4 to 6 months old. These "starter" strained foods are prepared as single foods so that the distinctive flavor of the food can be experienced. This also has the benefit of allowing a trial period of a couple of days to reinforce the flavor experience while verifying the lack of an allergic response to the food by the baby.

The next step for babies is the feeding of slightly more complex pureed foods, such as pureed apples and cherries. Consistent with the increasing capacity of infants older than 6 months, these foods are marketed in 4-oz jars. Commercial baby foods for somewhat older infants have distinct textural characteristics to promote chewing. These often are mixtures of foods and are in 6-oz jars.

When babies are first being fed strained fruits and vegetables, a very small amount is used. If strained canned baby foods are opened for feeding, shelf life is limited to only a couple of days in the refrigerator. The remaining food in the jar should be discarded because harmful levels of microorganisms may develop and infect the baby when food is stored more than two days. This waste adds to the cost of strained foods until a baby is eating about half a jar at a meal. The desire to avoid waste is likely to cause overfeeding; parents and other feeders often coax babies to eat more just to empty the jar. Overfeeding should be avoided.

PREPARING STRAINED FOODS AT HOME

Strained baby foods can be prepared at home with a little effort. If this is the plan, foods should be cooked until they are soft enough to be made into a puree, a process easily done in a blender or a food processor. These foods should be cooked without salt, MSG, or other flavoring agents. The simple flavors of the pureed foods themselves are quite palatable and do not require these ingredients to be acceptable to infants. Some of the

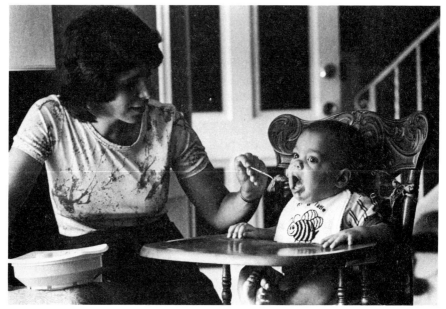

Pureed foods help to satisfy and add to the food experiences of babies.

water in which the food is cooked can be added to the puree if necessary to achieve desired viscosity for feeding.

A word or two of caution about preparing baby foods should be given. Pureeing food that has been prepared for adults is not satisfactory because of the likelihood of too much salt or other seasonings. Baby foods are simple foods. They will spoil quickly unless they are kept refrigerated from the time they are prepared until they are fed. They should be served within a maximum of two days and preferably the same day they are prepared. Pureed foods can be frozen into cubes in an ice cube tray and stored in the freezer for longer periods. These should, of course, be kept frozen and sealed in plastic bags with the air squeezed out of the bags until they are heated just before feeding.

PLANNING THE DAY'S MENUS

During the second half of the first year, babies are ready for a diet based on the Food Guide Pyramid, although the food will look quite different from what is served at the family table. Foods should be included from all the food groups during this period, even though the greatest portion is still provided by milk. At this age, many infants may be consuming about 1 qt of breast milk or formula daily. Until the age of 1 year, human milk or formula should be the only forms of milk fed. Cow's milk, because of its relatively high mineral content, places too great a strain on the kidneys of infants. Of course, formulas made with cow's milk are safe because of the changes that have been made in composition during preparation of the formula. Solid foods should vary from day to day to be sure the baby is experiencing many foods. However, the portions should generally not exceed 1 tablespoonful. Remember, the goal is to develop acceptance of a wide range of foods, not a huge capacity.

The daily diet should be examined to be certain that all necessary nutrients are being included. This is the responsibility of parents, physicians, and dietitians. Babies cannot be counted upon to indicate the foods they need. It frequently is said that babies have a sense of what they need to eat, but they apparently are no more gifted than adults in this regard. Their advantage is that they can eat only what is given to them. Impulse eating, which is the plague of many overweight adults, is an experience babies have not had.

The idea that babies can choose an adequate diet for themselves appears to stem from research done by Davis in the 1930s. She found that babies did select a reasonably adequate diet over a period of several days when they were given opportunities to choose. The limiting factor in this research is that only highly nourishing foods were offered. Candy and other low-nutrient-density foods were not included as choices. In the absence of proof that babies are capable of selecting a good diet for themselves, the person feeding the baby must assume responsibility for offering an adequate diet.

The size of a baby's servings will vary, depending on the infant's size and age as well as the variety and quantity of food planned for the day. The size of baby food containers is small enough to suggest to adults that they are intended as a single serving for babies. Actually, a considerably smaller serving will often be quite appropriate. The amount of food to serve needs to be gauged according to the infant's appetite and rate of gain. As babies grow, they gradually desire larger servings, and intake naturally will increase.

The primary limitation regarding serving sizes is that milk should be limited to 1 qt per day. This is not a negative comment about milk. It merely emphasizes the fact that some babies are so fond of milk that they may restrict their consumption of solid foods in favor of too much milk, which can lead to inadequate iron intake.

SCHEDULE FOR DAILY FEEDING OF SOLIDS

There is no particular time of day when solid baby foods need to be included in a feeding. The time to offer them depends on a family's schedule and routine. When solid foods are first being added, it is often convenient and practical to give cereal at the last feeding before the parents go to bed at night. Other solid foods can be added at other times during the day to provide the gradual addition of some solid food at each feeding. If a mother is involved in getting her husband and older children off to a job and school early in the morning, it is difficult to do a reasonable job of feeding the infant in the midst of the confusion. A quick milk or formula feeding at this time may be the best answer. Solid foods can be given at subsequent feedings during the day when things are less hectic.

Although it is not necessary to set up a rigid schedule for a baby's meals, both parents and baby will find mealtime smoother when a general feeding plan is followed. A regular meal pattern helps to promote a hearty appetite. A planned part of the day's solid food intake should be fed at each meal during the day. However, there may be quite a variation in the amounts of the solid foods that are eaten. A look at four days in the life of Lauren Elizabeth illustrates the fluctuations in quantity and eating time typical of babies in the second half of the first year.

LAUREN ELIZABETH'S FOUR-DAY DIETARY INTAKE AT 7 1/2 MONTHS AGE

DAY 1:
6:30   5 oz   formula
8:00   4 oz   formula
10:00 1 oz   applesauce
       3 oz   cereal
12:00 3 oz   formula
3:00   1 oz   puree of cottage cheese, pears, orange juice
4:45   5 oz   formula
6:30   1 oz   squash
       1 1/2 oz turkey dinner
7:30   3 oz   formula

DAY 2:
6:00   4 oz   formula
10:00 5 oz   formula
12:00 2 oz   sweet potato
       2 oz   turkey
       4 1/2 oz guava
3:00   6 oz   formula
4:30   6 oz   formula
6:00   1/2 oz   cereal
7:00   5 oz   formula

DAY 3:
6:00   6 oz   formula
8:00   4 oz   formula
9:45   6 oz   formula
11:00 5 oz   formula
1:30   4 1/2 oz squash
       2 oz   plantains
4:00   6 oz   formula
6:00   1 1/2 oz cereal

                  1/2 oz   applesauce
         7:00 4 1/2 oz formula

         DAY 4:
          6:00 5 oz   formula
          7:30 4 oz   formula
         10:30 5 oz   formula
                1 oz   cottage cheese
         12:00 4 1/2 oz applesauce
                4 1/2 oz vegetable beef
          1:35 6 oz   formula

          4:00 6 oz   formula
          6:00 1 oz   cereal
          7:30 1/2 oz   applesauce and cherries
                5 oz   formula

Note that Lauren Elizabeth generally ate eight times each day, although on one day she ate only seven times. She also shows a lot of variation in the amount of formula consumed in the morning. Note that her usual pattern is about 9 oz of formula by the middle of the morning, whereas she had already had 16 oz by 10 a.m. the third day. She drank 12 oz of formula in the afternoon on two days, but had only 6 oz and 5 oz the other afternoons. This variation might worry parents unless they take a look at the day's total intake. Note that Lauren Elizabeth's total formula intake for each day is between 20 and 31 oz for two days and 26 oz for one. Day 1 illustrates the shift in the amount of formula that occurs with increased solid foods, for she drank only 20 oz of formula. An analysis of Lauren Elizabeth's nutrient intake is presented in Table 6.5.

As can be seen in Table 6.6, the caloric content of Lauren Elizabeth's diet is significantly below the RDA. Interestingly, her nutrient intake generally exceeds RDA values. This illustrates the importance of maintaining a good intake of human milk or formula at this age. There is no reason to be concerned about the diet's low caloric content because she is growing well and is a happy baby. Although she could be given more food than at present, she is being fed a carefully selected and nourishing diet with many foods that reflect the priority being given to assuring varied food experiences in these early months. As meats are added in greater quantity and the transition is made to pasteurized whole milk in a few months, her caloric intake will increase accordingly. She can be expected to continue to grow well and to be receptive to many different foods.

TABLE 6.5 Analysis of Lauren Elizabeth's Nutrient intake for Four Days

Food	Measure (oz)	Cal	Protein (g)	Calcium (mg)	Iron (mg)	Vit. A (RE)	Thiamin (mg)	Riboflavin (mg equiv)	Niacin (mg)	Vit. C (mg)
Day 1										
Formula	20	395	8.9	271	7.5	378	0.3	0.4	4.4	33
Applesauce	1	27	0.1	1	0.1	—	—	—	—	10
Cereal	3	54	1.0	94	14.0	—	0.4	0.3	2.0	—
Cottage cheese w/ fruit	1	45	2.0	22	0.1	—	—	0.1	—	1
Squash	1	9	—	8	0.1	132	—	—	—	3
Turkey dinner	1.5	15	1.0	4	0.1	49	—	—	0.1	1
Total		*545*	*13.0*	*400*	*22.1*	*559*	*0.7*	*0.8*	*6.5*	*48*
Day 2										
Formula	26	512	11.5	352	9.7	491	0.4	0.5	5.6	42
Sweet Potato	2	14	0.4	12	0.2	67	—	—	—	4
Turkey	2	65	6.9	10	0.8	—	—	0.1	1.5	2
Guava	4.5	35	—	18	0.2	160	—	—	0.2	51
Cereal	0.5	9	0.1	15	2.4	—	0.1	0.1	0.3	—
Total		*635*	*18.9*	*407*	*13.3*	*718*	*0.5*	*0.7*	*7.6*	*99*
Day 3										
Formula	31.5	632	14.2	434	12.0	606	0.5	0.6	7.0	52
Squash	4.5	35	1.0	25	0.5	654	0.1	—	0.5	14
Plantain	2	50	0.5	5	0.4	—	—	—	0.4	6
Cereal	1.5	27	0.5	47	7.1	—	0.2	0.2	1.0	—
Applesauce	0.5	14	—	—	—	—	—	—	—	5
Total		*758*	*16.2*	*511*	*20.0*	*1260*	*0.8*	*0.8*	*8.9*	*77*
Day 4										
Formula	31	613	13.8	421	11.6	588	0.5	0.6	6.8	50
Cottage cheese	1	30	3.8	27	—	5	0.1	0.1	—	—
Applesauce	4.5	109	0.2	4	0.5	—	—	—	0.1	40
Vegetable beef	4.5	104	7.8	8	1.2	177	—	0.1	1.9	3
Cereal	1	18	0.3	31	4.7	—	0.1	0.1	0.7	—
Applesauce w/ cherries	0.5	12	—	1	—	6	—	—	—	2
Total		*886*	*25.9*	*492*	*18.0*	*776*	*1.5*	*0.9*	*9.5*	*95*

TABLE 6.6   Comparison of Lauren Elizabeth's Nutrient Intake for Four Days with the RDA

Day	Cal	Protein (g)	Calcium (mg)	Iron (mg)	Vit. A (RE)	Thiamin (mg)	Riboflavin (mg equiv)	Niacin (mg)	Vit. C (mg)
1	545	13.0	400	22.1	559	0.7	0.8	6.5	48
2	635	18.9	407	13.3	718	0.5	0.7	7.6	99
3	758	16.2	511	20.0	1260	0.8	0.8	8.9	77
4	886	25.9	492	18.0	776	1.5	0.9	9.5	95
Daily Average	706	18.5	452	18.4	828	0.9	0.8	8.1	80
RDA	1002	14.0	270	10	375	0.3	0.4	4	35

A LOOK AT WEIGHT

The importance of providing a broad range of foods in the diet without overfeeding is a key concept during the second half of the first year. Lauren Elizabeth's diet illustrated this point. Appropriate weight can be maintained without sacrificing good nutrition, even during infancy. If parents are aware of the relationship of their infant's weight to length, they will be able to adjust their feeding practices accordingly. The appropriateness of weight for length is far more important than striving to achieve as much weight gain as possible. Unfortunately, new parents easily slip into the attitude that a baby's rapid weight gain is an indication that they are doing a superb job of parenting. When parents with children at the same age get together, the conversation usually turns to a comparison of how much each baby weighs. Actually, abnormally large weight gain is not a reliable indication of the quality of parenting.

In addition to the desire to help a baby grow as much as possible, parents may be tempted to overfeed simply to avoid wasting food. This is not a problem with breast feeding, but bottle-fed infants are often urged to finish the last ounce or two of formula in a bottle just because it is there. The same behavior is seen frequently when solid foods are being fed. The bottom of a baby food jar may be the point at which feeding stops. Babies who lose their enthusiasm for eating while there is still some food in the jar may virtually be forced to empty the jar.

Excessive weight gain by infants is to be avoided, not encouraged. If parents and caretakers feed babies according to their appetites and not just to empty food containers, the problem probably can be avoided.

Appropriate weight is achieved by a two-pronged approach. Food intake is one factor, and exercise is the other. Of course, babies usually are not enrolled in exercise classes, but they can be given encouragement to exercise. A playpen may stifle the exploratory urge, whereas an infant loose on the floor can go roaming. A creeping or crawling baby uses considerably more energy in the course of a day than one restricted to a playpen. This freedom to explore may be inconvenient for parents, but it helps develop muscular coordination and physical activity in babies. A side benefit is the added exercise parents get while supervising walking or crawling babies.

Weight gain varies from baby to baby, but average weight gain is about 6 oz each week during the first six months of life; the rate gradually slows in the second six months. Height and weight gain tables for early childhood are presented in Appendix Tables A-1 and A-4. Although individuals grow at different rates, these tables are helpful in monitoring the growth pattern and weight of individual children.

THE TRANSITION

Babies are social creatures and great imitators. This can be helpful in making the transition to "adult" food. Babies will be ready to imitate adult feeding behaviors as they approach the end

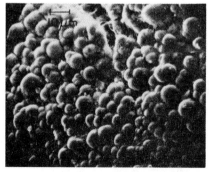 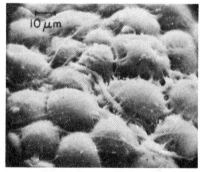

Scanning electron micrograph of adipose tissue from male Sprague-Dawley rats: left, 2 days old; right, 8 weeks old.

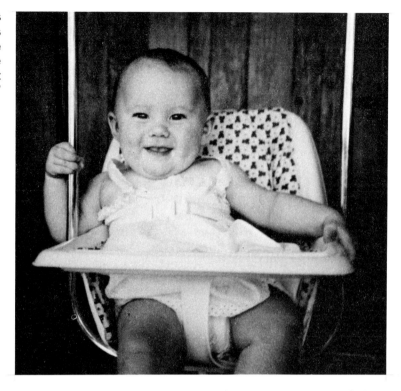

Well-nourished babies enjoy happy interludes with others and are responsive. Note the enthusiasm of this infant 'swinger."

of the first year. One of the early transitions is learning to drink from a glass or cup. Another is to hold finger foods in the hands and carry them to the mouth. Still another is to want to eat food from the table. By about 10 months of age, a gradual transition to chopped or coarsely mashed foods should be started to acquaint babies with textures that require more chewing than is needed for strained foods. These chopped baby foods can be purchased in commercially-prepared form, or they can be prepared at home.

With planning and care, it is possible to make the transition to table foods without buying many commercially-prepared chopped baby foods. This can be done at home by removing the baby's portion when the food is cooked, but before strong seasonings have been added, and chopping the food with a knife or the back of a fork until the pieces are small, but not pureed. Eggs, cheese, hamburger, boiled vegetables, carefully deboned fish, cooked fruits, avocados, bananas, and boiled pastas are examples of foods that can be easily converted into chopped foods at the family meal.

There are advantages to feeding chopped table foods to babies. When they see that they are being fed from the table at a family meal, they learn to eat new foods as a result of the socialization process. Their parents and others at the table serve as role models for them. Infants expand their food choices as they experience the wide range of foods eaten by others in the family.

Soups deserve special attention in children's diets at the end of the first year. If a baby has a large capacity and is eating numerous servings of meats, vegetables, fruits, and milk, soups may be appropriate in small amounts. However, some babies become so full with soup that they fail to eat the food they need to obtain adequate levels of the nutrients. These children should not be given soup until they are able to eat enough of the other foods along with a little soup. Some people serve babies undiluted commercial soup concentrates as a replacement for junior foods. This practice should definitely be avoided because of these soups' high salt concentration.

Infants preferably remain on human milk or on formula until the age of approximately one year, at which time they can usually be shifted to pasteurized whole milk. Milk reduced in fat should not be fed to children under the age of two.

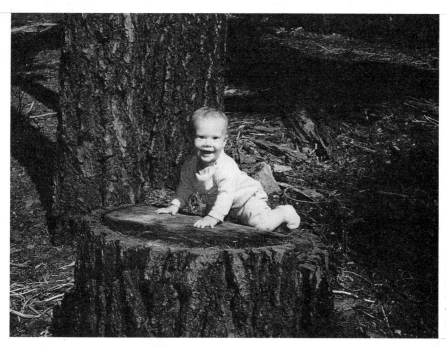

Unrestricted opportunities to explore not only stimulate babies, but also aid in using up energy and developing muscles and avoid excessive weight gain in later infancy.

SUMMARY

The first year of life is one of very rapid growth, particularly the first six months. This creates a significant demand for nutrients, almost all of which are adequately provided in human milk or in commercial formulas. Breast-fed infants require a vitamin D supplement from birth and an iron supplement or an iron-fortified baby cereal by the time they are six months old. Bottle-fed infants should receive an iron-fortified formula or a supplement by four months of age. Fluoride supplementation is needed throughout childhood if the water supply is not fluoridated, but the level must be carefully controlled to avoid excessive levels that can cause mottled teeth. Premature or small-for-date infants require special nutrition planning.

Eating frequency during the early weeks is greatly influenced by the size of the baby; very small babies may need to eat every two hours, whereas larger ones can wait three to four hours between feedings. Feeding should be done in a calm and quiet setting, an environment where babies can eat as much as they want without being interrupted. Other family members may want to participate in the feeding experience and can help create a happy social interaction without overstimulating the infant. To promote social interaction and reduce the likelihood of developing "nursing bottle syndrome," babies should never be put to bed with a bottle.

Solid foods are usually started between four and six months, depending on the baby's size and appetite. A plain cereal, usually rice cereal, is diluted to a thin gruel and fed without sugar as the first solid food. Only about 1/4 teaspoon cereal should be fed the first day. The amount can be increased gradually if the cereal is not causing any allergic reaction. Addition of cereal and other solid foods is important as a way to broaden a baby's food experiences as the physical developmental skills needed for eating gradually develop. These foods are also valued as sources of a variety of nutrients. Vegetables and fruits are added soon after cereals are established. Egg yolk and strained meats are the next type of food given to the baby. Breads and pastas are next. Desserts are not necessary in the baby's diet, but such items as fruits or custard are permitted.

Babies' first solid foods should be strained foods as they learn to chew and swallow. Commercial baby foods are one way to provide strained foods. Similar foods can be prepared at home, but it is important not to add salt or any other seasonings to pureed foods.

Once strained foods are added to the diet, meal planning is appropriate to be sure the right foods are being served. Strained foods should be served at various times throughout the day. It should be recognized that babies are independent beings, and their food intake patterns and desired eating schedule may vary from time to time, just like adults. Consumption of only small amounts of food or formula on a particular day is not a cause for alarm. Usually, the deficit will be made up quite soon. However, prolonged lack of appetite should be checked by a physician to rule out any possible physical problems. Over-feeding should be avoided and activity should be encouraged to help babies maintain a desirable weight for their length.

Near the end of the first year, babies are ready to learn how to drink from a cup and eat coarsely chopped food that requires more chewing than strained foods. The transition to table food can be made gradually by serving infants chopped foods that are not highly seasoned, but are tender enough to be chewed. Parents and others at the family table begin to serve as role models for eating patterns by the age of one year.

BIBLIOGRAPHY

AMERICAN ACADEMY OF PEDIATRICS COMMITTEE ON NUTRITION. Use of whole cow's milk in infancy. *Pediat. 89:* 1105. 1992.

AMERICAN ACADEMY OF PEDIATRICS Iron supplementation for infants. *Pediatr. 58:* 765. 1976.

AMERICAN ACADEMY OF PEDIATRICS COMMITTEE ON NUTRITION. Salt intake and eating patterns of infants and children in relation to blood pressure. Pediat. 53: 115. 1974.

AMERICAN ACADEMY OF PEDIATRICS COMMITTEE ON NUTRITION. Nutritional needs of low-birth-weight infants. *Pediat. 60:* 519. 1977.

ANONYMOUS Introduction of solid foods and total energy intake in exclusively breast-fed infants. *Nutr. Rev. 48:* 280. 1990.

ASHBROOK, S. AND M. DOYLE Infants' acceptance of strong- and mild-flavored vegetables. *J. Nutr. Ed. 17(1):* 1985.

BARNES, L.A. Fluoride in infant formulas and fluoride supplementation. *Pediatr. 67:* 582. 1981.

BARNES, L.A. Queries and minor notes: Then and now. Orange juice in infant feeding. *J. Am. Med. Assoc. 251:* 959. 1984.

BEAL, V.A. Termination of night feeding in infancy. *J. Pediat. 75:* 690. 1969.

BEE, D.E., T. BARANOWSKI, D.K. RASIN, C.J. RICHARDSON, AND W. MIKRUT Breast-feeding initiation in a triethnic population. *Am. J. Dis. Child. 145:* 306. 1992.

BHOWMICK, S.K., J.P. BLAIR, V.N. JONES, AND R.H. DURANT Infant feeding decisions among pregnant women from a WIC population in Georgia, *J. Am. Diet. Assoc. 90:* 255. 1990.

BIRCH, L.L. Children's food acceptance patterns. *Nutr. Today 31(6):* 234. 1996.

CHAN, G.J. Children's bone mineral status. *Am. J. Dis. Child. 145:* 631. 1991.

COMMITTEE ON DRUGS, AMERICAN ACADEMY OF PEDIATRICS. Transfer of drugs and other chemicals into human milk. *Pediat. 84:* 924. 1989.

COMMITTEE ON NUTRITION OF MOTHERS AND PRESCHOOL CHILD, FOOD AND NUTRITION BOARD *Fetal and Infant Nutrition and Susceptibility to Obesity.* National Academy of Sciences. Washington, D.C. 1978.

DALLMAN, P.R., M.A. SUMES, A. STEKEL Iron deficiency in infant and childhool. *Am. J. Clin. Nutr. 33:* 86. 1980.

DAVIS, C.M. Self selection of diets by newly weaned infants. *Amer. J. Dis. Child. 46:* 743. 1964.

EDININ, D.V. L.L. LEVITSKY, W. SCHEY, N. DUMBOVIC, AND A. CAMPOS Resurgence of nutritional rickets associated with breast-feeding and special dietary practices. *Pediatr. 65:* 232. 1980.

FENNER, L. Parents: Guard against food-related chokings. *FDA Cons. 18(9):* 21. 1984.

FINBERG, L. Human milk feeding and vitamin D supplementation. *J. Pediatr. 99:* 228. 1981.

FOMON, S.J. *Infant Nutrition.* Saunders, Philadelphia. 2nd ed. 1974.

FOMON, S.J., ET AL Human milk and the small premature infant. *Am. J. Dis. Child. 131:* 463. 1977.

FOOD AND NUTRITION BOARD, SUBCOMMITTEE ON TENTH EDITION OF THE RDAs. *Recommended Dietary Allowances.* National Academy Press. Wasington, D.C. 10th ed. 1989.

FORD, K. AND M. LABBOK Who is breast-feeding? Implications of associated social and biomedical variables for research on consequences of method of infant feeding. *Am. J. Clin. Nutr. 52:* 451. 1990.

GREENWALDT, E., ET AL Onset of sleeping through the night in infancy: relation to introduction of solid food in the diet, birth weight, and position in the family. *Pediat. 26:* 667. 1960.

HAYWARD, I., M.T. STEIN AND M.I. GIBSON Nutritional rickets in San Diego. *Am. J. Dis. Child. 141:* 1060. 1987.

HIRSCH, J. Cell number and size as determinant of subsequent obesity. In Winick, M., ed. *Childhood Obesity.* Wiley. New York. 1975.

ILLINGWORTH, R.S. AND J. LISTER Critical or sensitive period, with special reference to certain feeding problems in infants and children. *J. Pediat. 65:* 839. 1964.

JACOBSON, S.W., J.L. JACOBSON, AND K.F. FREY Incidence and correlates of breast-feeding in socioeconomically disadvantaged women. *Pediat. 88:* 728. 1991.

JARVIS, J.K. AND G.D. MILLER Fat in infant diets. *Nutr. Today 31(5):* 182. 1996.

JASON, J. Breast-feeding in 1991. *New England J. Med. 325:* 1036. 1991

JOHNSON, D.B. Nutrition in infancy: evolving views on recommendations. *Nutr. Today 32(2):* 63. 1997.

KELLY, V.J. Use of cereal grains in infant feeding. *Cereal Foods World 29:* 721. 1984.

KEMPER, K. B. FORSYTH, AND P. MCCARTHY Jaundice, terminating breast feeding and the vulnerable child. *Pediat. 84:* 773. 1989.

KNITTLE, J.L. Obesity in childhood: problems in adipose tissue cellular development. *J. Pediat. 81:* 1048. 1972

KURINI, J. AND P.H. SHIONO Early formula supplementation of breast-feeding. *Pediat. 88:* 745. 1991.

LAWLESS, H. Sensory development in children: research in taste and olfaction. *J. Am. Diet. Assoc. 85:* 577. 1985.

LIPSCHITZ, C.H. AND F. CARRAZZA Effect of formula carbohydrate concentration on tolerance and macronutrient absorption in infants with severe, chronic diarrhea. *J. Pediat. 117:* 378. 1990.

MACLEAN, W.C. Nutrition in Infancy. In *Present Knowledge in Nutrition,* ed. Olson, R.D., et al. Nutrition Foundation. Washington, D.C. 5th ed. 1984. p. 619.

MASON, J.O. Message to health professionals about fluorosis. *J. Am. Med. Assoc. 265:* 2939. 1991.

MCMILLAN, J.A., ET AL Iron sufficiency in breast-fed infants and the availability of iron from human milk. *Pediat. 58:* 686. 1976.

MENELLA, J.A. A cross-cultural perspective. *Nutr. Today 32(4):* 144. 1997.

MENELLA, J.A. AND G.E. BEAUCHAMP Maternal diet alters sensory qualities of human milk and nursling's behavior. *Pediat. 88:* 745. 1991.

MENNELLA, J.A. AND G.E. BEAUCHAMP Transfer of alcohol to human milk — effects on flavor and infant's behavior. *New England J. Med. 325:* 981. 1991.

MORALES, E., L.D. CRAIG, AND W.C. MACLEAN, JR. Dietary management of malnourished children with a new enteral feeding. *J. Am. Diet. Assoc. 91(10):* 1233. 1991.

NATIONAL ACADEMY OF SCIENCES. *Nutrition during Lactation.* National Academy Press. Washington, D.C. 1991.

NUTRITION FOUNDATION Overfeeding in the first year of life. *Nutr. Rev. 31:* 116, 1973.

O'CONNELL, J.M., M.J. DIBLEY, J. SIERRA, B. WALLACE, J.S. MARKS, AND R. YIP Growth of vegetarian children. Farm study. *Pediat. 84:* 475. 1989.

O'MALLEY, B., A.C. BROWN, M. TATE, A.A. HERTZLER, AND M.H. ROJAS Infant feeding practices of migrant farm laborers in northern Colorado. *J. Am. Diet. Assoc. 91:* 1084. 1991.

PAIGE, D.M. Infant growth and nutrition. *Clin. Nutr. 2:* 14. 1983.

PAYNE, M.L., ET AL Sorbitol is a possible risk factor for diarrhea in young children. *J. A. Diet. Assoc. 97(5):* 532. 1997.

PEEPLES, J.M., S.E. CARLSON, S.H. WERKMAN, R.J. COOKE Vitamin A status of preterm infants during infancy. *Am. J. Clin. Nutr. 53:* 1455. 1991.

PELTO, G.H. AND M.S. LUNG'AHO Weaning process. *World Health Oct.:* 5. 1984.

PENNELL, M.D., ET AL Infant fatness and feeding practices: a longitudinal assessment. *J. Am. Diet. Assoc. 79:* 531. 1981.

PERKIN, J.E. Maternal influences on development of food allergy in infant. *Topics in Clin. Nutr. 5(10):* 1. 1990.

PITTARD, W.B., III, K.M. GEDDES, T.C. HULSEY, AND B.W. HOLLIS How much vitamin D for neonates? *Am. J. Dis. Child.:* 1147. 1991.

POLLITT, E., J. HAAS, AND D.A. LEVITSKY International Conference on Iron Deficiency and Behavioral Development. *Am. J. Clin. Nutr. 50(Suppl.):* 565. 1989.

POSKITT, E. Infant feeding: a review. *Human Nutr.:* Apl. Nutr. 37C: 271. 1983.

ROLLAND-CACHERA, M.F., ET AL Adiposity rebound in children: a simple indicator for predicting obseity. *Am. J. Clin. Nutr. 39:* 129. 1984.

RYYAN, A.S., D. RUSH, F.W. KRIEGER, AND G.E. LEWANDOWSKI Recent declines in breast-feeding in the United States. 1984 through 1989. *Pediat. 88:* 719. 1991.

SAARININ, U.M., ET AL Iron absorption in infants: high bioavailability of breast milk iron as indicated by the extrinsic tag method of iron absorption and by the concentration of serum ferritin. *J. Pediat. 91:* 36. 1977.

SCHAEFFER, A. AND S. DITCHEK Current social practices leading to water intoxication in infants. *Am. J. Dis. Child. 145:* 27. 1991.

SCHAEFER, L.J. AND S.K. KUMANYIKA Maternal variable related to potentially high-sodium infant-feeding practices. *J. Am. Diet. Assoc. 85:* 433. 1985.

SERDULA, M.K., K.A. CAIRNS, D.F. WILLIAMSON, M. FULLER, AND J.F. BROWN Correlates of breast-feeding in a low-income population of whites, blacks, and Southeast Asians. *J. Am. Diet. Assoc. 91:* 41. 1991.

SKINNER, J.D., ET AL Longitudinal study of nutrient and food intakes of infants aged 2 to 24 months. *J. Am. Diet. Assoc. 97(5):* 496. 1997.

SMITH, C.A. Overuse of milk in the diets of infants and children. *J. Am. Med. Assoc. 172:* 567. 1960.

STIEHM, E. R. AND P. VINK Transmission of human immunodeficiency virus infection by breast-feeding. *J. Pediat. 118:* 410. 1991.

TAITZ, L.S. AND B.L. ARMITAGE Goat's milk for infants and children. *Br. Med. J. 288:* 428. 1984.

TATE, W.H., R. SNYDER, E.H. MONTGOMERY, J.T. CHAN Impact of source of drinking water on fluoride supplementation. *J. Pediat. 117:* 419. 1990.

THOMMENSSEN, M., G. RIIS, B.F. KASE, S. LARSEN, AND A. HEIBERG Energy and nutrient intakes of disabled children: Do feeding problems made a difference? *J. Am. Diet. Assoc. 91(12):* 1522. 1991.

VICTORIA, C.G., ET AL Is prolonged breast-feeding associated with malnutrition? *Am. J. Clin. Nutr. 39:* 307. 1984.

WEIL, W.B., JR. Current controversies in childhood obesity. *J. Pediat. 91:* 175. 1977.

YEUNG, D.L. Infant nutrition update. *J. Can. Diet. Assoc. 45:* 20. 1984.

ZACHMAN, R.D. Retinol (vitamin A) and the neonate: Special problems of human premature infant. *Am. J. Clin. Nutr. 50:* 413. 1990.

SECTION THREE

Emerging Individuals

CHAPTER SEVEN

Toddlers and Preschoolers

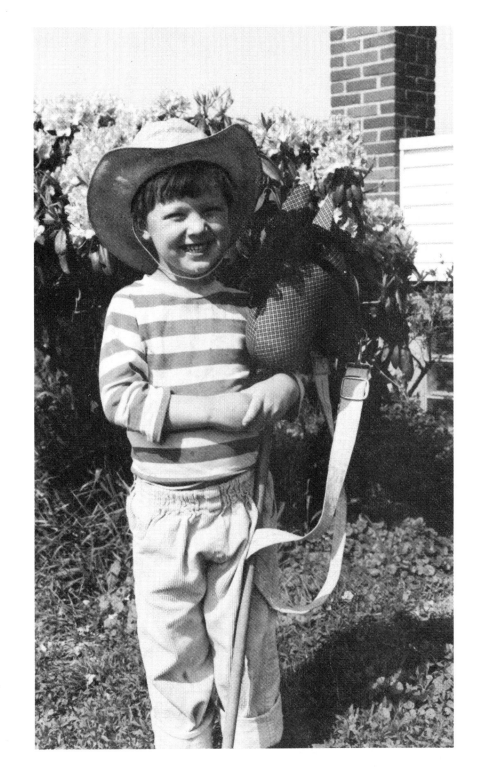

CHANGING EATING AND GROWING PATTERNS

Once babies celebrate their first birthday (or even a little earlier) changes begin to be evident. Ravenous is an apt word to describe babies' appetites much of the first year when growth is extremely rapid. After all, to grow enough in only twelve months to be half again as tall as at birth is a truly remarkable feat — yet that is just what happens from birth to the first birthday! Such tremendous growth requires plenty of raw materials — the nutrients. Appetite is the mechanism triggering babies to eat enough to accomplish this task.

TODDLERS

Period following infancy considered to be ages 1 to 3 in this discussion.

While they are eating so much, babies are also mastering physical skills to help them obtain their food with increasing ease. Formulas and bottles are replaced by milk from a cup. Self-feeding of some foods, or at least some disastrous attempts at self-feeding, become a part of the baby's mealtime experiences. Many babies start to join the family at the table when they are about one year old. Yes, change is the common denominator in feeding at this age.

Just when parents are beginning to think that there is no way to feed their babies enough to satisfy them, hearty appetites abruptly turn into small ones. Toddlers lose interest in eating

247

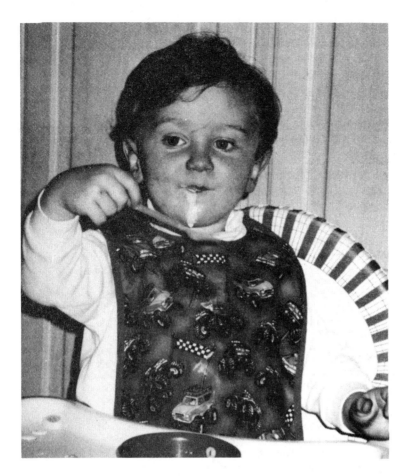

Self-feeding is a triumphant event for this 22-month-old boy and a bit of a challenge to his parents.

and may be quite selective about what they will eat. Such a change is quite understandable if it is viewed in relation to the growth pattern. Of course, growth continues during the second year, but it results in an increased height of only about 15 percent, a far cry from the 50 percent increase of the previous 12 months! With such a drastic reduction in growth, is it any wonder that babies, once eager for their food, are now easily distracted and eat only a small amount?

Although this drop in appetite and food intake is normal, parents may be concerned about this change. Parental worry over what a child is (or more accurately, is not) eating may cause considerable change in feeding dynamics. Some children quickly realize that they can manipulate parents with the food they ignore or choose to eat. Good nutrition continues to be an important part of life in this second year, but the reduced growth rate means that a drop in food consumption may spell trouble if parents coax or pressure their toddlers to eat. Worrying by parents can cause more problems than it solves.

NUTRITIONAL NEEDS OF TODDLERS AND PRESCHOOLERS

A reduced rate of growth and its accompanying reduction in appetite heightens the importance of wise food choices for these youngsters. Toddlers still need a well-balanced diet to supply the nutrients required for growth and maintenance; these nutrients have to be provided in a diet composed primarily of nutrient-dense foods because of the comparatively small volume that will probably be eaten. Although growth is not as dynamic between the ages of one and five, nutrient needs increase in quantity during this time, consistent with body size (Tables 7.1 and 7.2). Diet during these years is important to help instill sound dietary habits for a lifetime of healthful eating and to meet nutrient needs for growth and maintenance.

One of the big debates regarding nutritional needs for children between the ages of 2 and 5 has been the percentage of calories in the diet that should be derived from fat. Whereas there is consensus among nutrition researchers that fat intake should not be restricted prior to the age of 2, the merits of limiting fat intake after age 2 have been controversial. The numerous research studies springing from this question are beginning to point to possible benefits in limiting fat intake after age 2. Several agencies and organizations (including the American Academy of Pediatrics Committee on Nutrition, Healthy People 2000, American Heart Association Council on Cardiovascular Disease in the Young, the U.S. Departments of Agriculture and Health and Human Services, and the National Institutes of Health Consensus Development Panel 1985) now are recommending that total fat intake after age 2 and by age 5 should be limited to a maximum of 30% of the calories consumed and that saturated fat be less than 10% of total calories daily. These recommendations are based on anticipated health benefits and development of sound, healthy eating patterns for life.

Associated with concerns about fat intake is the question of total calories needed for optimal health. Evidence is accumulating that the energy needs of young children may not actually

DOUBLE LABELED WATER Technique for measuring energy expenditure by drinking water labeled with deuterium oxide and oxygen[18] and subsequently measuring levels of each in 2 urine samples (Hildreth and Johnson, 1995).

TABLE 7.1 RDA and AI for Children Ages 1–3 and 4–6[a,b]

Nutrient (daily amounts)	Ages 1–3	Ages 4–6[c]
Magnesium (mg)	**80**	**130**
Vitamin D[d] (μg)	5	5
Fluoride (mg)	0.7	1
Thiamin (mg)	**0.5**	**0.6**
Riboflavin (mg)	**0.5**	**0.6**
Niacin (mg equiv.)	**6**	**8**
Vitamin B_6 (mg)	**0.5**	**0.6**
Folate (μg)	**150**	**200**
Vitamin B_{12} (μg)	**0.9**	**1.2**
Calcium (mg)	500	800
Phosphorus (mg)	**460**	**500**
Pantothenic acid (mg)	2	3
Biotin (μg)	8	12
Choline (mg)	200	250

[a]Adapted from Food and Nutrition Board, Institute of Medicine — National Academy of Sciences Dietary Reference Intakes: Recommended Intakes for individuals. Washington, D.C. 2000.
[b]Adequate Intakes (AI). Bold values are RDA.
[c]Values in the table from which this is adapted cover ages 4–8.
[d]As cholecalciferol. 1 μg = 40 IU Vitamin D.

be as great as was accepted previously (Williams, et al, 1998). When Goran, et al (1995) measured total energy expenditure with doubly labeled water, total energy expenditure was found to be appreciably lower than had been estimated (up to 20% lower for infants to age 3 and 25% in children up to 10). Thus, present recommendations for calories may be too high for young children.

Milk continues to be an important source of calcium and phosphorus for bones and formation of teeth. The need for these minerals continues despite the normal slowing of growth at this time. Both growth and replacement demands mean that the calcium provided by milk, yogurt, and cheese is still necessary on a daily basis. Usually, children in the preschool years drink a little less milk than they did in infancy, but they need at least 1 pint each day; three glasses are preferable if they are active enough to drink this much milk and still eat the other foods recommended in the Food Guide Pyramid. Milk consumption

TABLE 7.2   Recommended Dietary Allowances for Children Ages 1–3 and 4–6[a,b]

Nutrient (daily amounts)	Ages 1–3	Ages 4–6
Protein (g)	16	24
Vitamin A (μg RE)[c]	400	500
Vitamin E (mg α-TE)[d]	6	7
Vitamin K (μg)	15	20
Vitamin C (mg)	15	25
Iron (mg)	10	10
Zinc (mg)	10	10
Iodine (μg)	70	90
Selenium (μg)	20	30

[a]Adapted from Food and Nutrition Board, Institute of Medicine — National Academy of Sciences, National Research Council Recommended Dietary Allowances, revised 1989 (abridged). Washington, D.C. 2000.
[b]Based on weight of 13 kg (29 lb) and 90 cm (35 in) for ages 1–3 and on weight of 20 kg (44 lb) and height of 112 cm (44 in) for ages 4–6.
[c]Retinol equivalents. 1 retinol equivalent = 1 μg retinol or 6 μg β-carotene.
[d]α-Tocopherol equivalents. 1 mg d-α-tocopherol = 1 α-TE.

should not take priority over other foods as long as children drink 1 pint each day.

Whole cow's milk can replace formula or human milk at about 12 months of age. Use of reduced fat or nonfat milks definitely is not recommended before at least 2 years of age or later. Toddlers continue to need the fatty acids and energy that are provided in whole milk. Unless a 2-year-old is definitely heavier than is appropriate for his height, whole milk continues to be a good choice throughout the preschool years. However, a shift to reduced fat (2%) milk is appropriate by the age of 5.

Meats and meat alternatives are sometimes difficult for toddlers to chew, and they may get so tired trying to chew a few bites that they lose interest and move on to other foods. This is a particular problem for children who are just beginning to eat from the family table. Eggs, fish, poultry, and cooked legumes provide alternatives that are usually easier to chew than red meats. Fish should be checked carefully to be sure there are no bones that might cause choking. Overcooking of eggs and fish should be avoided so that the protein will not toughen and make chewing difficult. Red meats can be fed when they are tender enough to be chewed easily.

As is true for older people, preschoolers need two servings of meat or meat alternatives daily, but the serving size is small — approximately 1 tablespoon for each year of life. By this standard, a one-year-old child will receive about 1 tablespoon meat, whereas a kindergartener will eat about 1/4 cup or slightly more. Eggs and cheese are especially useful during this period because they are fine sources of protein and are often accepted better than meats until chewing becomes easy for youngsters.

Five or more servings of fruits and vegetables are suggested. It is a good idea to have a good source of vitamin C daily and another rich in vitamin A. Serving sizes again are one tablespoonful per year. Some care is necessary in selecting fruits and vegetables to afford children good chewing experience without risk of choking. Carrot sticks can be a hazard when a child is a little over a year old, but can be chewed readily by the age of three. Almost any cooked fruits and vegetables can be managed by the time infants make the transition to the table around one year of age. As teeth erupt and children improve their

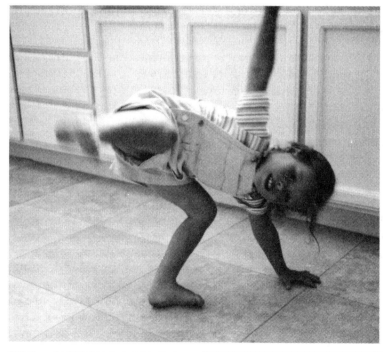

Plenty of exercise, whether indoors or out, helps to spur the appetite of this preschooler.

chewing skills, slightly crisp boiled vegetables and simmered fruits can be eaten easily. By the age of four, children should be able to eat any fruit or vegetable. A conscious effort should be made to increase the chewing challenge in this group between the ages of one and four. Habit can interfere with developing a wide array of fruits and vegetables. A familiar illustration is the parent who continues to peel apples for a four-year-old, not because the child cannot chew the skin, but because the peeling is done out of habit.

An effort should be made to expand the child's familiarity with a wide selection of fruits and vegetables during the preschool period to capitalize on the interest that children have in the world around them. If a variety of tastes, textures, and colors is part of the formative years, most children will develop a wide range of food preferences that will give them pleasure as they grow older. The textural qualities of different fruits and vegetables are experiences that youngsters enjoy. If they receive only soft foods for several years, they may be reluctant to accept coarser and tougher textures later. With a little effort, fruits and vegetables can be prepared in imaginative ways to make them an adventurous part of children's meals. Imagination in preparation is well rewarded.

The bread and cereal group is likely to occupy an excessive part of a toddler's diet. The tendency to serve too many cereals and breads is due to their convenience and ready acceptance by children. A cracker is a handy pacifier when a child is getting tired and it is not yet dinner time. Breads and dry, ready-to-eat cereals are finger foods many children love to hold in their hands and nibble. Whole-grain breads and cereals contribute excellent amounts of several vitamins and minerals and should be a part of the diet. The important point is to know just how much of the diet is breads and cereals.

How well does the Food Guide Pyramid provide a suitable guide for feeding a preschooler? First of all, a glass of milk (8 oz) contains approximately 9 g of protein, so a child drinking a total of 16 oz of milk receives 18 g of protein from the dairy group. Of course, this amount assumes that 16 oz of milk are consumed during the day, despite the fact that individual glasses of milk for preschoolers may contain 4 to 6 oz, making it necessary to serve milk perhaps four times a day to assure desired intake. If an egg is also a part of the day's food, another 6 g of protein will be provided. About 10 more grams of protein will probably be consumed as meat, for a total of about 35 g, and a child drinking three glasses of milk will receive about 42 g of protein daily. Because both these levels are above the 24 g of protein suggested for children ages 4 to 6 in the RDA, a protein deficiency for preschoolers in this country is not likely to occur.

Studies have shown that 1 pint of milk daily produces adequate growth in normal, healthy, preschool children who are eating a well-balanced diet. This is true despite the fact that calcium intake from 16 oz of milk is 576 mg, about 75 percent of the RDA for children in this group. However, some calcium is provided from other foods when a well-balanced diet is eaten. For preschoolers who are growing at a faster than average rate, as many as three glasses of milk (24 oz) may be preferable.

Iron requirements for preschoolers continue to test the mettle of nutritionists. The RDA for iron in children between the ages of one and six is 10 mg. This iron level is not provided in many preschoolers' diets, yet these children do not often show iron-deficiency symptoms. There are two plausible explanations for the failure to develop an iron deficiency on a seemingly inadequate diet. First, people who need iron usually absorb it more efficiently than those who have adequate iron in their bodies and diets. Second, many babies have excellent iron stores in their bodies by the time they are one year old because of the generous use of iron-fortified baby cereals during the second half of the first year. These stores can be drawn upon to maintain adequate hemoglobin levels for a time, even if iron-fortified cereals are eliminated from the diet. Thus, any iron-deficiency condition in these children would develop very slowly.

Although infant cereals are usually continued only to about one year, there are iron-fortified hot and cold cereals that are well suited to replace them in a preschooler's diet. Information regarding a cereal's iron content can be read on the label. One or more of these iron-rich cereals should be continued in the preschooler's diet. Some preschoolers may balk at eating a cereal that is "good for them." There is no reason to make an issue over this, for an iron supplement (ferrous sulfate, for example) can be a simple way to assure adequate iron intake.

Fluoride is an extremely important mineral in the preschool years because of its role in reducing the incidence of dental caries. Well-controlled studies, including the classic study conducted in Newburgh and Kingston, New York, have demonstrated that fluoridation of a city's water supply is an effective measure in protecting against caries if the fluoride is available from birth throughout the early years. Maximum protection of the permanent teeth is provided when fluoride is present in the diet at an optimal level no later than age two, continuing until the permanent teeth have erupted.

The most practical way to provide fluoride is to fluoridate a city's water supply (or use fluoridated water) so that the water children drink will contain neither too much nor too little fluoride. The level recommended for fluoridated water is 1 ppm (1 part fluoride per million parts water). This level has been proven effective in providing the desired protection against caries, and it is well below the level that can cause mottling of teeth. Mottling may occur when fluoride levels are very high for an extended period, but at levels below 2 ppm, mottling (fluorosis) does not occur. Fluorosis, the development of chalky and mottled teeth from excessive fluoride intake over an extended period, is only a possibility when fluoride levels are excessive during the time enamel is forming before a tooth erupts. Fluoride continues to be deposited as fluorapatite. The result is hard enamel (with large, well-shaped crystals) that makes the tooth

FLUOROSIS
Development of chalky, mottled teeth as a result of excessive intake of fluoride while enamel is forming.

FLUORAPATITE
Fluoride-containing crystals that result in acid-resistant tooth enamel, thus inhibiting formation of dental caries.

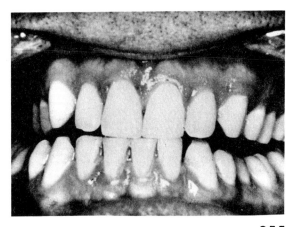

Fluoridated water during the early years is an aid in reducing the incidence of dental caries. This adult drank water with a fluoride content of 1 ppm in childhood. He has no decayed, missing, or filled teeth.

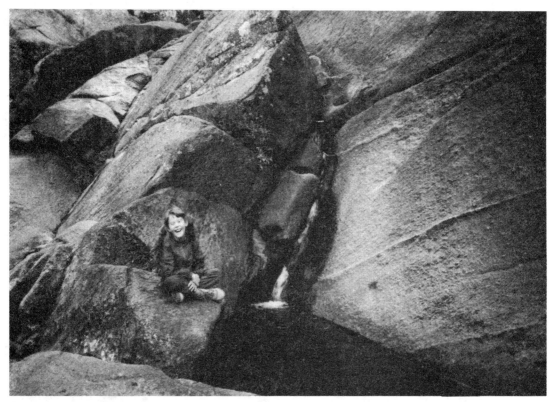
Even sparklingly clear mountain water supplies may lack the appropriate level of fluoride to protect developing teeth against caries.

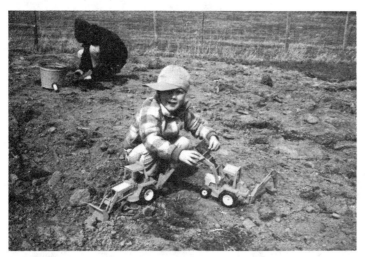
Construction projects help to sharpen appetites of these active preschoolers.

surface resistant to erosion by acid, thus protecting against dental caries.

Some communities have not yet elected to fluoridate their water supplies. While such communities are embroiled in discussions about whether or not fluoridation should be implemented in their city's water, children's teeth continue to form. For these children, alternative means of providing fluoride for optimal tooth health should be used. Topical applications of fluoride by dentists can be one approach. Other solutions are afforded by the use of fluoride toothpastes or fluoride drops and lozenges. For children under two years, 0.25 mg fluoride ion per day will provide suitable protection. At age 2 the level should be increased to 0.5 mg, and after age three, the level should be 1.0 mg per day. When a child is old enough to suck on a lozenge, this is the preferred way to administer fluoride; the lozenges bathe the teeth in fluoride and permit some of it to be absorbed into the system.

IMPROVING FOOD INTAKE

FOOD PREPARATION

It is not difficult to write a nutritionally-adequate plan for toddlers and preschoolers, but plan and actual intake may prove to be two different matters. Some of the factors that may determine what and how much a child eats deserve a close look. It may seem hard to realize, but a child is perfectly capable of deciding whether or not a food is good enough to eat. Therefore, food still need to be well prepared. There should be an attractive appearance, a tempting aroma, and an appealing flavor for a child's sensitive taste buds.

Toddlers are often quite experimental and interested in trying new foods. New flavors and textures may be greeted with approval. Parents can capitalize on this interest by expanding food experiences at the family table while children's minds are accepting and adventurous. Also, it is helpful to serve new foods more than once in the next couple of days to help toddlers become familiar with each food and to begin to add a variety of foods to broaden food acceptance during this formative period. Food preparation should focus on developing and maintaining color and beauty. Appearance can well be the key to getting a child to try a new food. Clearly, highly colorful foods have excellent visual appeal to children.

RESEARCH INSIGHTS

Bell, R.A., et al., Hispanic grandmothers preserve cultural traditions and reduce foodborne illness by conducting safe cheese workshops. *J. Am. Diet. Assoc. 99(9):* 1114. 1999.

This article is of interest in the context of this chapter because it emphasizes the importance of food safety, specifically in relation to the need for using pasteurized milk or assuring adequate heat treatment of foods being prepared with ingredients that are potentially unsafe. *Queso fresco,* a popular fresh, soft cheese particularly among the Hispanic population, commonly is made with raw milk. Serious bacterial infections sometimes have resulted from ingestion of live *Listeria* or *Salmonella* originating in the raw milk used to make *queso fresco.* A safe method for making this cheese which included adequate heating was developed and used for the research by Bell, et al.

Preparation of *queso fresco* can be incorporated into the curriculum of preschools and also elementary schools. The actual involvement of the children needs to be adapted to the specific school situation. Heating of the milk to a correct temperature and holding it there for the specified time allows children to learn about thermometers and timers or clocks. Use of vinegar to acidify the milk and promote curd formation affords a visual awareness of changes that occur in the milk because of acid. The most dramatic demonstration is afforded by squeezing the whey out of the curd, leaving the curd in the cheesecloth for the children to salt and squeeze again in the cheesecloth before sampling or refrigerating for snack time. The procedure is done as follows:

1. Place 1 tablet of rennet in cold water and set aside.
2. Heat together 2 quarts milk, 1 quart cultured buttermilk, and 7 teaspoons vinegar until the mixture reaches 90°F.
3. Remove from heat and stir in dissolved rennet.
4. Let stand 40 minutes before cutting into 1" cubes.
5. Place cheesecloth over large strainer before pouring the milk into the strainer and let it drain for 5 minutes before squeezing the curd tightly with the cheesecloth to squeeze out the whey.
6. Break up the curd and then salt it; let stand 5 minutes.
7. Twist the cheesecloth tightly again to eliminate as much whey as possible. Feed samples to the children. Be sure to keep any remaining cheese in the refrigerator until used.

The actual study reported by Bell, et al. involved training 15 female Hispanic volunteers to present a class (after they had been trained) to teach other Hispanic women how to make *queso fresco* using the procedure explained above. Evaluation of the project showed that 250 people had attended these workshops and that the number of cases of *S. typhimurium* (the food-borne bacterial contaminant in their local fresh cheese) dropped significantly. This was viewed as a very successful project that was well suited to the cultural needs of the area.

VEGETABLES   Problems of color and texture in poorly prepared vegetables can discourage children from even trying a bite. This is truly disheartening when you consider how naturally colorful vegetables are. When you also consider the fact that many of them have remarkable physical characteristics, you quickly see that vegetables could have tremendous appeal for children and adults alike. Nevertheless, talk about feeding toddlers and preschoolers often centers around problems in accepting vegetables.

Much of the lack of appeal in cooked vegetables is due to preparation techniques, and the most common offense is overcooking. When a dish of olive-drab, limp broccoli is brought to the table, visual appeal is poor. Add to that the strong, sulfur-like odor rising from the vegetable, and it is not surprising that preschoolers are assertive in their refusal to eat any of the vege-

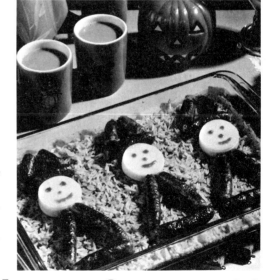

This Halloween main dish of rice, sausage links, and cheese rounds with faces creates a festive atmosphere, which helps encourage a child to get acquainted with new foods.

table. A sense of duty will not motivate a preschooler to eat poorly prepared vegetables. If an adult recognizes that this broccoli is not up to the desired standard of quality, the adult's negative feelings will be quickly mirrored by the youngster.

Overcooking not only harms color; it also has a negative impact on texture. Overcooked, mushy vegetables simply do not excite the palate with intriguing textures. Furthermore, aroma and flavor may be harmed by cooking vegetables too long. This is particularly true of those with cabbage-like flavors. Cabbage, Brussels sprouts, cauliflower, and broccoli gradually develop stronger flavors and odors with extended cooking. Although these vegetables are often well accepted by the preschool group when properly cooked, it is not unusual for enthusiasm to wane when they have been cooked too long. Their strong flavors and odors frequently repel, rather than attract.

The detrimental influence of strong odors on children's acceptance of vegetables is understandable. After all, youngsters' noses are usually so close to their plates that the aroma from a steaming vegetable engulfs them. Flavor expectations are quickly aroused — favorably or unfavorably — even before the food is tasted. The strong sulfur overtones of cabbage-like vegetables developed by prolonged cooking can be overpowering when the distance between the nose and the vegetable is only a few inches. Odor alone may be a sufficient reason for the child not to try the offending vegetable.

In contrast to strong-flavored vegetables, mild-flavored ones like carrots will be grudgingly accepted or ignored when overcooked, because their flavor becomes too weak. Mild flavor and aroma are gradually lost with extended cooking. Vegetables have the greatest textural appeal when they are cooked just until they can be easily cut. This degree of cooking makes bite-sized pieces of vegetables easy to pick up and eat as finger food, which adds to a child's interest in eating them.

A few cooking suggestions may be helpful in preparing vegetables that are enjoyed by the child and others in the family. Green vegetables retain their color best if they are cooked in an uncovered pan. By adding green vegetables when the water is already boiling, cooking time is kept as short as possible, an important aid in keeping the desired bright green color. Strong-flavored vegetables will have a milder, more pleasing flavor if they are cooked without a cover; this allows some of the strong, volatile flavoring compounds to escape while the vegetables are boiling. Conversely, mild flavors are optimized by cooking with a cover to keep the flavoring compounds inside the vegetable as much as possible.

Nutritive value is influenced a little by the techniques used in boiling vegetables. Some water-soluble vitamins will be lost in the cooking water, but the amount can be minimized by using just enough water to bubble up over the vegetable. However, additional water is needed for cooking strong-flavored vegetables to achieve as tempting a vegetable as possible. Even though the vitamin content may be reduced a little, the increased amount likely to be eaten will probably result in an excellent vitamin intake. If vegetables loaded with vitamins are unappealing, people will not be motivated to eat them.

Boiling is not the only way vegetables can be prepared. Steamed vegetables are very popular now. These retain their nutrients quite well and are often very appealing. Their disadvantage is that they require more time to become tender than boiled vegetables. Many homes have microwave ovens, and these can be used for cooking vegetables. Frozen vegetables are particularly appealing when cooked in a microwave oven. Color retention in fresh and frozen vegetables is excellent during microwave cookery; part of the reason for this is the comparatively short cooking time required. The texture of fresh vegetables prepared in a microwave oven is somewhat different, usually slightly tougher than boiled vegetables. Stir-frying is a technique particularly well suited to vegetable preparation. A very small amount of polyunsaturated vegetable oil can be used in a wok or a skillet to fry vegetables. Even though stir-fried vegetables are cut into thin pieces for stir-frying, nutrient retention is quite good as a result of the very short cooking time and the use of little or no water.

The preceding recommendations for vegetable cookery are designed to gain wide acceptance of vegetables. They are based on the premise that food left on the plate provides no nourishment for the child. In vegetable cookery, it is occasionally prudent to sacrifice a bit of the vitamin content to achieve greater palatability and acceptance.

By the time they are three years old, most children can chew quite well. This skill makes it possible to give raw vegetables to children, and not only carrot and celery sticks. Raw jicama, turnips, cauliflower, snap beans, peas, green peppers, and many other vegetables can be exciting discoveries to youngsters. To minimize the possibility of choking on these crisp, hard foods, children should sit while eating so they will not be distracted.

Another treat that may delight some preschoolers is a snack of a frozen vegetable just as it comes from the freezer. The cold ice crystals in frozen peas, beans, and other vegetables can make vegetables as exciting a snack as an ice cream cone!

FRUITS   Fruits require less comment and preparation, partially because children often consume fruits raw. Fresh fruits are generally a little softer than vegetables and are chewed more easily by young children. A possible exception to this is the skin of an apple, which can present a real chewing problem to a two-year-old. Occasionally, adults get in the habit of peeling apples for youngsters and then forget to break that habit as the children grow old enough to chew the peel. With the increased recognition of the importance of fiber in the diet, the roughage from apple peels and other edible fruit skins is clearly desirable when children are able to chew and swallow them safely.

MEAT   Preparation of meat for preschoolers requires some consideration in menu planning so that tender meats will ordinarily be fed. Chewing can be a real chore for toddlers. Pot roast and flank steak sound like chewy pieces of meat, but proper cooking can make them extremely tender. A long cooking time is needed to make these cuts tender enough for toddlers to chew easily. Otherwise, they may tire of chewing after a bite or two.

Meats have excellent flavor and maximum tenderness if they are cooked carefully at reasonably low temperatures. Unless they are ground, the less tender cuts of meats should be cooked for at least two hours in a covered pan with moisture added. The trapped steam slowly converts some of the tough connective tissue into gelatin, a change which obviously makes the meat very easy to chew. For variety, tomato juice, fruit juices, or even sour cream may be used as the liquid. These meats are done when they can be easily cut with a fork.

MILK   In most instances, milk is consumed as a beverage. However, there are several alternatives to fluid milk if a child happens to be in a period of saying "no" to drinking enough milk. Cream soups, usually popular with children, may be varied by using different vegetables to make a very appealing way of eating vegetables and milk. A considerable amount of milk is used in making baked custards, cornstarch puddings, and cream puddings (cornstarch puddings with egg yolks added). Cheese,

TABLE 7.3   Calcium Content and Caloric Contribution of Selected Foods[a]

Food	Measure	Calcium (mg)	Energy (kcal)
Milk, whole	1 c	288	160
Milk, low-fat (nonfat milk solids added)	1 c	352	145
Milk, nonfat	1 c	296	90
Milk, evaporated whole, undiluted	1/2 c	318	172
Milk, sweetened condensed, undiluted	1/2 c	401	460
Buttermilk	1 c	296	90
Cheese, cheddar	1 in^3	129	70
Cottage cheese, creamed	1/4 c	57	65
Cream cheese	1 in^3	10	60
Swiss cheese	1 in^3	139	55
Process cheese	1 in^3	122	65
Cocoa	1 c	295	245
Chocolate-flavored drink	1 c	270	190
Baked custard	1/2 c	149	153
Ice cream	1/4 c	49	64
Yogurt	1/2 c	147	63

[a]Adapted from *Nutritive Values of the Edible Part of Foods*, Home and Garden Bull. 72, USDA, Washington, D.C., Rev. 1971.

yogurt, and ice cream afford still other ways of augmenting milk intake. The calcium content of some milk and milk-based food is provided in Table 7.3.

MEALS FOR THE DAY

Regular meals scheduled at times when preschoolers are hungry can be a very sensible way of optimizing dietary patterns and maintaining good nutritional status. This schedule need not be completely rigid, but it should be maintained fairly well so that appetite will be good at meals.

Most families find it sensible to have a good breakfast in the morning. Preschool children usually have quite a long night's sleep and should be ravenous within half an hour of waking up. A hearty and appetizing breakfast should be served at that time. A typical menu might include: a glass of orange juice, a bowl of cereal, a soft-cooked egg, and a glass of milk. The size of the servings will vary with the size and age of the child, with orange juice probably ranging between 2 and 4 oz, cooked cereal between 1 and 4 tablespoons (or more if a ready-to-eat dry cereal), and milk from 6 to 8 oz.

If breakfast is eaten at 7:00 or 8:00 a.m., the preschooler will frequently be hungry and even tired and irritable between 9:30 and 10:30. When these signs appear, a snack is appropriate. This snack need not be large. A small glass of fruit juice or milk is suitable. Other good possibilities are fresh fruit or a slice of cheese. This mid-morning snack should be nourishing but small enough to leave the child hungry for lunch, which should be a well-balanced meal. If a child's appetite is poor at meals, snacks should be reduced or eliminated to improve eating at meals.

Usually, preschool children are hungry for a good lunch by noon, perhaps a grilled cheese sandwich, broccoli, apple wedges, and a glass of milk. If they are still hungry, a piece of sponge cake without icing may be added for dessert. This satisfying lunch sets the stage for a nap or rest time.

One of the happy traditions in some families is a light snack after the afternoon nap. This is a particularly nice time to have a little party with the toddler or preschooler. For most children, the afternoon snack should provide the lift needed to maintain a comfortable feeling until dinner, but should not interfere with the appetite for dinner. A suitable afternoon snack might be a small serving of gelatin with fruit in it.

With today's commuting families, the time for a very young child's dinner may fail to coincide with the parents' schedule. If a parent cannot be home at a time appropriate for the youngster's dinner, the preschooler may need to be fed before the family dinner, perhaps as early as 5:30. This should be a complete meal and might include meat loaf, baked potato, buttered carrots, sliced tomato, and a glass of milk. If the child is still hungry after eating small servings of all of these foods, a dessert (perhaps baked custard) may be served. Desserts are not necessary; if served, they should be either fresh fruit, a product high in milk, or perhaps a baked apple.

A suggested pattern for the preschooler is outlined below. It may need to be varied to fit the living pattern of the child and the family, but a day's total intake should approximate the total servings from the food groups suggested below.

Breakfast: 4 oz orange juice (or other good source of vitamin C)
Protein-rich food (1 egg or meat)
Cereal (whole grain or enriched) and 2 oz milk
Toast with a little margarine
6 oz milk

Snack: May be simply the toast from breakfast, if appetite at breakfast was not enough to finish the food on the suggested menu. If all of the breakfast was eaten, a few pieces of a raw vegetable and/or milk make a good mid-morning snack.

Lunch: Protein-rich food (poultry, meat, cheese, eggs, fish, or legumes may be used, often in a casserole made with large, identifiable pieces of foods)
Vegetable, either raw or cooked and selected to complement the main dish in color, flavor, and texture.
Fruit or a second vegetable
Bread, whole grain or enriched (unless an enriched pasta has been used in the main dish)
5 oz milk

Snack: Fruit
5 oz milk

Dinner: High protein food
Two vegetables or fruits (or one of each)
Bread with margarine
6 oz milk

In the above pattern, the meals suggested may be larger than some preschoolers wish to eat. However, the variety indicated is important to ensure that necessary nutrients are being consumed. Servings can be reduced in size for a child with a small appetite. Table 7.4 suggests typical serving sizes appropriate for toddlers and preschoolers. Note that a general rule of thumb of "one tablespoon per year of life" just about describes the amounts ordinarily consumed.

SNACKS

Both toddlers and preschoolers usually like and need a mid-morning and a mid-afternoon snack to help them last comfortably from one meal to the next. Snacks have a bad reputation in some parents' minds, but they can and should be part of a good nutrition plan for children in these early years. Their comparatively small capacities limit the amount toddlers and preschoolers can eat at a single time. Nourishing, well-timed snacks can be a good way to help youngsters be enthusiastic and hungry at meals.

The timing of snacks is important to the success of the total day's nutrition plan. If a snack is eaten at least two hours before the next meal is planned, appetites should be good at the meal. When eaten only an hour or less before the meal, a snack can have a damaging effect on appetite at the meal.

The choice of appropriate snack foods is often a concern to parents. Snack items are generally acceptable if they might be served as part of a meal's main course. For example, virtually any fruit or vegetable can make an interesting and pleasing snack. Sometimes a slice of cheese may be tempting. A glass of milk or juice can always be used as a snack. A "finger" sandwich of cheese spread on a quarter slice of toasted whole-wheat bread may fill the bill. In other words, snack foods should be of

TABLE 7.4   Suggested Serving Portions for Toddlers and Preschoolers

Type of Food	Suggested Portion for:					Number/day
	1 year	2 years	3 years	4 years	5 years	
Milk	4 oz	5 oz	6 oz	6 oz	6 oz	Total intake of 16–24 oz
Meats and alternatives	1 tbsp	2 tbsp	3 tbsp	4 tbsp	4 tbsp	2–3
Egg	1	1	1	1	1	0–1
Cooked legumes	1 tbsp	2 tbsp	3 tbsp	4 tbsp	4 tbsp	0–2
Fruits and vegetables						At least 5 total
Citrus juice/other vitamin C source	1/4 c	1/4 c	1/3 c	1/2 c	1/2 c	1
Dark green, leafy or yellow vegetable	1 tbsp	2 tbsp	3 tbsp	4 tbsp	5 tbsp	1
Other fruits and vegetables	1 tbsp	2 tbsp	3 tbsp	4 tbsp	5 tbsp	
Breads and cereals (enriched or whole grain)	1/4 sl	1/2 sl	1/2 sl	1/2 sl	1/2 sl	4 or more
Cooked cereal	1 tbsp	2 tbsp	3 tbsp	4 tbsp	4 tbsp	0–2
Ready-to-eat dry cereal	2 tbsp	1/4 c	1/3 c	1/2 c	1/2 c	0–2

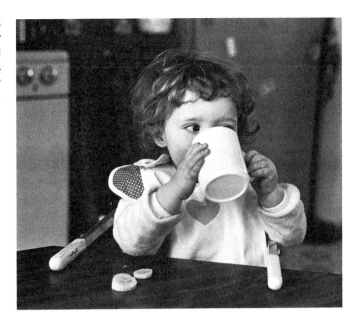

Success in self-feeding is aided by having a cup or glass which is easy to hold and difficult to tip over. This toddler confidently drinks by herself.

excellent nutrient density and not simply high-calorie treats that happen to be handy. Planned, nourishing snacks can be an effective way to introduce new foods and present familiar foods, too, while providing the nutrients needed each day.

PHYSICAL ARRANGEMENTS

Physical arrangements for feeding the preschool child should be carefully considered if the child is to establish good eating habits at this age. Usually, the preschooler will eat with the family each day. The sociability of family meals can be of great value to the developing child. To the rest of the family, however, the toddler or preschooler may be distracting unless physical arrangements have been worked out so that the youngster can sit comfortably with the group and eat easily.

There is nothing more annoying and chaotic than to have milk constantly spilled. One of the obvious ways of reducing this difficulty is to use a glass or cup that the child can manage easily. A small size and a weighted bottom are design features of considerable merit in solving the difficulty of "crying over spilt milk." Another practical fact of life is that the half glass of milk creates a smaller crisis than a full glass when it spills. Therefore, a pitcher at the table makes it easy to pour small amounts of milk at a time into the youngster's glass as refills are needed. A half-filled glass is easier for a young child to drink from than one that is filled to the top; the half-filled glass can be tipped to the lips with little or no spilling.

Table arrangements for young children should be simple and attractive, and chairs should be designed for comfort at the table. If adults had to eat a meal with their feet dangling in midair, they would soon realize the discomfort children feel when they are seated on chairs guaranteed to promote leg swinging. The preschooler's ideal chair meets two criteria: 1) it is the proper height for a preschooler to reach the table comfortably for eating unaided, and 2) it is equipped with a foot rest to hold the feet comfortably.

Silverware should be selected with the child's coordination and size in mind. Because a salad fork is smaller than a dinner fork, salad forks are often provided for preschoolers when they join the family table. Junior silverware sets are a comfortable size for preschoolers to use.

When children are eating at the family table, confusion and frustration at the beginning of the meal can be avoided by serving plates in the kitchen first. By doing this, there is little delay before they can start to eat. The distraction of passing serving dishes and the delay in getting some food may shift interest from eating to the general hubbub at the table.

MANNERS

Now that the physical arrangements at the table have been planned from the child's perspective, it is time to see how human interactions can influence nutrition. Clearly, the meal environment changes for the rest of the family when a toddler is present. Ideally, family meals are pleasant and comfortable social occasions with tempting, nourishing food. Unfortunately, this is not always true. In some families, the dining table might more accurately be described as the "dinning" table; parents may nag children about eating and manners, or arguments may be the featured conversation. Such situations are not conducive to good nutrition for anyone at the table, and they certainly fail to provide a good setting for helping youngsters develop optimal dietary habits.

When young children begin to eat at the family table, manners will not be perfect, but it is important that a child be accepted as just another family member and not be singled out for comments on what or how he/she is eating. Manners can be developed slowly. The first priority should be to set an example for eating and enjoying the various foods served at a meal and participating in the family fellowship. Refinements in manners can come as children's ability to feed themselves increases and as they become familiar with the family meal experience. Then they will not be quite as distracted as when they first joined the family table.

ENVIRONMENTAL INFLUENCES

Preschoolers are establishing food habits in these formative years that will be important influences on them throughout life. These habits are influenced in many ways, and parents are one of the most important influences. Whether they are conscious of it or not, parents influence their children's food patterns by their own attitudes toward food. When parents snack regularly, eat large amounts of sweets, or eat more than they need to maintain their weight, children are likely to mimic their parents and follow their lead.

The development of good nutrition for children begins with good nutrition for parents. First, food purchasing habits have a vital role in good nutrition. If high-calorie, low-nutrient foods are not purchased, the nutrient intake of both parents and children will probably be good. On the other hand, children quickly learn to clamor for sweets and desserts when they are available. In homes where parents obviously enjoy fruit or vegetable snacks, children are likely to want the same type of snack.

Television advertising is a familar part of many children's environment today. Young children watching television are subjected to numerous advertisements about food products directed specifically at them. This is particularly true on Saturday mornings, but it occurs throughout the week. These ads are directed solely at significantly influencing children's food choices, which is what the manufacturers are paying for when they purchase air time. Well before the age of four, children are influenced by food advertising on television. Parents are then faced with children appealing to them in the grocery store to buy the "rich," "sweet," or "chocolaty" cereal or other food item advertised on television. Who has not witnessed traumatic episodes in grocery stores in which parents and children argue about buying the advertised item?

Because children in their early years have a problem distinguishing fact from fancy, parents should have enough information and interest in nutrition to help children learn the truth about these compelling commercials and limit their exposure to them. Parents can help their children through this confusion by watching the ads themselves to know what their children are seeing. They can then discuss the nutrition available to them in related, but more nourishing foods. Samples of the nutritious food can be tasted right then, an advantage a television ad can never have. Another approach to countering negative nutrition messages on television is to limit television viewing by children, an act with consequences far beyond nutritional benefit to the child.

In addition to the influence of commercials, television has subtle effects on lifestyles. Adults often watch television while snacking. Children will observe this habit and quickly learn that they need to eat while watching television. In homes where television viewing is a favorite pastime, activity levels are likely to be low. Sedentary patterns enhance the likelihood of an imbalance between food intake and energy expenditure, thus promoting the possibility of gaining too much weight.

RESEARCH INSIGHTS

Van Itallie, T.B., Predicting obesity in children. Nutr. Reviews 56(5): 154. 1999.

Rolls, B.J., et al., Serving portion size influences 5-year-old but not 3-year-old children's food intakes. J. Am. Diet. Assoc. 100(2): 232. 2000.

Birch, L.L. and J.O. Fisher, Mothers' child-feeding practices influence daughters' eating and weight. Am. J. Clin. Nutr. 71: 1054. 2000.

The increasing problem of obesity in the United States presents challenges to health professionals to find the factors influencing this trend and define effective solutions for reversing it in individuals and society so that the negative health impact of overweight and obesity can be reduced. Various factors appear to be possible influences leading to overweight and obesity, but the extent of influence varies from person to person. Less than half of people who are overweight or obese in adulthood may have had this problem in childhood, although children with such weight problems in their teens have a greater risk for carrying this tendency to adulthood than do overweight 3-year-olds. If one or both parents are overweight or obese, the likelihood of this problem occurring in their children in adulthood is increased.

Various environmental factors may influence the incidence of overweight in children. Birch and Fisher (2000) explored the effects of mothers' child-feeding practices on their daughters' eating and overweight. These researchers measured 197 mothers for: relative weight, mothers' restrained eating behavior, perception of their daughters' risk of overweight, and restriction of daughters' eating. The 197 daughters (ages 4.6 to 6.4) were assessed for: relative weight, short-term control of energy intake in the absence of mothers' supervision, and 24-hour energy intake. Data analysis of the 156 mother-daughter pairs completing the study showed that the daughters ingested a large quantity of calories from free-access snack foods even though they had just eaten lunch and were not hungry. Mothers exercising higher degrees of restrained eating behavior were likely to place a higher degree of restriction on their daughters' intake. Girls having a high degree of maternal restriction on food intake were less able to regulate short-term intake than those girls having less restriction. These researchers found that maternal control of eating by daughters can increase risk of overweight in daughters. Possible reasons for the practice of controlling food intake of offspring include: strong parental concern about eating, perceptions that their children are at risk of eating or weight problems, and concern about maintaining an appropriate weight themselves.

Rolls, et al. (2000) examined the effect of portion size on food intake by 3- and 5-year-old children. Two classes of preschool children (16 in each class) were served portion-controlled lunches 3 times, with the portion of macaroni and cheese being varied (2/3 c, 1 1/6 c, and 1 2/3 c for the class of 3-year-old and 1 c, 1 1/2 c, and 2 c for the 5-year-old children). The amount eaten by the 3-year-old children was not influenced significantly by the portion size, but the amount eaten by the 5-year-old children increased as the portion size increased. A similar finding had been observed in adults previously. The possible implication of these findings is that large portions may be a contributing factor toward development of overweight and obesity, beginning near the age of 5 and continuing into adulthood.

The cultural food patterns of families will be strong influences in molding the food preferences and intake patterns of preschool children. When youngsters begin to join the family at the meal table, they usually will be served the foods that have been prepared for the rest of the family. As a result, food preferences of children from various cultural groups will often reflect the patterns typical of the group. For example, boiled rice will be a familiar food to many youngsters of Oriental heritage, whereas refried beans and rice would be found frequently in the preferences of many children with Hispanic heritage. Favorite foods often will be the familiar foods of early childhood. Even with the frequent moves of many families today, there still are many food ties with the heritage of the past.

PITFALLS IN FEEDING THE PRESCHOOLER

The importance of developing good dietary patterns in the preschool years is recognized by many parents, as well as by nutritionists and physicians. However, the day-to-day routine of child rearing masks subtle changes in feeding patterns. These subtle changes gradually become habits that may support good nutrition or hamper efforts to improve nutritional status. A look at some actual family situations and the resulting dietary patterns of the children will emphasize the need to review dining patterns periodically and to make conscious changes when warranted. The following case studies highlight some of the patterns and problems that have occurred in families.

EXCESSIVE INTAKE CASE STUDY

Beth is an alert child of 4 1/2 years. She weighs 42 lb and is 41 in tall. This places her in the 90th percentile for weight, but only in the 75th percentile for height. In other words, she is a bit heavier than is recommended for her height and age. Beth's father is a physician, and her mother is a teacher. Beth's care during the week is primarily the responsibility of a housekeeper.

A dietary record for a day showed the following food intake and nutrient consumption:

Breakfast: 3/4 c dry cereal with 1 tbsp sugar
             1/2 banana
             6 oz of milk

Morning snack:
             4 crackers
             1 orange

Lunch: 3/4 c spaghetti with tomato and meat sauce
             1 raw carrot
             1/2 c gelatin salad
             6 oz milk

Afternoon snack:
             2 oz cold roast beef

1 oz cheddar cheese
6 oz grape juice

Dinner: 3 oz meat loaf
1/4 c green beans
1/4 c green salad
1 1/2 tbsp blue cheese dressing
1/4 baked potato
1 tbsp butter
6 oz milk

Evening snack:
1/2 c vanilla ice cream

The nutrient contents of the above foods are listed in Table 7.5. A comparison of the nutrients provided by the foods with the recommended allowances for a child this age reveals that nutrient intake was more than adequate for all of the nutrients reported. Unfortunately, this is also true for the energy provided by the food. This pattern of frequent food intake and selection of items that are relatively high in fat and energy has been followed long enough to have already created a weight control problem for this young girl. Clearly, Beth and her parents now need to seek appropriate dietary modifications to alter this pattern of excessive consumption. Chapter 10 contains a discussion of weight control and various suggestions that could be given to Beth's parents to help control the situation.

VARIABLE APPETITE CASE STUDY

The typical preschool child will eat quite a large amount of food on some days, and on other days food intake will be surprisingly small in comparison with the average. An examination of the food eaten by Charlie during two consecutive days (Table 7.6) illustrates this point.

Charlie, a typical one-year-old, consumed the following foods on the first day:

Breakfast (9:00):1 tbsp applesauce
1 1/2 bananas
1/2 slice toast with jam
8 3/4 oz milk

Snack (10:15):   1 3/4 marshmallows

Snack (11:30):   8 3/4 oz milk

Snack (12:30):   1 3/4 doughnut

TABLE 7.5   Nutrient Content of Beth's Diet for a Day

Food	Cal	Protein (g)	Iron (mg)	Calcium (mg)	Vitamin A (IU)	Vitamin C (mg)
Wheaties (3/4 c)	82	2	1	0	0	0
Banana (1/2)	50	5	0.4	5	115	0
Milk, whole (6 oz)	120	6	—	216	258	Tr
Sugar (1 tbsp)	40	0	Tr	0	0	0
Crackers (4)	50	1	0.1	2	0	0
Orange (1)	65	1	0.5	54	260	66
Spaghetti, tomato, meat sauce (3/4 c)	195	9	2.4	39	500	24
Carrot (1)	20	1	0.4	18	5500	3
Orange gelatin (1/2 c)	70	2	—	0	0	0
Milk, whole (6 oz)	120	6	—	216	258	Tr
Roast beef (2 oz)	250	12	1.4	6	46	—
Cheese (1oz)	115	7	0.3	213	370	—
Grape juice (6 oz)	124	0	0.6	21	—	—
Meat Loaf (3 oz)	240	23	3.0	10	20	2
Green beans (1/4 c)	8	Tr	0.2	16	170	4
Blue cheese dressing (1.5 tbsp)	102	2	Tr	18	45	—
Baked potato (1/4)	75	5	0.7	2	—	0.5
Butter (1 tbsp)	100	Tr	0	3	470	0
Milk, whole (6 oz)	120	6	—	216	258	Tr
Ice cream (1/2 c)	95	2	Tr	73	220	1
Beth's Total	*2051*	*90*	*11.4*	*931*	*8734*	*105*
RDA	*1900*	*24*	*10*	*800*	*2500*	*45*

Lunch (1:30):   1 3/4 slice bread
                1 3/4 slice corned beef
                1 3/4 egg omelet
                1/4 cucumber

Snack (3:30):   8 3/4 oz milk

Snack (6:00):   8 3/4 oz milk
                1 3/4 banana

Dinner (6:30):   1 3/4 slice lamb roast
                   1/4 c potato salad
                   2 3/4 bananas

Snack (8:30):   8 3/4 oz milk
                   1 3/4 banana
                   1 3/4 cupcake

The following day Charlie's appetite was considerably smaller and his menu included:

Breakfast (9:30): 1/2 lamb patty
                   1 1/2 bananas
                   1/2 slice white enriched toast
                   6 3/4 oz milk

Lunch (12:30):   1 3/4 bananas
                   4 3/4 baby chicken sticks
                   4 3/4 oz apple juice

Snack (5:00):   3 3/4 marshmallows

Dinner (6:30):   1/2 c beef and egg noodle casserole
                   1/2 c banana pudding
                   4 3/4 oz milk

Of particular interest is a comparison of the caloric intake for the two days (Table 7.7) because it dramatically reflects the variation in a child's appetite at this age. The average caloric intake for the two days is higher than the recommendation. That Charlie is a little too heavy for his height (34 lb and 33 in) indicates that this average caloric excess is probably typical of his eating pattern. Charlie's nutritional status could be improved by increasing his physical activity, giving more careful attention to menu planning, and feeding him his dinner earlier. The use of cupcakes, marshmallows, and doughnuts should be curbed and a wider variety of fruits and vegetables introduced. It is not necessary, however, to try to get Charlie to eat the same amount of food each day, for this would focus too much attention on food and might cause Charlie to become a "problem eater."

A quick look at Charlie's menu also shows that children sometimes do go on food jags: bananas seem to play a significant role in Charlie's list of food likes at this time. Such food jags usually are short-lived and fade as quickly as they appear. To a point, it is all right to indulge these whims, but it is still important that a child eat a variety of foods each day to be well nourished. His low intake of iron should be corrected, preferably by adding an iron-fortified cereal.

TABLE 7.6   Nutrient Content of Charlie's Intake over a Two-Day Period

Food	Cal	Protein (g)	Calcium (mg)	Iron (mg)	Vit A (IU)	Thiamin (mg)	Riboflavin (mg)	Niacin (mg)	Vit C (mg)
First Day									
Apple sauce (2tbsp)	23	0.06	1.0	0.1	10	0.006	0.004	0.01	0.4
Bananas (5 1/2)	484	6.6	44.0	0.33	1265	0.22	0.25	0.385	55.0
Marshmallow (1)	22	0.2	0.0	0.0	0	0.0	0.0	0.0	0.0
Milk (40 oz)	830	42.5	1440.0	1.0	1950	0.45	2.1	1.5	15.0
Doughtnut (1)	136	2.1	23.0	0.2	40	0.05	0.4	0.4	0.0
Corned beef (1 slice)	37	3.4	8.0	0.4	Tr	0.007	0.045	0.7	0.0
Cucumber (1/40	12	0.8	10.0	0.4	0	0.04	0.04	0.2	8,0
Potato salad (1/4 c)	25	0.6	3.5	0.2	5	0.03	0.01	0.3	4.0
Lamb roast (1 slice)	115	10.0	0.5	1.3	0	0.06	0.11	2.2	0.0
Omelet (1 egg)	106	6.8	50.0	1.3	640	0.5	0.17	Tr	0.0
Cupcake (1)	161	2.6	58.0	0.2	50	0.01	0.04	0.1	0.0
Toast (1/2 slice)	31	1.0	9.0	0.2	0	0.02	0.02	0.25	0.0
Jam (1 tsp)	18	0.03	0.6	0.3	Tr	Tr	Tr	Tr	0.3
Bread (1 slice)	63	2.0	18.0	0.4	0	0.06	0.04	0.5	0.0
Total	*2063*	*76.69*	*1665.6*	*6.06*	*5055*	*1.003*	*2.869*	*6.045*	*82.7*
Second Day									
Lamb patty (1/2 med.)	178	10.0	5.0	1.15	0	0.07	0.08	2.3	0
Bananas (2 1/20)	220	3.0	10.0	2.2	575	0.07	0.17	4.0	0
Milk (10 oz)	208	10.5	360.0	0.3	488	0.10	0.52	0.4	4
Apple juice (4 oz)	62	0.1	8.0	0.6	45	0.025	0.035	Tr	1
Marshmallows (3)	65	0.06	0.0	0.0	0	0.0	0.0	0.0	0
Chicken sticks (4)	95	12.5	7.0	0.8	0	0.02	0.08	2.4	0
Pudding, banana (1/2 c)	141	6.1	141.0	0.6	420	0.06	0.25	0.1	0.5
Noodle casserole (1/2 c)	53	1.9	3.0	0.4	30	0.11	0.05	0.8	0
Toast (1/2 slice)	31	1.0	9.0	0.2	0	0.02	0.02	0.25	0
Total	*1053*	*32.16*	*543.0*	*6.25*	*983*	*0.475*	*1.205*	*10.25*	*5.5*

TABLE 7.7

TABLE 7.7 Comparison of Charlie's Intake with the Allowances Recommended for the One-Year-Old Child[a]

Intake	First Day	Second Day	Recommended Allowances
Calories	2063	1053	1300
Protein (g)	76.69	32.16	16
Calcium (mg)	1665.6	543.0	800
Iron (mg)	6.06	6.25	10
Vitamin A (IU)	5055	983	2000
Thiamin (mg)	1.003	0.475	0.7
Riboflavin (mg)	2.869	1.205	0.8
Niacin (mg equiv)	6.045	10.25	9
Vitamin C (mg)	82.7	5.5	40

[a]Adapted from Food and Nutrition Board, Institute of Medicine — National Academy of Sciences, National Research Council Recommended Dietary Allowances, revised 1989 (abridged). Washington, D.C. 1998; Food and Nutrition Board, Institute of Medicine — National Academy of Sciences, Dietary Reference Intakes: Recommended for Individuals. 1998. Washington, D.C.

INDULGENCE IN SNACKS CASE STUDY

Examination of several days' menus in the life of Karen, a two-year-old child, quickly reveals some of the problems that are common at this age when snacks are large and mealtimes erratic. In this particular example the problem was compounded because Karen was visiting relatives on one of the days, but the pattern tended to persist at home also.

Karen's menu the first day was as follows:

Snack (8:30):   6 potato chips
                  2 candy cigarettes (given to her by her aunt)

Breakfast (9:30): 1 egg and cheese omelet
                  1 piece of cheese
                  1/4 piece toast (white enriched bread) with jam
                       and peanut butter
                  4 oz milk

Snack (12:00):   5 marshmallows

Lunch (1:30):   2 all-beef frankfurters
                  2 baby all-meat franks (taken from brother)
                  1/2 dill pickle

| Snack (4:00): | 4 marshmallows |
| | 4 oz apple juice |

Dinner (6:30):   1/2 lamb taco
                    1/2 cheese enchilada
                    2 tbsp green salad
                    2 scoops vanilla ice cream

Snack (8:45):   3 marshmallows
                    2 oz milk

The menu for the second day, which was spent at home, again indicates Karen's tendency to consume excessively large quantities of food low in nutrients and high in calories.

The day's menu included:

Breakfast (9:00):1/2 sliced banana
                    1/2 slice toast with jam
                    4 oz milk

Snack (10:15):   4 marshmallows

Snack (12:30):   1 doughnut

Lunch (1:30):   1 slice corned beef
                    1/2 slice enriched white bread
                    1 egg omelet
                    1 dill pickle
                    1/4 cucumber
                    4 oz milk
                    2 pieces candy

Snack (3:30):   1 small piece celery

Snack (4:00):   2 pieces candy

Dinner (5:30):   1/4 c potato salad
                    2 small slices lamb roast
                    1/2 tomato
                    2 oz milk
                    1 scoop vanilla ice cream

Snack (8:30):   2 cupcakes

Tables 7.8 and 7.9 summarize the nutrients included in Karen's two-day diet. Karen is consuming more calories than she actually needs, yet she is not consistently meeting the recommended allowances for her age group. To overcome possible shortages of nutrients, she should eat more fruits and vegetables. Attention should be given to including a food high in ascorbic acid each day and an adequate source of iron. To promote good

TABLE 7.8

TABLE 7.8   Nutrient Content of Karen's Intake over a Two-Day Period

Food	Cal	Protein (g)	Calcium (mg)	Iron (mg)	Vit A (IU)	Thiamin (mg)	Riboflavin (mg)	Niacin (mg)	Vit C (mg)
First Day									
Potato chips (6 large)	100	1.0	5.0	0.3	9	0.03	0.02	0.5	2
Candy cigarettes (2)	31	0.4	13	0.25	9	0.0075	0.025	0.05	0
Toast (1/4 piece)	16	0.5	5.0	0.1	0	0.01	0.01	0.1	0
Jam (1 tsp)	18	0.0	0.6	0.03	Tr	Tr	Tr	Tr	0
Peanut butter (1 tsp)	30	1.4	4.0	0.1	0	0.007	0.007	0.9	0
Omelet, cheese (1 egg)	106	6.8	50.0	1.3	640	0.05	0.17	Tr	0
Milk (6 oz)	126	7.5	216.0	0.2	276	0.07	0.30	0.2	2
Cheese (1" cube)	105	6.6	191.0	0.3	370	Tr	0.12	Tr	0
Apple juice (4 oz)	62	0.1	8.0	0.6	0.025	0.035	Tr	0.0	1
Marshmallows (12)	264	2.0	0.0	0.0	0	0	0.0	0.0	0
Frankfurters (2)	248	14.0	6.0	0.12	0	0.16	0.18	2.6	0
Tomato (1/4)	8	0.4	4.0	0.2	416	0.02	0.015	0.2	8
Baby all-meat franks (2)	62	5.5	2.0	0.3	0	0.04	0.045	0.6	0
Pickle (1/2 large)	8	0.5	17.0	0.8	210	Tr	0.045	0.05	4
Enchilada, cheese (1/2)	267	16.5	236.0	1.7	7	0.085	0.25	2.7	6
Taco, lamb (1/2)	30	1.0	10.0	0.3	Tr	0.3	0.025	3.0	Tr
Lettuce salad (2 tbsp)	2	0.1	1.3	0.025	34	0.0025	0.005	0.05	0.5
Ice cream (2 scoops)	129	2.5	76.0	0.1	320	0.03	0.12	0.1	1
Total	1612	64.9	844.9	6.725	2336	0.7970	1.372	11.05	24.5

Food	Cal	Protein (g)	Calcium (mg)	Iron (mg)	Vit A (IU)	Thiamin (mg)	Riboflavin (mg)	Niacin (mg)	Vit C (mg)
Second Day									
Banana (1/4 piece)	22	0.3	2.0	0.15	107	0.01	0.01	0.2	3
Jam (1 tsp)	18	0.03	0.6	0.03	Tr	Tr	Tr	Tr	0.3
Toast (1/2 slice)	31	1.0	9.0	0.2	0	0.02	0.02	0.25	0
Ice cream (1 scoop)	64	1.25	38.0	0.05	160	0.015	0.06	0.05	0.5
Milk (10 oz)	208	10.5	360.0	0.3	488	0.10	0.52	0.4	4
Lamb roast (2 slices)	130	20.0	0.9	2.6	0	0.12	0.4	4.4	0
Doughnut (1 plain)	136	2.1	23.0	0.2	40	0.05	0.04	0.4	0
Tomato (1/2 med)	16	0.7	8.0	0.5	820	0.04	0.025	0.4	17
Pickle (1 large)	15	0.9	34.0	1.6	420	Tr	0.09	0.1	8
Egg omelet (1 egg)	106	6.8	50.0	1.3	640	0.05	0.17	Tr	0
Bread (1/2 slice)	31	1.0	9.0	0.2	0	0.02	0.02	0.25	0
Corned beef (1 slice)	37	3.4	8.0	0.4	Tr	0.007	0.045	0.7	0
Cucumber (1/4)	12	0.8	10.0	0.4	0	0.04	0.04	0.2	8
Cupcakes (2 iced)	262	5.2	124.0	0.4	100	0.02	0.06	0.2	0
Chocolate creams (4 pieces)	220	2.2	—	—	—	—	—	—	—
Marshmallows (4)	88	0.8	0.0	0	0	0	0	0	0
Celery (1 small piece)	3	0.2	8.0	0.06	0	0.01	0.006	0.06	1
Potato salad (1/4 c)	25	0.6	3.5	0.2	5	0.03	0.01	0.3	4
Total	*1424*	*57.78*	*688.0*	*8.59*	*2780*	*0.532*	*1.516*	*7.91*	*45.8*

TABLE 7.9   Comparison of Karen's Intake with the Allowances Recommended[a]

Intake	First Day	Second Day	Recommended Allowances
Calories	1612	1424	1300
Protein (g)	64.9	57.8	16
Calcium (mg)	844.9	688	500
Iron (mg)	6.7	8.6	10
Vitamin A (µg RE)	390	463	400
Thiamin (mg)	0.797	0.532	0.5
Riboflavin (mg)	1.372	1.516	0.5
Niacin (mg equiv)	11.05	7.91	6
Vitamin C (mg)	24.5	45.8	40

[a]Adapted from Food and Nutrition Board, Institute of Medicine — National Academy of Sciences, National Research Council Recommended Dietary Allowances, revised 1989 (abridged). Washington, D.C. 1998; Food and Nutrition Board, Institute of Medicine — National Academy of Sciences, Dietary Reference Intakes: Recommended for Individuals. 1998. Washington, D.C.

dental health and to avoid excessive weight gain, it would be wise to reduce markedly the amounts of candy in Karen's diet and increase the consumption of milk, fruits, and vegetables. The dietary patterns Karen is establishing as a pre-schooler are likely to persist unless she is helped to change them during this formative period.

Another area of concern when dietary patterns like Karen's develop is that there is an increased likelihood of developing dental caries. Carbohydrates, particularly sucrose, promote the formation of dental plaque by serving as food for *Streptococcus mitis*. These microorganisms convert dietary carbohydrates into glycogen-like polysaccharides that constitute a part of the plaque forming in the crevices along the gum line. Carbohydrate-containing foods that tend to stick to the teeth for a period of time present the greatest problem because of the length of time that they are present in the mouth. Caramels and other sticky candies are particularly noteworthy for their ability to adhere to the teeth.

The carious lesion in a tooth begins with decalcification of a small area of the enamel. This break permits the invasion of the tooth by *S. mitis*. Cavitation continues by this microorganism. The original decalcification is promoted by the presence of organic acids that are produced from sugars by bacteria. Dietary sugars are able to adhere to the plaque formed on the teeth so that the acids can be formed and then come in contact with the actual enamel of the tooth.

The protection of deciduous teeth against dental caries is important so that these teeth will remain in position and allow for normal development of permanent teeth. Young children are notably inept in doing a thorough job of brushing their teeth. Consequently, even this hygienic measure is not very effective in helping to remove food residues that would tend to contribute to formation of plaque and dental caries.

An important and effective means of helping to control dental caries in young children is through good dietary management. This means that fluoridated water should be used if at all possible, but it also means avoiding the use of sugar-containing snacks or prolonged use of bottle feedings in bed, a practice that bathes the teeth in sugar if the child falls asleep with the bottle still in the mouth. The intake of sucrose and other sugars should be infrequent and only in small quantities. Foods to limit include honey, raw sugar, sugar-coated cereals, and sugar-containing beverages such as soda pops and ades.

Sorbitol (a sugar alcohol used as a sweetener) is used in place of sucrose in the the coating mixture on some chewing gums, breath mints, and dietetic candies. Children do not have a nutritional need for any of these products, but sorbitol as a sugar replacement at least avoids the caries-promoting character of sucrose-containing products. People do not absorb sorbitol well, which means that consumption of it can lead to some intestinal discomfort from gas and diarrhea. For this reason, children who exhibit these symptoms after chewing sorbitol-coated gum or ingesting sorbitol from other sources, should have their intake of sorbitol reduced. Starch has been shown to be less caries-inducing in its action than sugars, but brushing teeth after eating is still an important protective measure. A classic study of the caries-inducing effect of various dietary regimens is the Vipeholm study, 1954, conducted in Sweden.

SORBITOL
Sugar alcohol sometimes used to sweeten chewing gum and other products; sucrose replacer that does not promote dental caries.

TOO MUCH MILK CASE STUDY

Suzie's eating haits are generally poor, but the most outstanding problem is that of unusually high milk consumption. Her meals are irregular in quantity and timing. Also, she frequently receives a bottle rather than a solid meal although she is 15 months old. Some of the causes of her poor eating habits are:

1. Because she is the youngest of six children, her mother is busy; it is quick and easy to give her a bottle.

2. Suzie is slow at teething and at present has only four teeth.

3. Suzie is at the point where she wants to try to feed herself. Her mother feels this is too time-consuming and messy. As a result, Suzie receives a scanty meal and a bottle.

4. Suzie's father is always concerned that she will choke on solid food. This is a major reason she did not begin solid foods at an earlier age to replace the bottle.

The examination of the menus for Suzie will quickly show the problems involved with excessive milk consumption.

Her menu for the first day included:

6:00 a.m.	2 oz milk in bottle
7:30	1 tsp tuna
8:00	1 soft-cooked egg 1/2 slice bread
10:30	4 oz milk in bottle
1:00 p.m.	8 oz milk in bottle 2 large jelly beans
4:30	2 tbsp chopped liver 5 oz milk 3 tbsp peas 1 diced apple 1 scoop ice cream
6:00	6 oz milk in bottle
7:30	8 oz milk in bottle
2:00 a.m.	8 oz milk in bottle

The menu for the following day was:

6:00 a.m.	3 oz milk in bottle

8:00	1 scrambled egg
	6 tbsp farina
	2 oz milk
9:30	4 oz milk in bottle
11:30	1/2 peanut butter and jelly sandwich
	2 oz milk
12:00 p.m.	8 oz milk in bottle
4:30	1 small bowl tomato soup
	1/2 peanut butter and jelly sandwich
	4 oz milk in bottle
7:00	1 scoop ice cream
	8 oz milk in bottle
12:00 a.m.	8 oz milk in bottle

The accompanying tables (Table 7.10 and 7.11) illustrate the problems present when milk occupies such a prominent place in the diet. Notice the low values for ascorbic acid and niacin intake. Notice also that, without farina in the diet, iron intake would be extremely inadequate. Niacin intake could be enhanced significantly, along with the iron, by increasing the use of meats and fortified cereals.

It is apparent that Suzie's diet is decidedly inadequate, but these simple suggestions for dietary modifications will not be sufficient to correct the problem. Before she can be helped, it is necessary to explain Suzie's nutritional needs to both her father and her mother in a clear and meaningful way. Her father will need to understand the importance of more solid foods to provide necessary iron and vitamins. It will also be necessary to allay his fear of Suzie choking because his anxiety will communicate itself to Suzie and make it difficult for her to adjust to a variety of solid foods. This adjustment in attitude may require some time and considerable patience.

Suzie's mother apparently does not realize that her child is not receiving an adequate diet. The importance of meat, fruits, vegetables, and cereals in the preschooler's diet should be pointed out to her. It also may be helpful for her to work out a schedule that encourages Suzie toward three meals and two snacks a day. Certainly it should be possible to eliminate the night feeding by changing the evening meal to 5:30 and offering a greater quantity of solid foods at that time. Suzie is old enough to be drinking from a cup. This transition should be accomplished as soon as possible. It is likely that the bottle is still being

TABLE 7.10 Nutrient Content of Suzie's Intake over a Two-Day Period

Food	Cal	Protein (g)	Calcium (mg)	Iron (mg)	Vit A (IU)	Thiamin (mg)	Riboflavin (mg)	Niacin (mg)	Vit C (mg)
First Day									
Milk (41 oz)	841	43.6	1476	0.5	1850	0.42	2.15	0.05	10.5
Tuna (1 tsp)	19	2.0	1	0.14	8	—	0.01	1.28	—
Egg, soft cooked (1)	77	6.1	26	1.3	550	0.05	0.14	Tr	—
Bread, enriched (1/2 slice)	31	1.0	9	0.2	—	0.03	0.02	0.02	2.0
Liver, chopped (2 tbsp)	17	1.7	1	0.6	3731	0.02	0.26	1.0	2.0
Peas (3 tbsp)	28	2.0	9	0.8	267	0.1	0.05	1.0	2.0
Apple, diced (1 tbsp)	7	—	0.04	11	Tr	Tr	0.02	0.13	4.6
Ice cream (1 scoop)	207	4.0	123	0.1	520	0.04	0.19	0.1	1.0
Jelly beans (2 large)	36	2.0	—	—	—	—	—	—	—
Total	*1263*	*633*	*1645*	*3.68*	*6937*	*0.57*	*2.82*	*3.92*	*20.1*
Second Day									
Milk (50 oz)	1000	56.0	1700	0.6	2290	0.50	2.57	0.6	12.5
Egg, scrambled (1)	110	7.0	51	1.1	690	0.05	0.18	Tr	—
Farina (6 tbsp)	50	1.7	71	6.0	—	0.07	0.01	0.2	—
Peanut butter and jelly sandwich (1)	243	8.2	49	1.1	Tr	0.14	0.10	3.6	—
Tomato soup (1/2 c)	45	1.1	12	0.5	615	0.01	0.50	0.3	5.0
Ice cream (1 scoop)	207	4.0	123	0.1	520	0.04	0.19	0.1	1.0
Total	*1655*	*78.0*	*2006*	*9.4*	*4115*	*0.81*	*3.55*	*4.8*	*18.5*

TABLE 7.11   Comparison of Suzie's Intake for Two Days with the Allowances Recommended[a]

Intake	First Day	Second Day	Recommended Allowances
Calories	1263	1655	1300
Protein (g)	63.3	78.0	16
Calcium (mg)	1645	2006	500
Iron (mg)	3.68	9.4	10
Vitamin A (µg RE)	6937	4115	400
Thiamin (mg)	0.66	0.81	0.5
Riboflavin (mg)	2.82	3.55	0.5
Niacin (mg equiv)	3.92	4.8	6
Vitamin C (mg)	20.1	18.5	40

[a]Adapted from Food and Nutrition Board, Institute of Medicine — National Academy of Sciences, National Research Council Recommended Dietary Allowances, revised 1989 (abridged). Washington, D.C. 1998; Food and Nutrition Board, Institute of Medicine — National Academy of Sciences, Dietary Reference Intakes: Recommended for Individuals. 2000. Washington, D.C.

used simply because Suzie's mother has not taken the time to wean Suzie to the cup. If Suzie seems to gain comfort from the bottle, some warm attention from her mother should facilitate the weaning.

PROBLEMS OF INTERACTION BETWEEN MOTHER AND CHILD CASE STUDY

The case of Gary is not a normal situation, but it does point out how complications may arise as a result of antagonism between mother and child. Gary is a four-year-old boy (height of 44 in and weight of 40 lb) whose parents expect a great deal of him. Throughout his lifetime there has been frequent occurence of forced feeding at mealtime. Feelings during meals have thus grown progressively stronger and more antagonistic between mother and son. The problem has deepened until, at the age of four, the boy is suffering from mild anemia and general lack of calories. Obviously, something needs to be done to correct this situation immediately.

The food ingested during one week is as follows:

Monday Breakfast: 1 scrambled egg
1 c milk

Lunch: 1 c chicken noodle soup
4 crackers

Dinner: 4 crackers
1 tbsp pork
2 tbsp broccoli
1 c milk

Tuesday Breakfast: 1 scrambled egg
1 c milk

Lunch: 1 c chicken gumbo soup
4 crackers

Dinner: 2 crackers
1 tbsp fried pork
2 tbsp broccoli
1 c milk

Wednesday Breakfast: 1 scrambled egg
1 c milk

Lunch: 1 c chicken gumbo soup
4 crackers

Dinner: 2 crackers
1 tbsp beef
2 tbsp cauliflower
1 c milk

Thursday Breakfast: 1 scrambled egg
1 c milk

Lunch: 1 c chicken gumbo soup
4 crackers

Dinner: 2 crackers
1 tbsp beef
2 tbsp broccoli
1 c milk

Friday Breakfast: 1 scrambled egg
1 c milk

Lunch: 1 c chicken gumbo soup
4 crackers

	Dinner:	2 crackers
		1 tbsp chicken
		2 tbsp broccoli
		1 c milk
Saturday	Breakfast:	1 scrambled egg
		1 c milk
	Lunch:	1 c chicken gumbo soup
		4 crackers
	Dinner:	2 crackers
		1 tbsp beef
		2 tbsp spinach
		1 c milk
Sunday	Breakfast:	1 scrambled egg
		1 c milk
	Lunch:	1 sliced chicken sandwich
		2 tbsp potato salad
		1 orange
		1/2 c ice cream
	Dinner:	2 tbsp rice
		2 tbsp turkey
		2 tbsp green peas
		1 piece apple pie
		1 c milk

Two observations can be made by examining the menus and information in Table 7.12. First, the menus throughout the week, with the exception of the last day, are extremely repetitious and monotonous for the child. This may be interpreted as a lack of interest on the part of his mother. The next point of interest is the food consumed at lunch and dinner on Sunday. Why is the food intake suddenly so much greater and more varied on that day? The answer is that Gary had gone to a friend's house after breakfast and had spent the rest of the day there.

The correction of the problems that exist in this family is not an easy matter. The attitude and habits of mother and son have been built up over a period of time and therefore will probably require a long time to correct. Since the boy did eat a reasonable amount of food when he was visiting others, it appears that food intake indicates a problem between him and his mother and is not an actual physical problem.

The most obvious changes to be made are an increase in the size of servings and greater variety in the menu. Gary needs

TABLE 7.12   Comparison of Gary's Intake for Seven Days with the Allowances Recommended[a]

Intake	1st	2nd	3rd	4th	5th	6th	7th	RDA
Calories	615	593	592	721	607	595	1322	1800
Protein (g)	37.3	38.3	36.5	38.5	36.4	37.3	69.5	24
Calcium (mg)	979	901	1139	952	999	1229	2526	800
Iron (mg)	4.9	4.57	5.67	6.27	4.94	6.26	7.36	10
Vitamin A (µg RE)	509	380	379	519	414	676	395	500
Thiamin (mg)	0.59	0.30	0.35	0.36	0.56	0.40	0.66	0.6
Riboflavin (mg)	1.73	1.11	1.19	1.25	1.61	1.26	2.38	0.6
Niacin (mg equiv)	4.97	4.74	4.67	4.55	5.14	4.46	8.67	8
Vitamin C (mg)	42	31	18	42	28	16	107	45
Vitamin D (IU)	200	200	200	200	200	200	200	500

[a]Adapted from Food and Nutrition Board, Institute of Medicine — National Academy of Sciences, National Research Council Recommended Dietary Allowances, revised 1989 (abridged). Washington, D.C. 1998; Food and Nutrition Board, Institute of Medicine — National Academy of Sciences, Dietary Reference Intakes: Recommended for Individuals. 2000. Washington, D.C.

to have many different foods included in his diet at this age. He particularly needs to be consuming a broader range of meats and other foods; his menu should be expanded to include a wider variety of fruits and vegetables. Fruits have been totally lacking in his diet at home. He should also receive various enriched cereal products rather than have his experience limited to crackers.

Such a problem is most readily remedied when an outsider helps to correct the situation. At the age of four, it might be possible for Gary to attend a nursery school where he would gradually learn to enjoy food by watching the example of the other children. The greater variety of food served at the school would also help to broaden his range of food preferences.

Nursery school personnel would help Gary's mother, too. She would be able to discuss her problem with the nursery school teacher and gain her counsel in coping with the problem. Nursery school can provide a valuable change in environment and routine from the situation that enabled this problem to develop in the first place.

If it is not possible to enroll Gary in a nursery school, perhaps Gary's mother could consult a dietitian or county nutritionist. In order to solve Gary's nutritional difficulties, it is necessary to help his mother understand the nutritional needs of her four-year-old and interpret these needs in practical terms. She may desire and need help with such facets of the total problem as: planning nutritious meals with child appeal; preparation techniques to make food more tempting; and understanding the abilitites and emotional needs of her child. Gary's situation can be corrected, but it will require considerable patience and time because the underlying attitudes have been developing over a period of many months.

SUMMARY

The preschool child will undergo periods of varying appetites; these changes in appetite should not cause concern because they are usually short-lived. The important thing to remember when feeding the preschool child is that this is a period when dietary habits are being firmly established. Efforts should be made to offer preschoolers a wide range of foods to broaden their experiences. The mealtime setting should be geared toward the comfort of the child.

Wise parents will periodically take time to analyze what their children are eating so that they can correct nutritional deficiencies that may occur. Such a check can be made by comparing the diet plan for the preschooler with the Food Guide Pyramid. If shortages appear to exist, an immediate effort should be made to correct the situation.

Frequently the parents themselves will be able to correct feeding problems that may exist for their children. Sometimes, however, outside help may prove to be the most suitable method for correcting existing conditions within the family.

BIBLIOGRAPHY

AST, D.B., ET AL Newburgh-Kingston caries — fluorine study. XIV: Combined clinical and roentgenographic dental findings after ten years of fluoride experiments. *J. Am. Dent. Assoc. 52:* 314. 1956.

BIRCH, L.L. Children's food acceptance patterns. *Nutr. Today 31(6):* 234. 1996.

BLAYNEY, J.R. Report of thirteen years of water fluoridation in Evanston, Illinois. *J. Am. Dent. Assoc. 61:* 76. 1960.

CHAN, G.M. Dietary calcium and bone mineral status of children and adolescents. *Am. J. Dis. Child. 145:* 631. 1991.

CHERY, A. AND J.H. SABRY Portion size of common foods eaten by young children. *J. Can. Diet. Assoc. 45:* 230. 1984.

CRYAN, J. AND R.K. JOHNSON Should the current recommendations for energy intake in infants and young children be lowered? *Nutr. Today 32(2):* 69. 1997.

CUMMINGS, N.P., ET AL Sensitivity to foods and additives: Effect on behavior. *J. Am. Med. Assoc. 251:* 1209. 1984.

DAVIS, C.M. Results of the self-selection of diets by young children. *Can. Med. Assoc. J. 41:* 257. 1939.

FENNER, L. Parents: Guard against food-related chokings. *FDA Cons. 18(9):* 21. 1984.

FRANKLE, R.T. Obesity a family matter: creating new behavior. *J. Am. Diet. Assoc. 85:* 597. 1985.

GALVIN, E.W., AT AL Children and allergies: Some effects and treatment. *Child. Today 13:* 31. 1984.

GARN, S.M., ET AL Lifelong differences in hemoglobin levels between blacks and whites. *J. Nat. Med. Assoc. 67:* 91. 1975

BORAN, M.I., ET AL Energy requirements across the life span: New findings based on measurements with doubly-labeled water. *Nutr. Res. 15:* 115. 1995.

GUSTAFFSON, B., ET AL The Vipeholm dental caries study: effect of different levels of carbohydates intake on caries activity in 436 individuals observed for five years. *Acta Odont. Scand. 11:* 232. 1954.

HADLEY, J. Facts about childhood hyperactivity. *Child. Today 13:* 8. 1983.

HAMILL, P.V.V., ET AL *NCHS Growth Curves for Children: Birth-18 Years. DHEW Publ. No. (PHS) 78-1650.* Washington, D.C. 1977.

HILDRETH, H. AND R.K. JOHNSON The doubly labeled water technique for the determination of human energy requirements. *Nutr. Today 30:* 254. 1995.

HOLMES, R.P. AND F. A. KUMMEROW Relationship of adequate and excessive intake of vitamin D to health and disease. *J. Am. Coll. Nutr. 2:* 173. 1983.

JOHNSTON, P.K. Getting enough to grow on. *Am. J. Nurs. 84:* 336 1984.

LAWLESS, H. Sensory development in children: research in taste and olfaction. *J. Am. Diet. Assoc. 85:* 577. 1985.

MASON, J.O. Message to health professionals about fluorosis. *J. Am. Med. Assoc. 265:* 2939. 1991.

McWILLIAMS, M. *Food Fundamentals.* Plycon Press, Redondo Beach, CA 7th ed. 1998.

MILLER, D.R., B.L. SPECKER, M.L. HO, AND E.J. NORMAN Vitamin B_{12} status in a macrobiotic community. *Am. J. Clin. Nutr. 53:* 524. 1991.

MORALES, E., L.D. CRAIG, AND W.C. MACLEAN, JR. Dietary management of malnourished children with a new enteral feeding. *J. Am. Diet. Assoc. 91:* 1233. 1991.

PAYNE, M.L. AND W.J. CRAIG Sorbitol is a possible risk factor in young children. *J. Am. Diet. Assoc. 97(5):* 532. 1997.

PEARSON, D.J., ET AL Food allergy: How much in the ind? *Lancet 1(4):* 1259. 1983.

POLLITT, E., ET AL Cognitive effects of iron-deficiency anaemia. *Lancet 1:* 158. 1985.

RICHMOND, V.L. Thirty years of fluoridation: a review. *Am. J. Clin. Nutr. 41:* 129. 1985.

SABATE, J., K.D. LINSTEAD, R.D. HARRIS, AND A. SANCHEZ Attained height of lacto-ovo vegetarian children and adolescents. *Euro. J. Clin. Nutr. 45:* 51. 1991.

SATTER, E.M. Internal regulation and the evolution of normal growth as the basis for prevention of obesity in children. *J. Am. Diet. Assoc. 96(9):* 860. 1996.

SAVAIANO, D., ET AL Lactose malabsorption from yogurt, pasteurized yogurt, sweet acidophilus milk, and cultured milk in lactase-deficiency individuals. *Am. J. Clin. Nutr. 40:* 1219. 1984.

SCHAEFER, L.J. AND S.K. KUMANYIKA Maternal variable related to potentially high sodium infant-feeding practices. *J. Am. Diet. Assoc. 85:* 433. 1985.

SHAPIRO, L.R., ET AL Obesity prognosis: Longitudinal study of children from age of 6 months to 9 years. *Am. J. Pub. Health 74:* 968. 1984.

SKINNER, J.D., ET AL Longitudinal study of nutrient and food intakes of infants aged 2 to 24 months. *J. Am. Diet. Assoc. 97(5):* 496. 1997.

SPLETT, P.L. AND M. STORY Child nutrition: Objectives for decade. *J. Am. Diet. Assoc. 91:* 665. 1991.

STORY, M. AND P. FAULKNER Prime time diet: Content analysis of eating behavior and food messages in television program content and commercials. *Am. J. Public Health 80:* 738. 1990.

TATE, W.H., R. SNYDER, E.H. MONTGOMERY, AND J.T. CHAN Impact of source of drinking water on fluoride supplementation. *J. Pediat. 117:* 419. 1990.

WILLIAMS, C.L., ET AL Dietary fat and children's health. *Nutr. Today 33(4):* 144. 1998.

CHAPTER EIGHT

Preadolescents

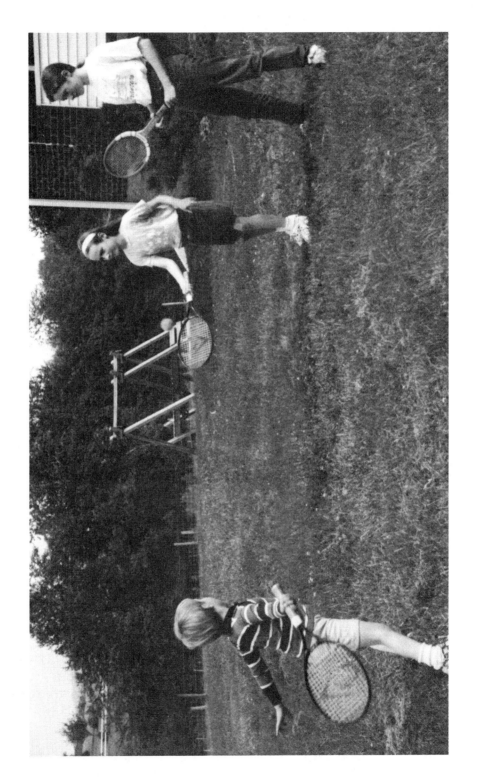

OVERVIEW

Latency, the term sometimes used to designate the elementary school years, is a period when growth continues, but with much less dramatic effect than the earlier years or the teens. In short, this phase of life is a rather quiet one physically, yet an important one from the perspective of nutritionists. This is the time when the body can build optimal stores of nutrients in preparation for the tumultuous growth of adolescence. Emphasis on nutrition education and the formation of good nutrition habits regulated by the children themselves are key aspects of preparing children to enter adolescence.

295

CHANGING NUTRITIONAL NEEDS

GRADUAL CHANGES

The elementary school child is growing, but the growth rate is distinctly less than that of infancy and certainly does not approach the spectacular change in height and weight that normally occurs in adolescence. If observable growth rates are used as the only criterion on which to base nutritional needs, one may erroneously conclude that nutrition does not play a significant role in the development of the child during this time. Actually, this is far from true. The elementary school child has a continuing need for an adequate diet to:

Plenty of exercise is important to help assure healthy appetites during the elementary school years.

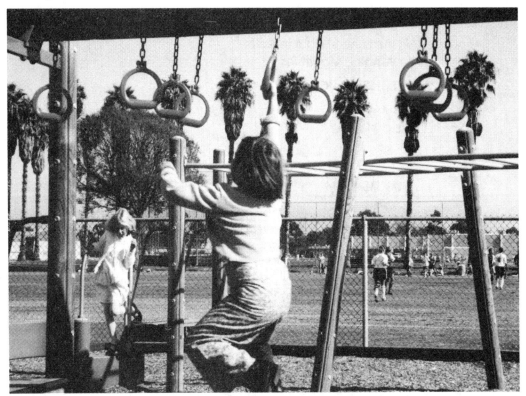

Boys and girls have similar nutritional needs until puberty. Then boys begin to require more food and its accompanying nutrients; girls' needs increase somewhat less.

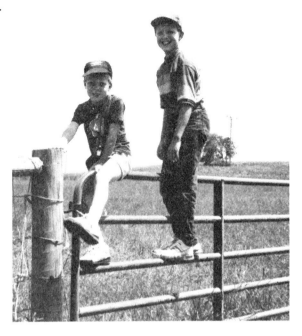

1. Provide building materials for growth.

2. Furnish the energy needed for the vigorous physical activities of this age group.

3. Help maintain resistance to infections.

4. Ensure that adequate body stores of nutrients are available for the future growth demands of the teens.

Attention should be given during these years to developing good dietary habits. By the time a child reaches adolescence, these habits should be well established; the reasons for eating a good diet should be understood. Good habits, coupled with knowledge, will help maintain good nutritional status during the teens.

From ages 7 through 10 of the elementary school years, nutritional needs are greater than the needs of the preschool child. An examination of the complete table of Recommended Dietary Allowances (Tables 1.8 and 1.9) reveals that there is a gradual increase in the need for calories from birth through the elementary school period, followed by an increasing need during the adolescent period. As one would expect, there is also an increased need for protein, calcium, phosphorus, iodine, magnesium, selenium, vitamin A, the B vitamins, vitamin C, vitamin E, and vitamin K. The recommended allowances for iron, zinc, and vitamin D remain the same for the elementary school child as they were for the preschooler.

It is apparent from this summary (see Tables 8.1 and 8.2) that the elementary school child needs more food than the preschooler, but the changes are not startling. The normal, healthy child will naturally increase food intake during this period if good nutrition habits are quietly encouraged and well-planned, tasty meals are served. It is appropriate to emphasize the importance of exercise in maintaining good appetites. Active

TABLE 8.1   RDA and AI for Children Ages 6–8 and Boys and Girls Ages 9–13[a,b]

Nutrient (daily amounts)	Ages 6–8[b]	Ages 9–13	
		Boys	Girls
Calcium (mg)	800	1300	1300
Phosphorus (mg)	500	1250	1250
Magnesium (mg)	130	240	240
Vitamin D[c] (μg)	5	5	5
Fluoride (mg)	1	2	2
Thiamin (mg)	0.6	0.9	0.9
Riboflavin (mg)	0.6	0.9	0.9
Niacin (mg)	8	12	12
Vitamin B_6 (mg)	0.6	1.0	1.0
Folate (μg)	200	300	300
Vitamin B_{12} (μg)	1.2	1.8	1.8
Pantothenic acid (mg)	3	4	4
Biotin (μg)	12	20	20
Choline (mg)	250	375	375

[a]Adapted from Food and Nutrition Board, Institute of Medicine — National Academy of Sciences Dietary Reference Intakes: Recommended Intakes for individuals. Washington, D.C. 1998.
[b]Values in the table from which this is adapted cover ages 4–8.
[c]As cholecalciferol. 1 μg = 40 IU Vitamin D.

TABLE 8.2   RDA for Children Ages 7–10 and Boys and Girls
             Ages 11–14[a,b]

| Nutrient (daily amounts) | Ages 7–10 | Ages 11–14 | |
		Boys	Girls
Protein (g)	28	45	46
Vitamin A (µg RE)[c]	700	1000	800
Vitamin E (mg α-TE)[d]	7	10	8
Vitamin K (µg)	30	45	45
Vitamin C (mg)	45	50	50
Iron (mg)	10	12	15
Zinc (mg)	10	15	12
Iodine (µg)	120	150	150
Selenium (µg)	30	40	45

[a]Adapted from Food and Nutrition Board, Institute of Medicine — National Academy of Sciences Dietary Reference Intakes: Recommended Intakes for individuals. Washington, D.C. 1998.
[b]Based on weight of 38 kg (62 lb) and height of 132 cm (52 in) for ages 7–10; weight of 45 kg (99 lb) and height of 157 cm (62 in) for boys 11–14; and weight of 46 kg (101 lb) and height of 157 cm (62 in) for girls 11–14.
[c]Retinol equivalents. 1 retinol equivalent = 1 µg retinol or 6 µg β-carotene.
[d]α-Tocopherol equivalents. 1 mg d-α-tocopherol = 1 α-TE.

physical play develops healthy appetites, but too much television viewing or other sedentary activity fosters poor nutrition. Frequently, children who watch television a great deal nibble while watching and spoil their appetites for meals.

The consumption of adequate amounts of nutrients without including too many calories and too much fat is important during latency. The data from the U.S. Department of Agriculture (1988) indicate that about a fourth of the boys and girls between the ages of 6 and 11 consumed less than 75% of the RDA for calcium and vitamin A. In contrast, total fat intake exceeded the recommended level of 30% of the calories in the diets of 81% and 91% of the boys and girls, respectively, in this same survey. Based on these findings, there clearly is a need to explore ways to increase the consumption of reduced fat, lowfat, and/or fat free milk and to reduce fat in the diet by these changes as well as choosing foods with fat substitutes or reduced fat.

SEX DIFFERENCES

Recommended nutrient intake is the same for both boys and girls until ages 9—11 (Tables 8.1 and 8.2). When children enter puberty, separate recommendations are made for the nutrient needs of girls and boys; this distinction continues in the RDA throughout the remainder of life. The recommendations for boys and girls at the time of puberty are quite similar with the exception of some of the minerals (notably iron, zinc, and selenium). The higher intake of iron that is suggested for girls is based on the iron losses that begin to occur during menstruation. Zinc is needed in larger amounts by pubescent boys than girls because of their greater growth in this period.

NUTRIENTS OF SPECIAL CONCERN

Nutritional status, a matter of considerable importance to individual health, is also vital to the collective health of the nation. In fact, nutritional status of the population as a whole is of such significance to the nation that the Federal government has conducted broad nutrition surveys at various times during this century. One of the signficiant studies was the Ten-State Nutrition Survey, conducted in 1969 in the states of California, Kentucky, Louisiana, Massachusetts, Michigan, New York (including a special survey in New York City), South Carolina, Texas, Washington, and West Virginia. This study, which was directed toward districts within these states where many families were living on low incomes (the majority with incomes of less than $3,000 per year at the time of the study), revealed a number of nutritionally-based problems for individuals of all ages and helped document the need for increased national attention to nutrition. Dental problems, retarded growth, and evidence of low serum levels of vitamin C were found in many individuals. Tangible evidence of improved nutritional status (increased stature, body weight, advanced skeletal and dental development, and earlier maturation) was correlated positively with increased per capita income.

The data collected in the Ten-State Nutrition Survey were evaluated in relation to the 1968 revision of the Recommended Dietary Allowances. Results indicated that elementary-age school children until the age of 9 were receiving adequate amounts of protein, calcium, iron, vitamin A, thiamin, riboflavin, and vitamin C. Between the ages of 9 and 11, boys were found to be better nourished than girls; girls were considerably lower than boys in their intake of calcium, and boys were consuming less

TEN-STATE NUTRITION SURVEY
National survey of nutritional status of low-income populations in selected states, conducted in 1969; documented the need for increased emphasis on nutrition in the United States.

NHANES I, II, AND III
National Health and Nutrition Examination Surveys I, II, and III conducted by the Department of Health Education and Welfare in 1971–75, 1976–80, and 1988–91, respectively. The surveys were done to determine nutritional status of a broadly-based population.

Preadolescent boys often are more active and have higher energy needs than their female counterparts. This boy studiously flips a pancake in a class at school. Later he enthusiastically devoured "his" pancakes.

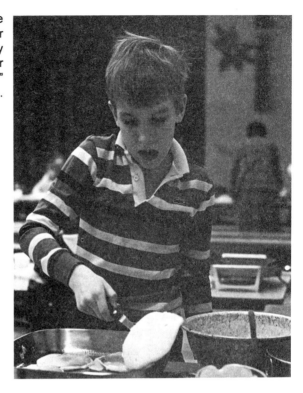

calcium than recommended. Girls also had very low intakes of iron and a slightly low intake of thiamin.

Three National Health and Nutrition Eduction Surveys (NHANES I, II, and III) were conducted by the Department of Health Education, and Welfare in 1971—75, 1976—80, and 1988—91, respectively). They were designed to obtain detailed information on nutritional status of a broad population.

NATIONAL FOOD CONSUMPTION SURVEY, 1977–1978. Study of Americans' food intake by age and sex in 1977–1978.

The National Food Consumption Survey was another governmental study to obtain information regarding nutrient levels in the diets of a broad sample of people of all ages and both sexes in 1977—78. Again, this study demonstrated that elementary school children generally ate very adequate diets. Exceptions were calcium and vitamin B_6, which boys consumed at levels between 90 and 99 percent of the RDA, and magnesium, with an intake of between 80 and 89 percent of the RDA. Girls between the ages of 9 and 11 consumed only 80 to 89 percent of the RDA for calcium, magnesium, and vitamin B_6, and from 90 to 99 percent of the RDA for iron. According to these data, girls start to consume diets somewhat inferior to the quality of boys' diets by the age of 11. Even though many youngsters, both boys and girls, eat very adequate diets during the elementary years, attention to strengthening good dietary patterns is appropriate at this time.

FAMILY RESPONSIBILITIES FOR NUTRITION

MEAL PREPARATION

The nutritional needs of large numbers of elementary school children will be met only partially at home because most rural and city schools have a lunch program. Families still maintain an important role, because they usually are responsible for two meals and an after-school snack each day. It is essential, however, that the school recognize its responsibility at lunchtime.

If a child is to be well nourished during the elementary school period, it is essential that a conscientious effort be maintained in the home toward planning and serving organized meals. Appetizing, nourishing meals should be served on a schedule convenient to most family members. Unfortunately, in today's urban societies, there appears to be a growing tendency for family meals to be less and less a family affair. With fathers and mothers often gone from the home many hours a day and children involved in numerous activities outside the home, there is not much incentive to prepare the family fare that was traditional in the past. Despite all the convenience foods available today, much time is still required to plan and prepare meals that will meet families' nutritional and social needs. For mothers working away from home, this time may be difficult to find. The temptations are great for modern families to let children help themselves to ready-to-eat convenience foods that they can fix for themselves whenever they are hungry. Unfortunately, this type of helter-skelter approach does not lead to optimal nutrition for elementary school children (or other family members).

Parents likely would find it illuminating — perhaps even frightening — if they would have their elementary-age children keep an accurate record of everything (including amounts) they eat for a week. Comparison of this actual account with the recommendations of the Food Guide Pyramid can provide sobering evidence of the need for family involvement in the eating patterns of the children (and also their parents)! A week's record for Lisa (age 10) is as follows:

Breakfast	Lunch	Snack	Dinner	Snack
Sunday Waffle Hot Chocolate	Hamburger French fries	Nachos Soda	Chicken stir-fry Rice Green salad Apple pie Iced tea	Soda
Monday Cold cereal Milk Orange juice	Pizza Soda	Popcorn Soda	Lamb chops Baked potato Sour cream Spinach salad Chocolate cake Apple juice	Chips Soda
Tuesday Cold cereal Milk	Spaghetti Meat balls Tossed salad Milk	Snow cone	Chicken Red beans & rice Roasted peppers	Bagel Soda
Wednesday Bagel, peanut butter Orange juice	Grilled cheese sandwich Banana Chocolate bar	Snow cone	Hot dog Chips Ice cream Cake Soda	Chips Soda
Thursday Cold cereal Milk	French fries Milk	Bagel	Pasta & tomato sauce Garlic bread Green salad Strawberry shortcake	Apple
Friday Cold cereal Milk	Turkey sandwich Carrot sticks	Granola bar	Beef fajita vegetables Caesar salad	Chips Soda

	Fruit roll-up Grape juice		Lemon pie	

Saturday

French toast	Tuna sandwich	Pizza	Snow
Orange juice	Celery sticks	Apple	cone
Milk	Baked custard	Soda	

Table 8.3 reveals the need for some definite changes to improve Lisa's diet (and probably her parents' diet, too). Her intake of grain products is almost up to the recommendation, but her vegetable and fruit consumption should include about twice as many vegetables and more whole fruits rather than mostly in the form of juice. A particular problem is her very inadequate intake of milk and large consumption of sodas. Nonfat or lowfat milk at all of her meals at home would improve the picture greatly and reduce sweets. Meat does need to be included daily.

Few elementary school children are capable of planning a well-balanced diet each day without some adult assistance, nor are they able to prepare complete meals that will meet their needs. Parents still need to retain the final responsibility for family meals. If the mother is working outside the home, it may be appropriate to have school-age children or a domestic helper do some meal preparation. However, parents should still be certain that the meals are nutritionally adequate and appetizing.

It is as important for children to have a nourishing breakfast and lunch as it is for them to have a good dinner. In the modern family, the greatest tendency toward skimping on

TABLE 8.3   Comparison of Lisa's Intake for Seven Days with the Food Guide Pyramid (FGP) Recommendations

Intake	1st	2nd	3rd	4th	5th	6th	7th	Avg.	FGP
Grain products	5	4	7	6	6	5	4	5.3	6–11
Vegetables	2	2	2	0	2	3	1	1.7	3–5
Fruits	1	2	0	2	2	1.5	2	1.5	2–4
Milk products	1	1	2	0.5	2	1	1.5	1.3	2–3
Meat and beans	2	1.5	2.5	1.2	0	2	2	1.6	2–3
Fats, oils, sweets[a]	1	2	1	4	0.5	2.5	1	1.7	Sparingly

[a]Does not include diet sodas in Lisa' intake. However, Lisa would have added 11 more servings for the week if they contained sugar, bringing the average intake for fats, oils, and sweets to 3.3.

nutrition probably occurs at breakfast and lunch. Because parents are ordinarily home for dinner, the evening meal is usually far more adequate than other meals. Good breakfast habits are likely to be maintained in families who have a formal breakfast together. Unfortunately, the staggered scheduling in some families may make this arrangement impractical. Parents, however, can still encourage children to eat a good breakfast by preparing an appetizing meal and eating with them, both on school mornings and during vacations.

SUPERVISORY CAPACITY

The parents' role now assumes a slightly different character from that performed when the child was younger. The supervisory role begins to gain in importance as children go through elementary school. During the elementary school period, there is an increasing tendency to consume more foods that are low in nutritive value and high in calories. Children of this age become increasingly independent, particularly in regard to snacks. The small amount of financial independence resulting from allowances, odd jobs, and paper routes enables boys and girls to buy candy or pop, both of which fill little nutritional need and are superfluous in the elementary school child's diet.

It is the conscientious parents' responsibility to be certain that school-age children have an adequate diet. It will be necessary to make a deliberate effort to be aware of the foods a child actually consumes during the entire day, including school lunches and snack foods. Many schools regularly have their school lunch menus published weekly in the local newspaper, a practice that makes it easier to coordinate family meals with those eaten at school.

Children are usually very hungry after school and do need a snack. The snack, however, should be eaten as early as possible and should be sufficient to ease immediate hunger without interfering with the appetite for dinner. When necessary, children should be given help in planning more nourishing food for snacks, and they may also need suggestions regarding the quantity of the snack eaten after school. The amount of the after-school snack is impossible to suggest here because of individual variation in children's appetites and differences among families in their traditional time for the evening meal. It is important, however, that snacks not interfere with dinner appetites, because a well-planned dinner will provide many necessary nutrients that may be lacking in a snack.

ROLE MODEL

Parents have a strong influence over their children's dietary patterns in the elementary school period, just as they do in the earlier years. When food is eaten with enthusiasm by parents, children will usually follow suit. Favorable comments about the pleasing aspects of food served at the meal also create pleasure in eating (and encourage the cook toward continuing efforts in the kitchen). Creation of a warm and sociable family meal environment is a helpful step toward promoting good nutrition for all family members.

Another important example to set is that of regular physical activity. Elementary school children need considerable exercise, and so do their parents. The entire family will benefit if parents can establish regular patterns of physical activity for themselves, particularly if children are included in these activities. For example, bicycle riding on a regular basis by the entire family is an excellent form of exercise for people of all ages. Jogging is another popular activity. The increased caloric expenditure will be significant in maintaining a desirable weight. Exercise is also essential for maintaining good muscle tone.

Parents can also aid their children in achieving good nutritional status if they watch their own dietary patterns, particularly if they eat for weight control. If parents are overeating, either for social or psychological reasons, children are likely to adopt this practice. The acceptance of a wide range of foods by parents encourages children to have broad tastes, too. The likelihood of achieving good nutrient intake is enhanced greatly by the practice of eating a wide variety of foods on a regular basis.

Fat free or lowfat milk at all family meals is a good beverage for all family members, not just the children. Parental example in drinking milk is invaluable in helping to establish and maintain adqeuate calcium intake throughout life to help protect against osteoporosis later. Emphasis on a wide variety and frequent service of vegetables and fruits not only enhances nutrient intake of vitamins and minerals, but also increases fiber intake to help protect against some cancers.

RESEARCH INSIGHTS

Falciglia, G.A., et al., Food neophobia in childhood affects dietary variety. *J. Am. Diet. Assoc.* 100(12): 1474. 2000.

This study addressed the question of whether children who are unwilling to try new foods (a condition termed neophobia) eat diets that are more restrictive than do neophilic children. After completion of screening using the Food Neophobia Scale, 70 4th and 5th grade students in Cincinnati, Ohio were grouped into 3 categories based on their responses to the screening tool. Each student completed a 3-day (2 weekdays and 1 weekend day) dietary record obtained first through an interview to elicit dietary information for the first day conducted by trained graduate students in nutrition and in the presence of a parent. Then each participant was asked to recall food intake on 2 other days with assistance from the parent. These diets then were assessed by Nutritionist V (version 2.2, 1988) software. Demographic data were analyzed using descriptive statistics. Comparison of categorical data among groups was done using chi square, and differences for continuous variables among groups were calculated using 1-way analysis of covariance.

Results of demographic analysis showed that whites (75%) comprised 75% of the neophobic group and 70% of the neophilic group, but only 48% of the average group, which corresponds to 18, 11, and 16 whites in the respective groups. In contrast, 12 of 20 African American children were in the average group, with the other two groups each having 4 each. Of the 4 Asian children in the study, 1 was considered neophobic and 3 were neophilic. The only Hispanic was in the neophobic group. Although these are very small numbers of subjects, they do suggest the need for further research studies regarding variety in diet according to ethnic backgrounds.

Nutritional analyses indicated that the students in this sample study did not meet the RDAs/DRIs for energy, vitamin E, folate, calcium, and zinc. Also, fiber intake was low. However, total fat and saturated fat intakes were above Dietary Guidelines recommendations. Children in the neophobic group were less likely to meet vitamin E recommended intake than were the children in the other 2 groups, but overall the intakes still were too low. No significant differences in meeting recommendations for the other nutrients were found between the 3 groups, thus failing to support the hypothesis that neophobic children would be more likely to have inadequate intakes of essential nutrients. Neophilic children tended to have the highest caloric intake. The foods eaten most frequently by all 3 groups were white bread, ready-to-eat cereals, 2% white milk, nondiet soft drinks, ice cream, hamburgers/cheese-burgers, mashed/baked/fried potatoes, cookies, and fried chicken. Intakes of vegetables in all 3 groups were very low compared with the Food Guide Pyramid recommendations, and fruit, meat, and cereal servings were low. Fortified cereals were found to be important in improving the children's intake of the nutrients included in the fortification.

PRACTICAL APPLICATIONS

BREAKFAST

The dietary pattern for the elementary school child should include a broad variety of foods selected to meet the child's needs for growth, maintenance, and activity. Attention should certainly be given in the home to eating an adequate breakfast. Children will perform better in school when they have an adequate breakfast before starting the day's school work. This should include a citrus fruit or other good source of ascorbic acid, a good source of protein such as an egg, cereal or toast, and a glass of milk. This breakfast is adequate for the elementary school child, but quantities will need to be increased considerably to satisfy a boy's appetite by the time he reaches sixth grade. A typical sixth-grade boy's breakfast might include a 4-oz glass of juice, an 8-oz glass of milk, a large bowl of cereal and milk, two pieces of toast, and bacon, wiener, or egg.

LUNCH

Whether lunch is eaten at home or at school, it is again important that a good source of protein be available in adequate quantities. The protein at lunch could be from either animal or vegetable sources; cheese, eggs, meat, poultry, fish, kidney beans, lima beans, or other legumes are all appropriate. It is important to realize that soups containing a small amount of meat are definitely inadequate as the sole source of protein at a meal. Soups have their place, but they should be supplemented by another food high in protein to meet the need for protein at the lunch meal. Soup, combined with a meat sandwich, would adequately meet the body's need for protein at lunch. The lunch menu should also include two or more vegetables and/or fruit, a serving of bread or bread substitute, and a glass of milk. Many elementary school children, particularly older boys, may need more food than this; they may desire additional servings or a greater variety of food at lunch.

If a child brings lunch to school, it is still important that the lunch be well prepared and appetizing. Simply taking a jelly sandwich and calling it lunch is not adequate for any elementary school child. Again, protein should be included in the sack lunch every day. The protein food can be varied from day to day by including such foods as cold fried chicken, a slice of cold meat loaf, cold cuts, peanut butter, pizza, a hard-cooked egg, or cheese. Sack lunches often contain a high proportion of bread and baked products and inadequate amounts of protein foods, fruits, and vegetables. Fruits and raw vegetables are quite adaptable to use in a sack lunch. Milk can usually be purchased at school, but it could be taken in a thermos bottle when necessary. Table 8.4 includes menu ideas for sack lunches.

When preparing sack lunches, the safety of the food must be borne in mind. Many protein-rich foods are possible sources of food poisoning unless lunches are kept cold during the morning. If lunches cannot be kept refrigerated, potentially dangerous items should not be included in the lunches or they should be frozen when packed at home. For example, fried chicken should be frozen solid when it is packed in the morning.

TABLE 8.4   Menus for Sack Lunches[a]

Day	Entree	Fruits/Vegetables	Other
Monday	Sliced ham on French roll, w/ mustard and lettuce	Raw cauliflower, Tokay grapes	Pickle
Tuesday	Mixed bean (kidney, garbanzo, wax, and string beans) salad	Celery sticks, Apple	Bran muffin
Wednesday	Meat loaf on whole-wheat bread, w/ dash of catsup and lettuce	Raw zucchini sticks, d'Anjou pear	
Thursday	Celery sticks stuffed w/ peanut butter	Cherry Tomatoes, Orange	Banana nut bread w/ cream cheese
Friday	Sliced chicken on cracked wheat bread, w/ butter and lettuce	Raw broccoli spears, Tangerine	

[a]Menus are listed assuming milk will be available at school and that portions will be sized to meet the appetite of the individual child.

Frozen sandwiches are also possibilities. Use of insulated bags or lunch boxes provides further protection against food spoilage during the morning. Also, frozen cold packs can be added to the lunch container.

DINNER

Dinner in most families is probably adequate. Attention should be centered on pleasant service of an attractive, well-balanced meal. Dinner usually provides the best opportunity for being creative in the kitchen and attempting to expand a child's experiences with new foods, including a variety of seasonings and spices. Children of elementary school age are able to experiment with a wide range of seasonings because the gastrointestinal tract is less easily irritated and they are able to digest more highly seasoned foods than preschoolers.

This is a good time to expand the family menus to include many things that may not have been prepared previously for the children. Families may wish to establish the tradition of having a meal typical of a different foreign country one night each week. The children will learn about the various countries in this way, and the entire family will enjoy such a project. Appropriate table decorations can be made by the children. Menus and recipes from foreign countries are readily available, and most of the ingredients needed can be found in supermarkets or specialty shops.

THE SCHOOL LUNCH

Although the school lunch is a government-subsidized program operated in the public schools, it still seems wise for parents and teachers to learn something about the purpose of the program and its operation. Interested involvement by parents in the community is vital to a vigorous, effective school lunch program. The ensuing discussion pinpointing some of the key factors involved in successful operation of school lunch programs is intended to develop a greater understanding of some of the problems schools face in this area.

LEGISLATION

The National School Lunch Program developed from a Federal program that was launched in 1935 to distribute surplus foods to schools to be used in free lunch programs. Eight years

NATIONAL SCHOOL LUNCH PROGRAM
Federal lunch program established in 1935 to provide lunches at school using surplus foods.

later, in 1943, schools received payments through the United States Department of Agriculture to meet part of the cost of foods that were purchased locally for school lunches. Formal support of the concept of the school lunch program was provided in 1946 when the National School Lunch Act was passed. Its purpose was defined: "to safeguard the health and well-being of the Nation's children and to encourage the domestic consumption of nutritious agricultural commodities and other food, by assisting the States, through grants-in-aid and other means, in providing an adequate supply of foods and other facilities for the establishment, maintenance, operation, and expansion of nonprofit school lunch programs." Subsequent legislation has added to the program to improve the nutrition of the nation's children. An amendment in 1970 stipulated that every American school child who was needy (according to specified guidelines) should be served meals free or at a reduced cost. States were charged with the responsibility of bringing this program to every school.

The Child Nutrition Act of 1966 was significant because it authorized a two-year pilot program for a School Breakfast Program. Funds to extend this effort were provided in 1968 and 1971. In 1973, the breakfast program became available to all schools wishing to apply. The reimbursement rate for the program provides Federal funds for each free and reduced-price breakfast and limited support for each paid breakfast. Participation in the aspect of school feeding programs had expanded to about 1.5 million children, with more than 60% receiving free breakfasts in 1982.

The Special Milk Program was a part of the Child Nutrition Act of 1966. This legislation was implemented to provide as much as 1 pt of milk daily for children from needy families. By 1978, more than two million children were benefiting from this legislation.

The National School Lunch Program is now operated under the original act with a number of amendments extending and modifying the original legislation. The 1973 amendment authorized Federal reimbursement to the states at the rate of 10 cents per lunch, with an additional 45 cents average for free lunches served. With an eye toward the inflationary trend in food prices that was evident in 1973, the legislation provided for semi-annual review of costs and adjustments to be made as necessary. About 25 million children participate in the National School Lunch Program, with about one-third receiving free or reduced-price lunches.

Another aspect of Federal support for nutrition is found in the 1968 amendment to the National School Lunch Act, establishing a three-year-pilot Special Food Service Program for Children. Under this amendment, the program was extended to cover day care centers, settlement houses, and recreation programs operated as public and nonprofit institutions. Summer recreation programs for school children in low income areas were included. Year-round programs for preschool as well as older children of needy working mothers are included for support. Coverage may include support for breakfast and/or lunch and/or dinner and/or between-meal supplements. Up to 100 percent of the daily dietary allowances may be provided under this program. This program has been extended beyond the original three-year period.

The 1977 Amendment to the Child Nutrition Act represented an exciting and challenging opportunity to begin an intensive program of nutrition education in the schools. This was made possible by the requirement that $.50 per child be allocated for nutrition education. Considerable activity in generating curriculum and teaching aids resulted, but the funding was reduced to less than a third of the initial allocation (actually less than 15 cents per child) in 1981. This reduction has had a strong negative impact on the evolving nutrition education programs, although rather strong efforts are continuing in some programs.

The deadline for incorporating the U.S. Dietary Guidelines into school lunch programs around the nation was 1996. This

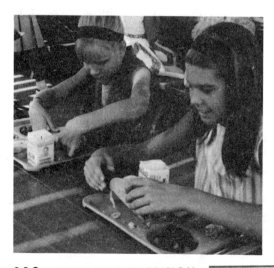

Two eager consumers prepare to enjoy their tacos, which are part of the Type A school lunch menu.

Children partici-
pating in the
National School
Lunch Program
enjoy helping
themselves to this
wide array of salad
ingredients.
Creative presen-
tation and menu
planning are
important compo-
nents of today's
school lunches.

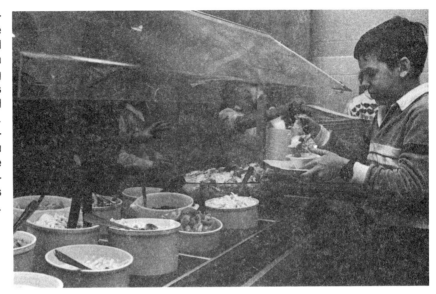

federal mandate has focused considerable attention on finding
acceptable ways to modify menus and recipes to bring the fat
content of the menus to about 30 percent of the calories over the
course of a week's menus. Various techniques and ingredients
have been tried, including reducing the fat content of ground beef
by a 2-step cooking and washing process, adding applesauce to
replace some of the fat in cake recipes, and similar modifications
in other baked products. The U.S. Department of Agriculture has
taken a leadership role in making such information available to
school lunch personnel. The acceptance of reduced fat items has
been good (Borja, et al, 1996). This clearly is a major concern
because of the importance of attracting students to participate in
the Nationl School Lunch Program in order to help assure good
nutritional status for school children.

PLANNING THE MENUS

Planning a school lunch is a real challenge for any nutritionist despite the fact that the school lunch supervisor is
assisted in the planning by the requirements set forth under the
National School Lunch Program. The regulations, as modified in
1978, specify guidelines for Type A lunch that must be followed if
the program is to qualify for Federal reimbursement. The lunch
requirements now provide for different amounts of food for
different ages (Table 8.5), a modification aimed at reducing plate

TABLE 8.5   Type A School Lunch Requirements[a]

Food Group	Preschool		Elementary School		Secondary School
	1–2 yrs	3–5 yrs	6–8 yrs	9–11 yrs	12+ yrs
Meat and Meat Alternates[b]	1 oz[c] equiv	1 oz equiv	1.5 oz equiv	2 oz equiv	3 oz equiv
Vegetables and Fruits[e]	1/2 c	1/2 c	1/2 c	3/4 c	3/4 c
Bread and Bread Alternates[f,g]	5 slices or alt/wk	8 slices or alt/wk	8 slices or alt/wk	8 slices or alt/wk	10 slices or alt/wk
Milk, Fluid	1/2 c	3/4 c	3/4 c	1/2 pt	1/2 pt

Meat and Meat Alternates[b]

A serving (weight amounts given for portions as served) of cooked lean meat, poultry, or fish, or alternates.

The following alternates for 1 oz cooked lean meat may be used:[d]
    Cheese (1 oz)
    Eggs (1 large egg)
    Cooked dry beans or peas (1/2 c)
    Peanut butter (2 tbsp)

Vegetables and Fruits[e]

Two or more servings consisting of vegetables or fruits or both. A serving of full-strength vegetable or fruit juice can be counted to meet not more than half the total requirement.

Bread and Bread Alternates[f,g]

A serving (1 slice) enriched or whole-grain bread; or serving of biscuits, rolls, muffins, etc. made with whole grain or enriched meal or flours; or a serving (1/2 c) cooked enriched or whole grain rice, macaroni, or noodles or other pasta products[h]

Milk, Fluid

Two types of milk must be offered, one of which must be unflavored, fluid low-fat milk, skim milk, or

[a]From school lunch pattern requirements, Federal Register 43, No. 163 919780.
[b]Equivalents determined and published in guidance materials by FNS/USDA.
[c]It is recommended that in schools not offering a choice of meat/meat alternates each day, no one form of meat (ground, sliced, pieces, etc.) or meat alternate be served more than three times per week. Meat and meat alternates must be served in a main dish or in a main dish and one other menu item.
[d]When it is determined that the serving size of the meat alternate is excessive, the meat alternate shall be reduced and supplemented with an additional meat/meat alternate to meet the full requirement.
[e]Cooked dry beans or dry peas may be used as part of the meat alternate or part of the vegetable/fruit component, but not as both in the same meal.
[f]One-half or more slices of bread or an equivalent amount of bread alternate must be served with each lunch, with the total requirement being served during the 5-day period. Schools serving lunch 6 or 7 days per week should increase this specified quantity for the 5-day period by approximately 20% (one-fifth) for each additional day.
[g]Bread alternates and serving sizes published in guidance materials by FNS/USDA.
[h]Enriched macaroni products with fortified protein may be used as part of a meat alternate or as a bread alternate, but not as both in the same meal.
[i]A half pint of milk may be used for all age groups if the lesser specified amounts are determined by the school food authority to be impractical.

waste. Another change is represented by the policy of "offer versus serve." This policy requires that children be offered all five foods specified in the Type A lunch, but they need to take only three for the lunch to qualify for Federal reimbursement. "Offer versus serve" is an option available to junior and senior high school students, but not to younger children. This option clearly provides a less appropriate balance of nutrients than is provided by the complete Type A meal, but it has been implemented on the premise that students will leave the food they do not like on their plates, even if it is served to them. The option of taking at least three out of the five items offered should help reduce plate waste, which helps keep costs under control.

Planning a menu that meets the preceding government specifications, contains at least 80 percent locally-available food, fits the required cost limitations, and can be prepared within the physical setup of the school kitchen is only part of the problem. Perhaps the most difficult facet of the menu to predict is acceptance of the meal. Even when a menu meets all other criteria for a good lunch, it can be considered a failure if many children do not eat the food. Menus should be planned to include not only variety, but also enough familiar foods so that they will be accepted and eaten by the children. Anyone could plan a lunch of hamburgers and potato chips day after day, and the acceptance would be relatively high, at least for a time. One purpose of the school lunch, however, is to encourage children to eat a variety of foods, and repetitious menus are not in concert with this objective. It is necessary to find other foods that children of this age enjoy and that the cook can prepare satisfactorily.

To develop a set of menus that will be suitable for use in a particular school system, the school lunch supervisor must test many different recipes and be on the alert to locate suitable recipes for the lunch program. The only realistic way of evaluating the new food is to see how the "judges" rate it in the lunchroom. The most practical way to determine consumer acceptance is to visit the school lunch scene where it is possible to overhear children's candid comments on the food and to observe the food that is left on the plates. Such visitations are essential to correct gross errors in expected acceptance.

When planning school menus, it is wise to consider the racial and cultural backgrounds of the children in the school and to include regularly some foods typical of the groups represented. Familiarity with foods helps increase acceptance of the lunch program. Then some new, closely related foods may be added.

This approach is especially important when most of the children are from homes where a limited menu is usually served.

PHYSICAL FACILITIES

Once the menus have been determined, it is also necessary for the school lunch supervisor to view the setting in which the children eat. Although children may seem to ignore the physical arrangements for a meal, a comfortable, pleasing environment will promote acceptance. Such influences are subtle and can best be assessed by a well-trained, sensitive individual. It may seem unimportant, but children will eat a meal more eagerly when they are able to use the silverware. Bent fork tines or very cheap stainless steel utensils with sharp edges do not feel comfortable in the hand or mouth and so discourage consumption of food. Ideally, younger elementary children will have smaller silver to use.

Food should be served neatly and carefully to make each plate attractive. Many children like to have their food arranged on the plate so that the different foods are not overlapping or running together. Distinct servings have far more appeal to children than do jumbled plates. It is also desirable to have the food hot when it is served, but this factor appears to be less important to children than to adults.

Efficient service is essential because there are ordinarily many children to feed, and school schedules usually allow only a short lunch period. Inefficient service will cause some children to have a long wait in line and a very short time for eating.

In addition, tables should be comfortable for children, of a convenient height and equipped with movable benches or chairs. If fixed benches are used, they should be close enough to the table so that the smaller youngsters can reach their plates without difficulty. Tables should be located in a pleasant room or in a shady area outdoors. In a noisy, very hot setting the consumption of food becomes a chore to be avoided or cut to a minimum.

SCHEDULING

Cooperation is needed from the school administration if a really smooth-running lunch program is to be achieved. The time schedule for the school day should include a reasonable time for serving and eating food. Many schools allow such a limited lunch time that children literally have to gobble their food to finish in the allotted time. Slow eaters simply cannot consume a complete meal in 10 minutes, yet this is the amount of time available if they happen to be near the end of the lunch line.

This is a very real problem in many schools. It would seem far wiser to avoid such a chaotic lunch break by adding approximately 10 minutes to the lunch hour.

In schools having two or more shifts for lunch service, it is advisable to serve the younger children first. An early lunch helps keep the younger children from becoming too tired to eat.

THE LUNCH ROOM IN ACTION

Supervision of the lunch area should be undertaken with the idea of making the lunch time as pleasant as possible for all the children. A few suggestions may solve most of the problems that arise in the typical school lunch program.

One suggestion that could be used to advantage by many schools is to allow the children to sit where they wish, whether they have brought their own lunch or are participating in the hot lunch programs. When "hot lunch children" and "cold lunch children" have to sit in different areas, acceptance of the hot lunch program diminishes. Children who otherwise would be participating in the hot lunch program may elect to bring a cold lunch just so they can eat with their friends who regularly bring sack lunches. Certainly, it is desirable to do everything possible to encourage participation in the hot lunch program. Unless parents are careful about its contents, the sack lunch is likely to be less adequate nutritionally than the hot lunch available at school.

An adult monitoring the school lunch situation can be quite effective in controlling food trading. Children in elementary school seem to thrive on the bargaining that can take place at lunch time if trading is permitted. Some children may be particularly clever at this and end up with three or four desserts for which they may have bartered the rest of their meal. Not only do these entrepreneurs end up with a poorly balanced diet, but changes also take place in the meals of the children with whom they have been trading. Menus in the school lunch program are designed to provide an adequate meal when each child receives the planned portions of each of the foods on the menu. Obviously, when trading occurs, lunches will bear little resemblence to the original menu.

VENDING MACHINES

Vending machines are not actually a part of the lunch program, and yet they have a significant influence on the food items eaten by children while they are at school. Many schools have vending machines available on school grounds, and these machines make selected food items available to students. The presence and contents of vending machines have been the subject of hot debates in communities. One of the loudest arguments in favor of vending machines has been the money raised by student groups who receive a portion of the machines' profits. On the opposite side is the concern that vending machines are contrary to good nutrition because they compete directly with the Type A lunch offering.

There is no single answer to the issue. Vending machines can be stocked only with items of high nutrient density to eliminate complaints of the nutritional crimes they perpetrate. However, sales may plummet when this is done, and this could result in a canceled school excursion because of fewer funds from the vending machines. Conversely, favorite snack items may be the only items in the machines; this may bring in plenty of money for trips but limit the opportunity for good nutrition. Some schools lock their vending machines until after the lunch period. Various solutions have been found in different localities. Persons interested in promoting good nutrition among elementary school children should be aware of vending machines, as well as the school lunch room and the nutrition education program in the classroom.

Good nutrition at lunchtime also is threatened when schools have open campuses and students can leave to eat at fast food outlets or other nearby facilities. Although fast food chains have been working to improve the nutrient content of their menu items, the usual choices made by customers provide a less adequate nutrient intake and often more calories than would be available in the Type A lunch. For school children who cannot go home for lunch, selection of all five items in the Type A lunch definitely is the wisest choice nutritionally.

NUTRITION EDUCATION

The elementary grades are an important time to emphasize nutrition education in the classroom, as well as in the lunchroom. An enthusiastic, imaginative approach is essential.

The study of nutrition need not be a regimented, dull routine done entirely with a book, but can take on many forms. After an adequate elementary introduction to nutrition has been given, this subject can be integrated very effectively with other courses throughout the school year. The program should be based on a study of the food groups, and this theme should be developed carefully with the students.

To supplement classroom work, field trips might be taken. The five food groups could be given emphasis if the class made five field trips, one to study some specific aspect of foods in each of the food groups. For instance, a trip to the dairy to observe the milking of cows and the subsequent pasteurization and bottling of milk could be a very informative nutrition lesson for elementary school children. If possible, slightly older children could be taken to watch cheese-making; many dairies make

A vegetable garden on the school grounds can become a valuable laboratory for teaching about nutrition and some of the sources of nutrients.

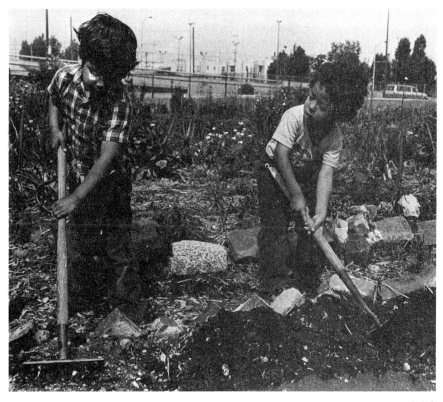

cottage cheese, and some classes probably could observe the more complex manufacturing of cheddar and other cheese. In lieu of such opportunities, interest in dairy products could be stimulated by making cottage cheese or ice cream in the schoolroom. This type of lesson can be reinforced by summarizing the field experiences and including a discussion of the value of such foods in the diet.

Another interesting field trip is a tour to a local cannery or freezing plant to observe the processing of fruits or vegetables. An alternative to emphasize the value of fruits and vegetables would be to plant a small vegetable garden at the school so that the children could observe the transition from seed to the mature food. The vegetables could then be cooked and served to the children as a culmination of this project.

Another project to stimulate interest in fruits and vegetables is to have the class dry fresh produce. If the group has grown produce in a small garden, some of the food can be washed, sliced, blanched (if necessary), and dried. In some areas, the food can be placed on drying racks and covered with cheesecloth before being placed in the sun to dry. However, oven-drying at the lowest possible temperature setting of 140°F is an overnight method of drying fruits and vegetables. If grapes are available, children would find it very interesting to make raisins from the grapes. These dried foods not only make nourishing snacks for elementary school children, but they also provide the opportunity to teach the structure of plant foods and aid students in understanding the role of water in cells.

The bread and cereal group gains considerable interest when a class visits a flour mill or a cereal manufacturer, but a trip to a local bakery is suitable when mills or manufacturing plants are not accessible. Various baking projects could be accomplished effectively in the classroom with the use of a portable electric oven or frying pan.

The meat category might be studied by visiting a farm, a large aquarium, an egg ranch, stock yards, or a fish hatchery. Students will gain a greater appreciation of the diversity of foods that are good sources of protein if more than one of these trips can be taken. If time and facilities for field trips are limited, this might be accomplished effectively by a trip to the meat market of a large grocery store.

Children in the upper elementary grades can undertake the project of keeping a week's record of their individual food intake. These records can then be analyzed to see whether individual children are consuming adequate diets. The Daily Food Guide is a convenient standard for this evaluation. When shortages have been assessed, suggestions can be worked out for improving dietary habits. Obviously, such an ambitious project is for the upper elementary grades.

In conjunction with a nutrition unit in the fifth or sixth grade, a dentist could talk about the roles of the various nutrients in promoting sound teeth. An additional perspective can be added by inviting a physician to visit the class to discuss the importance of good dietary habits for optimal growth and physical performance. Dietitians can provide sound information to the class about recommended dietary patterns and other ideas on how to be well nourished.

Another project for the upper elementary grades is a careful study of the school lunch program, in which students keep a record of the food eaten at lunch time. With this information, they begin to consider and appreciate the influence of food preferences and prejudices on nutrition of the individual and the group. After studying the consumption patterns at their school, the older elementary children could work with the school lunch supervisor and plan a week's menus for the school lunch program. Such a project is more educational and meaningful when it is possible to use these menus in school. The class can learn a great deal from eating the meals they have planned and from observing the reactions of other children to the menus.

Nutrition can be brought very effectively into social studies units because malnutrition is commonplace in some parts of the world. For example, protein-calorie malnutrition is found in some areas of India, Africa, Central America, and South America. Some children are blind as a result of a severe vitamin deficiency. United Nations films are available that will show such conditions of the people as well as their nutritional problems.

Social studies units on the locale in which school children live may also include some nutrition work. For example, a fourth-grade class in California was studying California Indians of the past. When the diets of early Indians in various sections of California were studied, nutrition began to assume greater importance in the eyes of the students. The class found that the Indians along the coast had a more prosperous, flourishing civilization than did those living in the desert regions. There were several reasons for this, but one significant contributing factor certainly was the diet of the Indians along the coast. These Indians were somewhat larger in stature and a bit more advanced

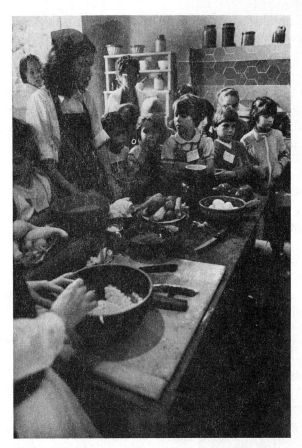

This lesson on Creole cookery and the exotic ingredients used in the recipes adds an exciting realism to the study of these people in Social Studies.

in their civilization than the inland Indians, a difference that could be explained by the large amount of fish and shellfish in the diet of the coastal Indians. This provided considerably more protein than was available to the inland Indians, who had a limited vegetarian diet.

It is an interesting sidelight to note that nutrition can be drawn into an amazing variety of disciplines. For instance, nutrition knowledge was one avenue explored by archaeologists in an attempt to estimate the population of an extinct Indian population group. By measuring the quantity of shells thrown into refuse dumps by these ancient people after they consumed the shellfish and figuring the minimum amount of fish that would be needed by each person each day, a rough estimate of the population was determined. If a teacher can find such information in the library, it can be brought to the classroom; this will help the study of nutrition come to life and make it fascinating and challenging to the elementary school child.

These examples of nutrition projects have been mentioned to stimulate thought on how nutrition can be made more interesting and meaningful to the elementary school child. Parroting nutrition education information to children is a waste of time; no subject is interesting when it is taught in such an unimaginative manner. it is the responsibility of the teacher to plan and carry out projects that graphically illustrate the importance of nutrition for children in this age group.

One of the goals of nutrition education programs for elementary school children is the development of a basic, elementary knowledge of nutrition. Evaluation of the effectiveness of educational programs indicates that well-planned units of study can be valuable in teaching knowledge of nutrition. Difficulty is encountered in achieving a second goal: accomplishing behavioral change to modify dietary patterns consistent with the knowledge acquired.

Fisk (1979) effectively cited the problem that plagues nutrition educators continually; specifically, the difficulty lies in motivating people, whether children or adults, to apply basic nutrition information to their daily food choices. This area of nutrition education has been drawing increasing attention from researchers. In assessing approaches toward this end, Fisk describes three categories of people seeking nutrition infor-

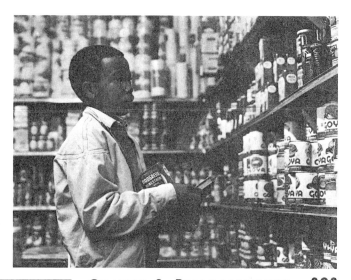

Nutrition education in school is important to help preadolescents begin to gain the knowledge they will need to select good nutrition in the grocery store.

mation: 1) those seeking just enough nutrition information to be able to select the basic necessities of a diet for good health, 2) persons desiring to obtain additional information along specific lines of nutritional knowledge, and 3) people preparing for careers as professionals in this field. According to Fisk, nutrition education has focused too much on the needs and interests of the second and third group, leaving a paucity of material designed to meet the basic needs of the vast majority of consumers of nutritional information (which includes elementary school children). Tests in the field throughout California have served as the basis of Fisk's conclusion regarding the need for nutrition education for daily living and food choices. Despite the considerable debate conducted among nutritionists about the adequacy of the food groups as a teaching tool, Fisk strongly endorsed the use of this approach in food selection and menu planning. In several states extensive educational programs based on application of the food groups to daily living have been shown to be effective in initiating changes in food selection. Nutrition educators also need to be aware of the current "nutrition" messages being received by elementary school children from television, particularly television commercials. Children viewing advertisements will pressure parents to buy the featured food, a choice that may not be consistent with the best nutritional patterns for children or parents. Parents may welcome information from professional nutritionists about the actual nutritional impact of foods currently being marketed on television. Such information will aid parents considerably when they are being pressured by their children to buy advertised products. In fact, elementary school children can be encouraged to examine the facts behind advertised foods and determine whether or not the items are good choices for them. This can be the beginning of developing informed consumers. Clearly, nutrition education must occur in the context of the lives of the people involved in the learning process, whether they are elementary school children or older persons.

SUMMARY

The nutritional needs of elementary school children gradually increase as they continue to grow and prepare for the adolescent growth spurt. The needs of boys, beginning at approximately 11 years of age, increase more rapidly than those of girls. The elementary school period is particularly important as a time to learn about and develop an enduring interest in applied nutrition. A firm foundation in good nutrition practices at this age will greatly facilitate the achievement of good nutrition during the demanding adolescent period.

Parents need to work with their children as individuals to improve the nutritional status of elementary school children. It is certainly true that the final responsibility for helping each child to be well nourished lies with the parents. Examples set in the home will mold, to a great extent, the dietary habits of children in a family. It is important that parents recognize the exemplary influence that they exert and make every effort to establish healthful dietary patterns in their children. Parents also need to be aware of the nutrition "education" their children receive from television.

By implementing an effective nutrition education program in both classroom and lunchroom, the school can also be an important influence on the lives of its students. Creative teachers will find ways to bring nutrition into the classroom in an interdisciplinary presentation when appropriate, thus giving nutrition a broader and deeper meaning to the children. This interest aroused in school can serve as the foundation for continuing nutrition projects in the home.

BIBLIOGRAPHY

AMERICAN ACADEMY OF PEDIATRICS Ten-state nutrition survey: pediatric perspective. *Pediat. 51:* 1095. 1973.

AMERICAN HEART ASSOCIATION Committee report: Diet in the healthy child. *Circulation 67;* 1411A. 1983.

ANONYMOUS Timely statement of the American Dietetic Association: nutrition guidance for child athletes in organized sports. *J. Am. Diet. Assoc. 96(6):* 610. 1996.

ANONYMOUS Position of ADA, SNE, and ASFSA: school-based nutrition programs and services. J. Am. Diet. Assoc. 95(3): 367. 1995.

BARANOWSKI, T., ET AL Low validity of a seven item fruit and vegetable food frequency questionnaire among third-grade students. J. Am. Diet. Assoc. 97(1): 66. 1997.

BORJA, M.E., ET AL New lower-fat dessert recipes for the school lunch program are well accepted by children. *J. Am. Diet. Assoc. 96(9):* 908. 1996.

CROSS, A.T., ET AL Snacking patterns among 1800 adults and children. *J. Am. Diet. Assoc. 94(12):* 1398. 1994.

DWYER, J.T. AND J. MAYER Beyond economics and nutrition: Complex basis of food policy. *Science 1888:* 566. 1975.

FISK, D. Successful program for changing children's eating habits. *Nutr. Today 14(3):* 6. 1979.

FOLEY, C.S., ET AL Establishing need for nutrition education: III. Elementary students' nutrition knowledge, attitudes, and practices. *J. Am. Diet. Assoc. 83:* 564. 1983.

FRANKLE, R.T. Obesity a family matter; creating new behavior. *J. Am. Diet. Assoc. 85:* 597. 1985.

GETLINGER, M.J., ET AL Food waste is reduced when elementary school children have recess before lunch. *J. Am. Diet. Assoc. 96(9):* 906. 1996.

GUARINO, M.A., ET AL Program of nutrition education for school and community. *J. Nutr. Ed. 16:* 125. 1984.

GUSSOW, J.D. Counternutritional messages of TV ads aimed at children. *J. Nutr. Ed. 4:* 48. 1972.

HERTZLER, A. Children's food patterns — a review: I. Food preferences and feeding problems. *J. Am. Diet. Assoc. 83:* 551. 1983.

HERTZLER, A. Children's food patterns — a review: II. Family and group behavior. *J. Am. Diet. Assoc. 83:* 555. 1983.

HURD, S.L., ET AL Evaluation of implementation of the U.S. Dietary Guidelines into the child nutrition programs in Texas. *J. Am. Diet. Asoc. 96(9):* 904. 1996.

LOWENBERG, M.E. Development of food patterns. *J. Am. Diet. Assoc. 65:* 262. 1974.

NICKLAS, T.A. Dietary studies of children: the Bogalusa Heart Study experience. *J. Am. Diet. Assoc. 95(10):* 1127. 1995.

NOVOTNY, R., ET AL Adolescent milk consumption, menarche, birth weight, and ethnicity influence height of women in Hawaii. *J. Am. Diet. Assoc. 96(8):* 802. 1996.

PLINER, P. Family resemblance in food preferences. *J. Nutr. Ed. 15(4):* 137. 1983.

POLLITT, E. Does breakfast make a difference in school? *J. Am. Diet. Assoc. 95(10):* 1135. 1995.

SHAPIRO, L.R., ET AL Obesity prognosis: longitudinal study of children from age of 6 months to 9 years. *Am. J. Pub. Health 74:* 1984.

SNYDER, M.P., ET AL Reducing the fat content of ground beef in a school food service setting. *J. Am. Diet. Assoc. 94(10):* 1135. 1994.

CHAPTER NINE
Adolescents

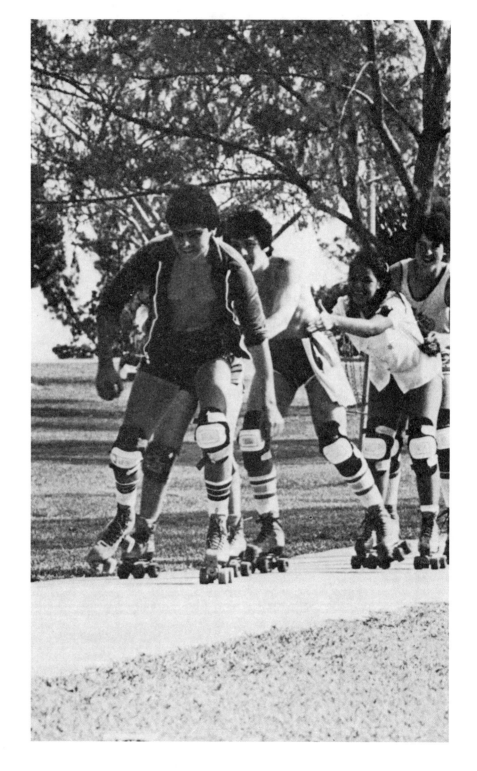

ADOLESCENCE — A PERIOD OF CHANGE

The adolescent period is a time of significant change, both physically and psychologically. The physical changes of sexual

329

maturation are accompanied by impressive growth, particularly in some boys, necessitating a careful examination of nutritional needs and the selection of foods to provide needed nutrients. At the same time, psychological and social pressures begin to interact to influence food behaviors. From the period of latency, young people emerge into a time when they have high nutritional needs and increasing independence in deciding how to meet these demands. No wonder this stage of development is viewed with both amazement and concern by adolescents and parents alike!

ADOLESCENCE
Usually designates the period from the time sex hormones are secreted, secondary sex characteristics develop, and sexual maturation is completed, until growth stops.

The adolescent is viewed by psychologists and nutritionists in different ways, yet they find certain similarities. Psychologists identify this period as a time when the individual is attempting to develop an understanding of himself and find a way

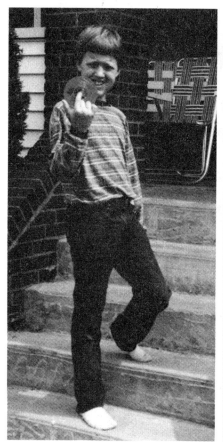
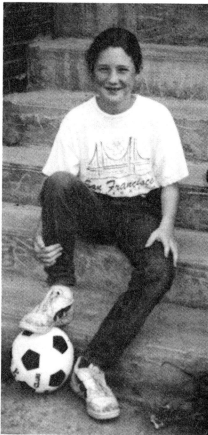

Teenagers (especially boys) have high nutrient needs.

of relating to the adult world. The nutritionist views this period also as a time for significant growth in a physical sense. Adults tend to be concerned about the adolescent period because behavior patterns at this age are often different from any other time in life. The teenage period frequently brings considerable concern with appearance and desire for a high degree of conformity to the peer group. These two aspects of development may manifest themselves in nutritional problems for a number of adolescents.

The nutritional status of teenagers influences their own sense of well-being and affects relationships with family and friends. People have long recognized that proper diet promotes a general sense of well-being, a contribution of importance to teenagers and persons of all ages.

NUTRITIONAL NEEDS OF THE TEENAGER

The tremendous growth typical of the adolescent dictates changes in nutrient needs after the period of latency in the preadolescent years. The mean peak rate of height gain for boys (Tanner, 1966) was measured at 4.06 inches per year, whereas the mean peak rate for girls was 3.54 in! No wonder trouser legs and jacket sleeves shrink as if by magic during the adolescent growth spurt. Weight increases are also a normal part of adolescent growth, with boys gaining an average of about 21.6 lb per year during their peak growth period, and girls gaining about 19.4 lb during a comparable time.

The timing of these spectacular growth spurts differs with each sex (see Chapter 2). The average boy will begin his adolescent growth spurt when he enters puberty at about 13, and peak growth period will occur when he is 14. The rate slows at about 15.5 years, but growth usually continues until boys are at least 18 years old. In contrast, girls usually begin their rapid growth spurt at about 11 years of age, and experience their peak rate at age 12; their growth rate begins to slow by the age of 13. Most girls finish their growth by age 17. However, there are wide individual differences in the growth patterns of both boys and girls. Some girls do not reach their peak rate until 13 or 14 years of age, and some boys begin their peak growth rate around age 12.

As noted in Chapter 1, the growth pattern in the teens assumes different dimensions from the preteen period. From the first year of life to adolescence, the legs grow faster than the trunk, accounting for about two-thirds of the body's growth. However, this situation changes in the teens and the trunk's growth comprises about two-thirds of the total growth occurring during adolescence, bringing the body's proportions to those found in adults.

The RDA for boys and girls (Tables 9.1 and 9.2) are reflective of the dynamic nature of growth during the teens. The allowances for energy, vitamin A, thiamin, riboflavin, niacin,

PUBERTY
Period of sexual change and growth, beginning with the secretion of sex hormones and development of secondary sex characteristics, until sexual maturity has been reached.

TABLE 9.1   RDA and AI for Boys and Girls Ages 11–13 and 14–18[a,b]

Nutrient (daily amounts)	Ages 11–13		Ages 14–18	
	Boys	Girls	Boys	Girls
Calcium (mg)	1300	1300	1300	1300
Phosphorus (mg)	**1250**	**1250**	**1250**	**1250**
Magnesium (mg)	**240**	**240**	**410**	**360**
Vitamin D[c] (μg)	5	5	5	5
Fluoride (mg)	2	2	3	3
Thiamin (mg)	**0.9**	**0.9**	**1.2**	**1.0**
Riboflavin (mg)	**0.9**	**0.9**	**1.3**	**1.0**
Niacin (mg)	**12**	**12**	**16**	**14**
Vitamin B$_6$ (mg)	**1.0**	**1.0**	**1.3**	**1.2**
Folate (μg)	**300**	**300**	**400**	**400[e]**
Vitamin B$_{12}$ (μg)	**1.8**	**1.8**	**2.4**	**2.4**
Pantothenic acid (mg)	4	4	5	5
Biotin (μg)	20	20	25	25
Choline (mg)	375	375	550	400

[a]Adapted from Food and Nutrition Board, Institute of Medicine — National Academy of Sciences Dietary Reference Intakes: Recommended Intakes for individuals. Washington, D.C. 1998.
[b]Adequate Intakes (AI). Bold values are RDA.
[c]Values in the table from which this is adapted cover ages 9–13.
[d]As cholecalciferol. 1 μg = 40 IU Vitamin D.
[e]In view of evidence linking folate intake with neural tube defects in the fetus, it is recommended that women capable of becoming pregnant consume 400 μg of synthetic folic aicd from fortified foods and/or supplements in addition to intake of food folate from a varied diet.

vitamin B$_6$, vitamin E, vitamin K, magnesium, and zinc are notably higher for boys than for girls between the ages of 15 and 18.

The distinct difference in protein recommendations for the two sexes between the ages of 15 and 18 is an indication of the difference in growth patterns. The high iron intake for adolescent girls reflects the needs of menstruation.

Even when the rapid growth period slows down, there is a continuing need for calcium; this mineral continues to be laid down in the body to enhance the bone mass of both young men and women. Increase in bone mass continues well beyond adolescence, and in fact, even into the fourth decade of life. This fact emphasizes the need for adolescents and young adults to continue conscientious patterns of milk consumption to provide enough calcium, even though their height no longer increases.

Other noteworthy changes in body composition occur during the teens. Of special interest is the increasing difference in body composition between boys and girls during the adolescent growth period. Boys tend to develop more lean body

TABLE 9.2   RDA Boys and Girls Ages 11–14 and 15–18[a,b]

Nutrient (daily amounts)	Ages 11–14		Ages 15–18	
	Boys	Girls	Boys	Girls
Protein (g)	45	46	59	44
Vitamin A (µg RE)[c]	1000	800	1000	800
Vitamin E (mg α-TE)[d]	10	8	10	8
Vitamin K (µg)	45	45	65	55
Vitamin C (mg)	50	50	60	60
Iron (mg)	12	15	12	15
Zinc (mg)	15	12	15	12
Iodine (µg)	150	150	150	150
Selenium (µg)	40	45	50	50

[a]Adapted from Food and Nutrition Board, Institute of Medicine — National Academy of Sciences Dietary Reference Intakes: Recommended Intakes for individuals. Washington, D.C. 1998.
[b]Based on a weight of 45 kg (99 lb) and height of 157 cm (62 in) for boys 11–14; weight of 46 kg (101 lb) and height of 157 cm (62 in) for girls 11 –14; weight of 66 kg (145 lb) and height of 176 cm (69 in) for boys 15–18; and weight of 55 kg (120 lb) and height of 163 cm (64 in) for girls 15–18.
[c]Retinol equivalents. 1 retinol equivalent = 1 µg retinol or 6 µg β-carotene.
[d]α-Tocopherol equivalents. 1 mg d-α-tocopherol = 1 α-TE.

mass than girls; girls have about two-thirds the lean body mass that the average teenage boy has. Girls in this same age bracket usually develop between 1.5 and 2 times as much body fat as boys.

The teenage girl may well envy her male peers during this period, because the number of calories a boy can consume to provide the recommended nutrients permits more frivolous choices than are available to her. She requires considerably fewer calories than a boy of the same age; hence, she must provide herself with all the nutrients she needs in a more restricted quantity of food. To provide the necessary calcium, iron, and vitamins for her body, she must concentrate on eating a well-balanced diet with only a few frills. The teenage boy, on the other hand, is confronted with the delightful responsibility of consuming a large number of calories, and it is likely that many boys will unconsciously meet their needs for the various nutrients simply by attempting to satisfy their ravenous appetites. Conscious menu planning is certainly still advisable for boys, but it is less critical than for girls at this time.

NUTRITIONAL STATUS OF ADOLESCENTS

Various nutritional status studies have been conducted in recent years in an attempt to determine more fully the role of nutrients in the body and establish the extent of nutritional deficiencies in the American population. The conclusions reached regarding the nutrition of teenagers in the United States have long been a source of great concern.

The U.S. Department of Agriculture's Continuing Survey of Food Intake by Individuals revealed that in 1989 adolescents were not eating as well as young children (Table 9.3). A particular concern for teenage girls was their intake of calcium. For the entire group between the ages of 12 and 18, the mean intake of calcium was only 65 percent of the RDA. In view of the importance of building the body's calcium deposits throughout childhood and early adulthood, this inadequate intake is a likely prelude to osteoporosis later in life.

Another major concern for both boys and girls was their high mean intake of total fat and saturated fat; the mean percent of the RDA for total fat intake was 36 for boys and 35 for girls. The survey showed that 93 percent of the boys and 85 percent of

TABLE 9.3   Intake of Selected Nutrients by Boys and Girls ages 6–11 and 12–18[a]

Nutrient (daily amounts)	Ages 6–11		Ages 12–18	
	Boys	Girls	Boys	Girls
Mean % of RDA				
Energy	87	82	84	73
Protein	226	215	167	141
Iron	116	109	137	72
Calcium	107	103	87	65
Vitamin A	138	134	114	113
Vitamin C	211	165	185	151
Vitamin B_6	110	99	109	96
Niacin	132	123	129	114
Mean % of calories from				
Total fat	34	35	36	35
Saturated fat	13	13	14	13
% meeting 75% of RDA				
Protein	100	100	99	96
Iron	84	90	89	39
Calcium	76	70	66	31
Vitamin A	74	76	54	55
Vitamin C	89	89	80	68
Vitamin B_6	89	74	69	68
Niacin	97	98	85	85
% exceeding guidelines from				
Total fat	81	91	93	85
Saturated fat	88	97	94	91

[a]Adapted from USDA's Continuing Survey of Food Intake by Individuals, 1989. Figures rounded to next whole number.

the girls exceeded the recommended level of 30 percent of calories from fat.

FAMILY INCOME AND NUTRITIONAL STATUS

In general, increasing income increases the likelihood that families (including teenagers) will have an adequate diet, but a high income is not a guarantee of adequate nutrition. In fact, anorectic teenagers are often from families with high incomes. The ability to buy food does not guarantee wise choices. However, families with incomes below the poverty line may have difficulty in buying the foods needed to assure dietary adequacies of all nutrients.

DIETARY PATTERNS

The eating pattern of numerous teenagers today can perhaps best be described as "grazing;" that is, they tend to skip meals and then eat whatever is available when they are hungry. Teenagers may be breakfast skippers, although the vast majority do eat breakfast, according to the USDA Food Consumption Survey. However, there is an increase in breakfast skipping as boys and girls move through the teens. Only one percent of boys between the ages of 11 and 15 skipped breakfast, whereas five percent missed this meal between the ages of 15 and 19. For girls, the incidence of breakfast skipping was somewhat higher — three percent between the ages of 11 and 15 and eight percent between 15 and 19. These figures are defining breakfast as any morning meal, regardless of the menu. Lunches may also be skipped; dinner is the meal eaten most regularly by teenagers.

Snacking is an established part of teenagers' diets. This does not automatically mean that teenagers are poorly nourished. The key to the role of snacks in dietary patterns is the food choices made. Snacks are useful in contributing nutrients not provided by meals when nutrient-dense foods are selected wisely. For example, selection of orange juice as a snack is a good way for a teenager who has skipped breakfast to be sure to get the vitamin C needed.

The popularity of various snack foods has an influence on teenagers because of peer pressure to conform. In fact, snack trends rise and fall, depending on advertising and availability of specialized promotional items, such as the craze for chocolate chip cookies and a few other "homemade" commercial cookies. Pizza has long been a popular choice. Soft drinks are showing continuing growth in consumption by both male and female teenagers, and teenage boys choose soft drinks at a rate far in excess of girls. Unfortunately, some of the growth in soft drink consumption has been at the expense of milk intake. The decrease in milk consumption by adolescents is contrary to providing the necessary nutrients, particularly calcium. Another aspect of this shift in beverage choices is that phosphorus intake in relation to calcium becomes less favorable from lack of calcium and the presence of phosphate, making calcium absorption occur at a reduced level.

Personal food preferences are also reflected in adolescents' choices of snack foods. Young people like more intense flavors and sweeter and saltier foods than adults. These preferences lead to candies, other sweets, and various salty snack foods currently on the market. The food industry has been quite creative in developing snack foods geared toward these preferences.

HEALTH PROBLEMS INFLUENCED BY NUTRITIONAL STATUS

AMENORRHEA
Cessation of menstruation; may be caused by excessive weight loss and resultant depletion of body stores of fat.

Poor nutrition has the potential for causing nutrient-deficiency conditions as well as other health problems. Tuberculosis may be a problem for underweight teenagers. Anorexia nervosa and bulimia (see Chapter 10) are such severe conditions that some teenagers have died from these nutrition-related behaviors; many other teenagers are isolating themselves from family and friends as they pursue the goal of being thin. Amenorrhea develops when fat deposits become seriously depleted. These related problems have come to the fore in the past few years, although they have been in existence for some time previously. Overweight presents added health risks to adolescents, as well as older people. Diabetes is more prevalent in obese people.

NUTRITIONAL DEFICIENCIES

Inadequate calcium intake by teenage girls poses a potential problem for them because of low stores of calcium in the bones. However, frank problems of calcium deficiencies are not evident physically by the assessment techniques used in studies at present. With the increasing concern about the high incidence of osteoporosis among post-menopausal women, this low intake of calcium in the teens had commanded attention among nutritionists; they view the current dietary practices of adolescent girls as an indication of problems in later life.

Low iron intake, particularly among adolescent girls, may result in anemia and accompanying problems of fatigue, lassitude, and general disinterest in school and social interactions. Boys may also have an iron-deficiency problem during their teens as a consequence of the demand for iron for the increasing blood supply and physical changes associated with sexual maturation. Table 9.3 clearly identifies the discrepancy between the RDA and iron intake for adolescent boys and girls. However, iron-deficiency anemia is not automatically a consequence of an iron intake less than the RDA level. Individual cases of anemia can only be determined through careful blood analyses. Iron supplementation will raise the hemoglobin level rather quickly if a teenager has iron-deficiency anemia.

NUTRITIONAL EXCESSES

Protein intake in the form of meats tends to be high in the United States; this is particularly true of adolescent athletes, who have been persuaded that athletic prowess and high protein intake are synonymous. High meat intakes are of concern because they provide not only high protein intakes, but also fat. The full significance of a high intake of fats from meat in heart disease is not yet known. Adolescents, in many instances, could reduce their intake of meat without a detrimental effect on nutrition; they might actually improve their diets because of the consequent reduction in fat.

The balance between food intake and energy expenditure is important to teenagers. Overweight (see Chapter 10) is the result of an imbalance between energy available from food and energy expended. For overweight teenagers, excessive weight is likely due to a comparatively inactive lifestyle. In other words, overweight or obese teenagers may be eating about the same amount of food as their counterparts of normal weight, but their comparatively low energy expenditure as a result of inactivity results in their excessive weight. For these adolescents, a conscious change to a more active lifestyle may be all that is needed to achieve normal weight. For others, dietary changes are also necessary if normal weight is the goal.

RESEARCH INSIGHTS

Stang, J., et al., Relationships between vitamin and mineral supplement use, dietary intake, and dietary adequacy among adolescents. *J. Am. Diet. Assoc.* 100(8): 905. 2000.

Stang, et al. analyzed data from 423 adolescents ages 13–18 who had participated in the Continuing Survey of Food Intakes of Individuals (CSFII), the national study in 1994 that used a 2-day self-reporting of food intake based on the 24 hour recall method and personal interviews, which included questions on use of nutrient supplements. Patterns of nutrient supplement use among the adolescent subjects and determination of a possible relationship between their dietary intake and supplement use were the foci of this study.

About one-third of the adolescents indicated they took nutritional supplements daily or occasionally; within this group, approximately half of the subjects reported daily supplementation, and roughly one-third of users took individual nutrients. Examination of actual food intakes revealed that supplement users were more likely to be eating a nutrient-dense diet than those not taking nutrient supplements. However, more than 30% of the females and a somewhat smaller percentage of males ingested less than 75% of the RDA for vitamins A, B_6, C, and E and for calcium and zinc. Although this study reviewed data on a rather small sample of adolescents, it serves to underline the fact that this population group likely is setting the stage for less than optimal health later because of the relationships between calcium and osteoporosis and possible influences of vitamins on development of cancer and heart disease. Stang, et al. emphasized the importance of developing preventive programs to influence adolescents' nutrition positively so their future health may be enhanced.

ADOLESCENT CONCERNS AND THEIR RELATION TO NUTRITION

From the preceding discussion, it is apparent that inadequate nutrition can complicate the adolescent period in a variety of ways. The nutritional status of many teenagers, particularly girls, in the United States is less than optimal. Before it is possible to overcome inadequacies, however, it is necessary to identify the factors that contribute to the problem.

PHYSICAL IMAGE

An important problem for adolescents is the need to achieve a desirable body size. Height is perhaps of more concern to teenage boys than girls because, as interest in the peer group and the opposite sex increases, a certain amount of prestige is given to taller boys. An atypical height is a matter of grave concern for many teenagers.

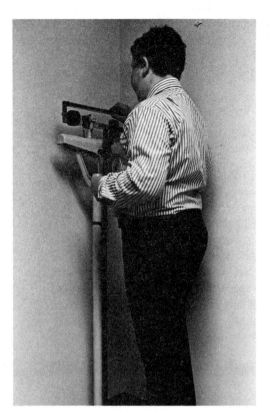

Adolescents are particularly concerned with physical image, making weight control a serious problem for some.

Physical growth is one way in which adolescents assess their own and their peers' maturity. It is true that growth patterns are variable, but proper nutrition throughout childhood and adolescence is essential if one's own growth potential is to be achieved. Adjustments to adolescence can be helped by proper nutrition throughout childhood and the teens, so that normal physical growth occurs.

The teenager must achieve not only the desired physical height, but also the appropriate weight for height. For boys, this usually means large quantities of food must be eaten daily to fill out their frames during this period of rapid growth. The problem of eating enough food is reduced for many adolescent girls because of the minimal physical activity.

Two important motivating forces that are directly opposed to sensible nutrition in girls of this age are a desire to be slim and a desire to be independent. The motivation for slimness apparently stems, at least in part, from the desire to be attractive to

Teenage girls are sometimes extremely thin as a consequence of anorexia nervosa. Even when anorectics become painfully thin, they may still be eating very little food to attempt to lose still more weight.

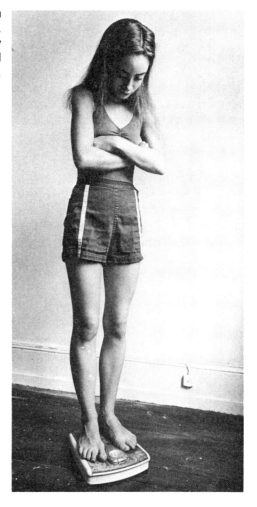

boys. The desire for independence may lead teenage girls to attempt to achieve the desired slim figure by completely ignoring sound advice on nutrition.

The common problem for the teenage girl is usually that of fulfilling the body's nutritional requirements without consuming excessive calories. Two factors complicate the achievement of good nutrition by many female adolescents: a penchant for snacks (regardless of nutritive value) and a preoccupation with being thin. Snack foods are often high in calories and low in nutrients. When food is served at gatherings, it is common for many teenage girls to eat the snack and then reduce their intake at mealtime. The result is that they consume close to the recommended number of calories each day, but they may not receive adequate amounts of vitamins and minerals.

The second obstacle to good nutrition is the teenager's concept of a beautiful figure. To fit the expected figure pattern of slenderness, bordering on skinniness, many teenage girls feel that they must severely limit their caloric intake each day. Unfortunately, such a restriction usually means that important nutrients will be consumed in inadequate amounts.

INDEPENDENCE

One of the key tasks of adolescents is to become independent, a relationship quite different from the dependence on parents that characterizes earlier stages of childhood. Independence tends to be an elusive goal in some aspects, such as financial independence, during the teens. However, adolescents normally seek independence in areas where they believe they can be autonomous. Diet is one of the areas chosen as a point for exhibiting independent behavior. A loose translation of independent behavior is that some teenagers eat whatever and whenever they choose. Others may make choices very much in line with the dietary patterns they learned before entering the teens.

Fortunately, there are many nourishing ways of eating. Teenagers are not required to eat exactly as their parents do. Fast foods and wisely selected snacks can be readily incorporated into a nourishing diet that is consistent with the teenager's need to be different from parents and at ease with peers. However, wise selections on the part of an independent teenager require a functional knowledge of applied nutrition. Fast food restaurants are an important part of many teenagers' domains. Teenagers who rely on these restaurants should be aware of the nutritional benefits and pitfalls associated with the choices they make at fast food establishments. A summary of the nutritional value of selected fast foods is provided in Table 9.4. Summaries of the nutritional value of selected meals at an American fast food restaurant are presented in Table 9.5.

TIME PRESSURES

In the hectic life of the typical city teenager today, one of the biggest obstacles to meeting nutritional needs is the problem of finding time to eat. If an individual is active in school affairs, it may be necessary to leave for school very early in the morning

TABLE 9.4   Nutritional Contribution of Selected Food Items Commonly Available at a Fast Food Operation[a]

Nutrient	Egg McMuffin		Hamburger		Cheeseburger		1/4 lb Burger		1/4 lb Cheeseburger		Big Mac	
	Actual	%[b]	Actual	%	Actual	%	Actual	%	Actual	%	Actual	%
Calories[c]	310	—	250	—	310	—	415	—	520	—	560	—
Protein (g)	18	27	13	20	16	25	27	41	41	48	26	40
Fat (g)[c]	11	—	10	—	14	—	19	—	28	—	32	—
Carbohydrate (g)[c]	35	—	28	—	20	—	33	—	36	—	41	—
Vitamin A (μg RE)	460	9	165	3	315	6	260	5	395	8	210	4
Vitamin D (μg)	80	20	17	4	25	6	45	11	50	13	33	8
Vitamin E (mg)	0.7	2	0.3	1	0.2	1	0.3	1	0.5	2	1.3	4
Vitamin C (mg)	4	6	4	6	4	6	3	5	5	9	5	8
Folacin (mg)	0.02	5	0.02	5	0.02	6	0.02	7	0.03	8	0.03	8
Niacin (mg)	3.1	16	3.7	19	3.9	20	6.5	32	7.1	36	6.3	32
Riboflavin (mg)	0.5	27	0.4	21	0.5	30	0.6	37	0.7	42	0.6	38
Thiamin (mg)	0.4	25	0.2	12	0.2	13	0.2	15	0.3	17	0.3	18
Vitamin B_6 (mg)	0.14	7	0.14	7	0.15	7	0.30	15	0.31	16	0.24	12
Vitamin B_{12} (μg)	0.9	15	0.8	13	1.0	17	1.9	31	2.3	39	1.5	26
Calcium (mg)	0.17	17	0.05	5	0.14	14	0.07	7	0.23	23	0.16	16
Phosphorus (mg)	0.38	38	0.12	12	0.19	19	0.23	23	0.37	37	0.29	29
Iodine (μg)	27	18	47	31	47	31	66	44	84	56	77	51
Iron (mg)	2.5	14	2.6	14	2.3	13	3.8	21	3.9	22	3.8	21
Magnesium (mg)	0.02	4	0.02	4	0.02	4	0.03	7	0.03	8	0.03	8
Sodium (g)[c]	1.3	—	0.5	—	0.8	—	0.7	—	1.2	—	1.1	—

[a] Adapted from *Nutritional Anaylsis of Food Served at McDonald's Restaurants*, McDonald Corp., Oakbrook, IL.
[b] Percent of US RDA.
[c] — (em dash indicates) no US RDA established.

TABLE 9.5   Nutritional Contributions of Various Menus Available at a Fast Food Operation[a]

Nutrient	Percent of US RDA Provided by French Fries, Chocolate Shake, and:						
	2 Hamburgers	1/4 lb Cheeseburger	1/2 lb Hamburger	Big Mac	Filet of Fish	Cheeseburger	Hamburger
Calories[b]	1030	1055	950	1090	940	840	780
Protein	62	70	63	62	45	47	42
Vitamin A	7	8	5	4	2	6	3
Vitamin D	17	22	20	17	18	15	13
Vitamin E	2	2	1	5	4	1	1
Vitamin C	28	24	20	23	17	21	21
Thiamin	32	30	28	30	28	26	24
Riboflavin	78	78	73	73	57	66	57
Niacin	51	50	47	46	29	34	33
Vitamin B_6	27	29	28	26	19	21	20
Folacin	16	14	12	13	11	12	11
Vitamin B_{12}	52	65	57	52	39	43	39
Calcium	52	65	48	58	51	55	47
Phosphorus	65	78	64	60	65	60	53
Iron	22	23	22	23	20	19	19
Magnesium	35	29	28	28	16	20	21
Iodide	156	149	137	145	169	125	125

[a]Adapted from *Nutritional Anaylsis of Food Served at McDonald's Restaurants*, McDonald Corp., Oakbrook, IL.
[b]There is no US RDA for calories. Figures represent actual calories available rounded off to nearest 5.

and stay until suppertime for sports, music, and play practice. Additional time is required for commuting to and from school. These demands may mean that the adolescent finds it difficult to have meals with the rest of the family. All too often this leads to informal snacking rather than consumption of a good meal when there finally is time to eat.

FINANCIAL LIMITATIONS

Some teenagers live in families with incomes so low that good nutrition is almost an unattainable goal. Insufficient money is often coupled with inadequate knowledge of nutrition and marketing, with the result that problems in feeding the family become even more complex than they need to be. In some areas, for example, children from low-income families may have money to purchase food at the school lunch program; but they often use it to buy soft drinks rather than milk or other nourishing foods available at the nutrition period and at lunch.

LIMITED KNOWLEDGE OF NUTRITION

Another problem that may lead to poor nutrition is inadequate knowledge of nutrition and lack of appreciation of good nutrition habits. Teenagers frequently have little understanding of what nutrients are contained in different foods and of the role of these nutrients in their bodies. When a person does not understand basic nutrition principles and is unaware of the nutritional content of various foods, it is difficult to choose foods that supply all the body's needs. Deficiency conditions may gradually develop.

Some teenagers are misinformed in matters of nutrition. This can be a real problem for them; they may be pursuing a diet with considerable dedication and enthusiasm, but the diet they think they need may not be nutritionally sound. A familiar example is the high school athlete who religiously consumes protein supplements in his diet, which is already unnecessarily high in protein, while ignoring the fruits and vegetables needed for vitamins and minerals not supplied in meat. Fad diets printed in magazines and books provide another familiar example of nutrition misinformation which can motivate well-intentioned adolescents to follow poor or unsafe reducing diets. These are two examples of the gross nutrition misinformation that can assault teenagers (as well as the rest of the population). Unless they have had a sound nutrition education, adolescents (and possibly their parents) are at risk of poor nutrition as a result of

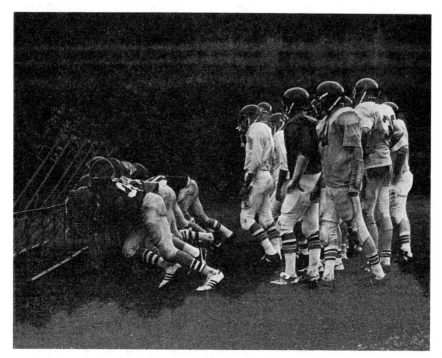

faulty nutrition information. They are also likely to waste money on supplements or other costly and unnecessary items in their efforts to be well nourished.

DIETARY TRENDS OF ADOLESCENTS

SNACKING

Teenagers have a strong need to be accepted by the group. Peer approval is essential, for this is an indication that they are appreciated for being themselves. Feelings of insecurity can be put aside when the group is reinforcing the fact that they measure up to the group's expectations and requirements. A normal part of teenage camaraderie is eating. Thus, snacking is an expected and enjoyable part of everyday life during the teens. Whether snacking is good or bad nutritionally depends on the quality and quantity of foods consumed as snacks. The frequent choices of easy snacking items, such as soda pop, potato chips, and candy, can result in weight problems and less than desirable intakes of several vitamins and minerals. On the other hand, a snack consisting of nonfat milk and raw vegetables can be an important source of essential nutrients without providing excessive calories.

Snacks can provide the relaxing atmosphere important for group interactions in the teens. Elimination of snacks may be detrimental from the perspective of developing satisfying personal relationships. Adolescents should not feel they must avoid snacking if they wish to be well nourished. The key to the situation is to choose snack foods wisely. Foods that complement those eaten at regular meals without resulting in too high a caloric intake for the day are the preferred choices for snacking toward good nutrition. The importance of wise choices is underscored by findings from the Ten-State Nutrition Survey. From a large population sample, specifically black and white teenagers (12 to 14 years old, and 15 to 16 years old) from both low and high income families participating in the study, Thomas and Call (1973) reported that inadequate levels of calcium and iron were the most fequent dietary problem among adolescents who snacked. The snacks themselves were low in these two nutrients, and intake was also insufficient at meals to meet the recommended allowances.

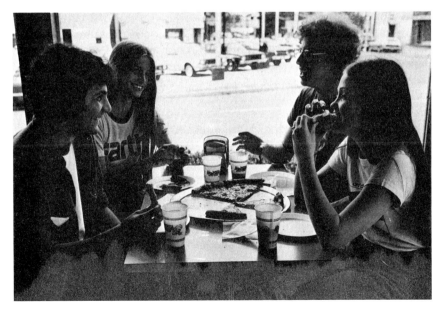

Snacking is an important part of the social scene for adolescents. The choices of foods for snacks need to be made wisely to fit in with the food intake the rest of the day, yet peer pressure may interfere with sensible selections.

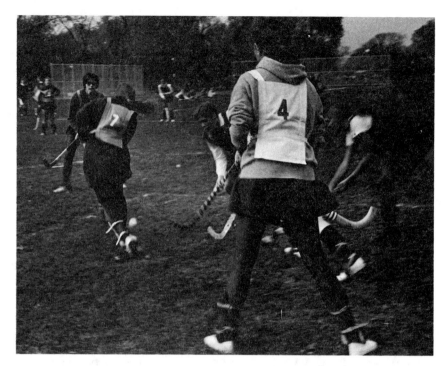

Increased emphasis on active sports is wise for adolescent girls to help maintain good muscle tone and an appropriate weight.

The idea of fortifying popular snack foods to enhance their nutrient contribution to the nutrient intake has been widely discussed. This might be an approach toward assuring adequate nutrition. However, calcium fortification is difficult in these types of foods, and greater stress on use of dairy foods for snacks might be a more practical approach. Amidst the "hand wringing" of concerned nutritionists, there has been some discussion of adding protein to snack foods to fortify them. On the basis of the findings of the Ten-State Nutrition Survey, there is little justification for adding protein to the so-called "empty calorie foods." The intake of protein, riboflavin, ascorbic acid, and thiamin was found to be adequate when total intake of snacks and meals was analyzed.

ERRATIC EATING PATTERNS

The increasing emphasis on independence during the adolescent years is reflected in the eating patterns of many teenagers. When children are young, parents usually structure the family meals tightly; all meals are eaten each day. In contrast to this practice, teenagers begin to run their own schedules.

Breakfast may drop out of the daily routine. This practice may be triggered by other influences, too, such as the example of other family members (particularly the mother) skipping breakfast. Teenagers may also find a few extra minutes of sleep can be more appealing than getting up for breakfast.

Regardless of the reason for missing breakfast, it is clear from the standpoint of the day's total nutrient intake and from performance expectations during the morning hours that an adequate breakfast each day is a sound idea. The problem is one of motivating teenagers to make breakfast a regular part of the day. For girls who are skipping breakfast as a weight control measure, breakfast suggestions for menus that are high in nutrients and low in calories may be the answer. For example, a glass of juice, a glass of nonfat milk, and a bowl of cereal provide a good balance of nutrients with only a modest portion of the day's total calorie requirement. For teens who are struggling to keep their weight down, some attention to planning the entire day's menus can be helpful in demonstrating that there is room within the day's plan to eat a good breakfast. Some teenagers may enjoy a family breakfast with some conversation; others might prefer a solitary breakfast with music to help them wake up slowly. Still others may be skipping breakfast because they are tired of the usual breakfast menus. A hamburger or a hot dog in a bun might be just the answer to starting the day. Creativity in breakfast menus can be encouraged. Bacon and eggs and other typical foods do not have to be the sole selections for breakfast.

VEGETARIAN DIETS

VEGETARIAN DIET
Any of several different diets that omit red meat from the menu.

LACTO-OVO-VEGETARIAN
Person who eats a diet that includes milk (lacto), eggs (ovo), and any foods of plant origin, but excludes meats.

TYPES   Various social movements have had an impact on the dietary patterns of some Americans in the past few years, and some teenagers have been among the population adopting various forms of vegetarian diets. Lacto-ovo-vegetarian diets are rather broad in definition and provide animal foods (in the form of milk and other dairy products, as well as eggs) to round out the nutrients provided by vegetables and other plant foods. This type of vegetarian diet can be very adequate nutritionally. However, some persons practice vegetarianism on a much more narrowly defined dietary basis. The most extreme position is that taken by the vegans, who consume no food of animal origin.

An extreme form, which is even more restricted than the vegan diet, is the fruitarian diet. People practicing this form of vegetarianism eat only fruit, although some also include nuts in the menu. There appear to be far fewer fruitarians than lacto-ovo-vegetarians.

MOTIVATIONS FOR VARIOUS FORMS OF VEGETARIANISM The reason for adopting a diet that contains no animal flesh foods or fish may be religious in origin. Long-established religions with specified meat avoidance include Seventh Day Adventist and Hindu. Seventh Day Adventists have conducted extensive research studies to work out adequate dietary patterns without the use of flesh foods. In contrast, extreme positions on the use of animal foods without appropriate dietary modifications have been adopted by some recent religious cults.

Other vegetarians may espouse this dietary pattern because of concern for the agricultural space required to raise the food to feel animals, space that some feel should be used for raising plants to feed people. Some people refuse to include meat in their diets because of their distaste for killing animal life. Others hold that meats are sources of toxins and other impurities that are not compatible with their philosophy of life.

Vegetarianism is not always a dietary pattern pursued by its followers merely because of attitudes toward meats. There is an emotional value that some vegetarians place on the importance of eating plant foods in their most natural form. This branch of vegetarians has been loud in its criticism of pesticides and chemical fertilizers. Their vegetarian foods are touted to be "organically grown" and free of any type of refinement or chemical (or nutritional) additives. (This "chemical concern" has, of course, drawn many meat eaters into a small corner of the vegetarian philosophy, even though meats continue to occupy a place in their diets.)

Vegetarians in the adolescent and early adult years are described by Erhard (1973) as "usually well educated, self-reliant, socially mobile, and reflect a middle- and upper-class background that is not strongly influenced by ethnic origins." Some are living in communities that follow the vegetarian dictates.

NUTRITIONAL IMPLICATIONS Although properly planned vegetarian diets can provide excellent nutrition, nutritional consequences of more narrowly defined vegetarian diets have been experienced by many teenagers. If all animal products are excluded, devotees of vegan diets may develop pernicious anemia (Chapter 1) from lack of a dietary source of vitamin B_{12} on their

VEGAN
Strict vegetarian diet that eliminates all foods from animal sources, thus eliminating both milk and eggs.

FRUITARIAN
Person who eats only fruits although some also eat nuts.

ZEN MACROBIOTIC DIET

Extreme vegetarian diet with progressive levels of dietary restriction. At the final level, only brown rice is eaten; death can be the result.

strict vegetarian diet. Lacto-vegetarians may develop anemia due to a deficiency of iron. Vegetarian diets that do not include milk may result in deficiences of calcium and riboflavin. The narrow restrictions of the Zen macrobiotic diet lead to possible scurvy, anemia, and lack of protein and calcium, leading to starvation and kidney failure in extreme cases. These extreme diets are particularly harmful if imposed by pregnant and lactating teenagers on their children.

Vegetarian diets, when carefully planned and consumed, can provide excellent nutritional intake (with the possible exception of vitamin B_{12}) if milk and eggs are included. Therefore, adolescents who have elected to become vegetarians have a particular need to study nutrition so that they will be able to formulate menus for themselves that will maintain adequate levels of all essential nutrients. A few nutrition suggestions can be the basis for such planning:

1. Inclusion of milk, cheese, or eggs on a daily basis ensures that the protein provided will have adequate levels of all the essential amino acids.

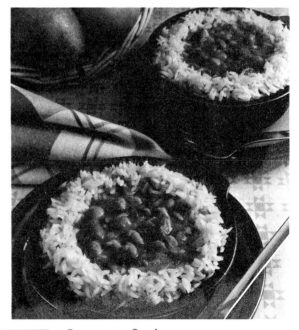

Vegetarian menus need to include protein from complementary sources. In this meal, the limiting amino acid in the beans is offset by the abundance of that amino acid (methionine) in the rice. Conversely, the relatively high level of lysine in the beans complements the low level in the rice.

2. Selection of protein from two complementary plant protein categories (i.e., legumes, cereals, or nuts) at each meal will improve protein utilization.

3. Attention is needed in selecting adequate sources of iron, such as sunflower seeds, nuts, baked beans with molasses, dried fruits, greens, and enriched cereals and bread products.

4. A continuing awareness of weight is necessary to avoid undesirable weight loss on a vegetarian diet.

The first suggestion, that of including some non-meat animal sources of protein, provides insurance for the availability of vitamin B_{12} and the essential amino acids in amounts necessary for maintaining good nutritional status. Milk and cheese have the added advantage of providing important amounts of calcium, a mineral that is deficient in the diets of some teenagers.

The second suggestion is based on the fact that plant proteins individually do not contain the essential amino acids in proper proportions, but they do vary somewhat in their amino acid pattern. One way of handling this blending of protein sources is to combine rice and beans in a ratio of three parts rice to one part beans (on a dry basis). Rice is low in lysine and high in methionine, whereas beans show the reverse pattern; they are high in lysine and low in methionine.

The reason for emphasizing the selection of foods high in iron is twofold. Iron intake, even on a mixed diet, often falls short of the Recommended Dietary Allowances. Second, when meat and meat products are excluded from the diet, these relatively rich sources of iron are also eliminated from the diet. Therefore, it is essential to plan meals to utilize available sources of iron.

Lacto-ovo-vegetarians are less likely to be overweight than people eating a mixed diet in the United States, because the caloric contribution of plant foods tends to be low, owing to low fat content. However, there are some foods, notably nuts and avocados, that are rich in fat. Persons on vegetarian diets having unusually high intakes of these foods or consuming large amounts of fats and oils as table spreads, fried foods, salad dressings, or rich desserts could have a problem with being over-weight. The far more usual problem on vegetarian diets is main-tenance of normal weight. Fruits and vegetables are quite bulky in relation to their caloric content. This characteristic favors a diet with too few calories rather than too many for maintaining desirable weight. If weight is monitored when one is on a vegetarian diet, any significant caloric deficiency will be apparent; minor adjustments can be made to increase fat or carbohydrate in the diet.

Teenagers following a carefully planned lacto-ovo-vegetarian diet will be well nourished and are likely to be a desirable weight. Unfortunately, teenagers who do not have good nutritional guidance from a qualified dietitian or nutritionist (identified ordinarily as a Registered Dietitian or R.D.) may have trouble choosing an adequate vegetarian diet if they exclude milk and eggs. The inclusion of these two foods will help them achieve their goal of being well nourished.

FAD DIETS

The concern with overweight that many teenagers have and the need for establishing independence are key factors in triggering adolescents to follow fad diets. There are many fad diets available in the popular press, and daily conversations on nutrition and dieting contribute still more suggestions for special diets to vulnerable teenagers. Their desire to achieve a more beautiful physical figure causes some girls to try many of these diets, often to the detriment of their mental and physical well-being. A few even develop anorexia nervosa (Chapter 10).

Teenagers with dietary concerns that lead them to unusual intakes of a few selected foods can improve their nutritional status by gaining more knowledge of nutrition and structuring their dietary plans to achieve desired results. Suggestions for weight control diets are made in Chapter 10. The management of diets for athletes is discussed in the next section. Because many adolescents are strongly independent, they are more likely to improve their dietary practices when they are given the knowledge necessary to plan their own diets than when they are harangued to eat what somebody else dictates.

DIETARY NEEDS OF ATHLETES

MEETING NUTRITIONAL DEMANDS

The influence of nutritional status on athletic performance has been the subject of considerable research, as well as myths. Many teenagers are interested in nutrition as a means of improving athletic prowess. The athletic training table has been a long-standing tradition that exemplifies the importance that coaches attach to diet for their teams. Clearly, an adequate diet is necessary for athletes, just as it is for all teenagers, if the body is to have all nutrients present in the diet in sufficient quantities to meet physical needs. Athletes expend more energy in physical activity than many of their more sedentary peers. This increased need for energy requires a larger food intake, commensurate with total energy expended. Since thiamin, niacin, and riboflavin are required to release energy from food, the additional quantity of food will require somewhat more than the recommended intake of these B vitamins. However, the extra food that is selected for the athlete's diet can easily provide this.

On a day-to-day basis, it is not necessary to increase the protein intake of the athlete, because extra physical activity in a day does not increase the body's need for protein. Persons who are very active as a regular way of living will develop more muscle mass than the average person, a physical characteristic that does increase protein need slightly. However, the practices of feeding athletes diets high in protein and of providing them with protein supplements are not warranted. The diet pattern recommended for athletes is the same as for nonathletes; only the quantities need to be changed.

ENERGY NEEDS

The actual need for energy for athletic events is determined by the type of activity as well as its duration. Some sports have a comparatively low energy cost, either because they require only limited muscular effort or they last for only brief periods. Examples of this type of sport activity include archery, horseback riding, and golf. Some sports require endurance and result in a higher energy expenditure. Examples of such activities are skin diving, long- and middle-distance running, and hockey. If sports in the first category are practiced for less than an hour daily, they make only a small increase in the body's need for energy. Sports classified in the category of higher energy expenditure may increase the body's need for energy to a daily total of between 4,000 and 5,000 cal. Table 9.6 lists the energy cost per kilogram of body weight per minute spent in selected sports activities.

The management of food to supply energy during athletic events is often based on misconceptions and superstition rather than demonstrated effect. If an athlete is well nourished, there will be sufficient stores of glycogen and glucose available for immediate energy needs created in a strenuous, short-term

TABLE 9.6 Energy Expended in Selected Sports Activities[a]

Sport	kcal/kg/min[b]	Sport	kcal/kg/min[b]
Badminton	0.097	Skiing, level moderate rate	0.119
Basketball	0.138		
Boxing, sparring	0.138	Skin diving, moderate motion	0.206
Climbing hills			
no load	0.121	Swimming	
11-lb load	0.129	backstroke	0.169
22-lb load	0.140	breast stroke	0.162
		crawl, fast	0.156
Bicycling		crawl, slow	0.128
5.5 mph	0.064	side stroke	0.170
9.4 mph	0.100	treading, normal	0.062
Field hockey	0.134	Table tennis	0.068
Running, cross country	0.163	Tennis	0.109
Running		Walking, normal pace	
9 min/mile	0.193	asphalt road	0.080
7 min/mile	0.228	fields, hillside	0.082
6 min/mile	0.252		

[a]Adapted from Katch, F. and W. McArdle. *Nutrition, Weight Control, and Exercise.* Lea and Febiger. Philadelphia. 2nd ed. 1983.

[b]Obtain body weight in kilograms by dividing weight in pounds by 2.2. Multiply kcal times kg weight times minutes of activity. Kcal figure is the figure in the table. The result of this calculation is the energy expenditure in the activity.

CARBOHYDRATE LOADING Dietary manipulation in which the body is first depleted of glycogen, and then a high-carbohydrate diet is eaten to build glycogen stores to an abnormally high level; this is not recommended at present time.

sports event. Some people think that eating candy will give them quick energy just before a competition. In fact, sucrose or glucose may have the opposite effect, because their presence triggers digestion, absorption, and metabolism of these sugars. Actually, fructose is the best choice of the sugars if sugar in some form is eaten before a competition; but it is only useful for an event that extends over a fairly long period of time, such as cross country or a basketball game. Fructose is preferred because it causes less of a drop in blood sugar level than glucose, which triggers insulin secretion.

For special athletic competitions, some athletes have followed a special dietary regimen — carbohydrate loading — in an effort to produce artifically high levels of glycogen in muscles at the time of an athletic event. This is because glycogen can be used to fuel the body for a longer time than normal before the body's fat stores have to be broken down for energy. This actually can be accomplished, but it places a strain on the body; athletes, particularly adolescents, are being encouraged to avoid carbohydrate loading. To carbohydrate load, an athlete has to follow a low-carbohydrate diet (usually for three days or so) and then exercise so hard that essentially all of the body's glycogen stores are eliminated. The regimen is then reversed by eating very high carbohydrate foods like pasta and baked potatoes to provide abundant starch the day before the competition. Carbohydrate loading is a strain on any athlete and probably should not be done. Clearly, no athlete should follow this stressful diet more than twice a year. Adolescent athletes should definitely avoid carbohydrate loading. The stress of growth and athletic demands are as much as should be asked of any teenager.

A well-balanced diet in sufficient quantities to maintain a desirable weight is considered the best approach to feeding athletes. Emphasis should be put on consuming a diet somewhat higher in starch than often is eaten in the United States and decreasing fat to between 30 and 35 percent of the calories. In contrast to the former image of athletes devouring large steaks while training, the recommendation now is to have small servings of meat and very large baked potatoes or pasta, plus other vegetables, fruits, bread, cereals, and milk needed for their nutrient contributions.

LIQUIDS

One of the important considerations in meeting nutritional needs of athletes is to be sure that adequate liquids are included in the diet. Milk is an appropriate beverage in athletes' diets; alcoholic beverages should definitely be avoided because of their depressant effect and effect on coordination. Tea and coffee may be used in moderate quantities. Their caffeine content has a stimulating effect on athletic performance for some, but there is considerable individual variation.

Replacement of water lost during sports activities is vital to an athlete's well-being. Water is the best liquid to use for fluid replacement. The use of special fluid formulations with added minerals is not recommended because the large amounts of fluid usually required for replacement can alter the normal mineral balance of the body significantly. The amount of water that needs to be replaced can be accurately determined by weighing before and immediately after exercising or participating in a competition. A rough guide is that 1 qt of water is needed to replace every 2 lb lost. Despite the fact that sodium and chloride are lost when an athlete perspires greatly, there is ordinarily no need to provide a salt supplement for replacement. The next meal will normally provide replacement of sufficient salt and lost minerals. The problem immediately following sports activities is water replacement, not mineral replacement.

THE PRE-COMPETITION MEAL

Individual athletes may have special pre-game meals that they find work best for them. However, some general suggestions for most athletes begin with the recommendation that a cup of bouillon be drunk at least three hours before the competition is scheduled to begin. This is because bouillon provides salt far enough in advance so that the thirst it creates can be satisfied with a big drink of water, which is excreted before competing.

The meal itself should also be eaten about three hours before the event. Ideally, this meal will be high in carbohydrate and low in fat and cellulose. Vegetables with a high fiber content are usually deleted from the diet about two days before the game. A spaghetti dinner with crusty French bread and very little butter is a typical pre-game menu. Milk can be the beverage for this meal unless the athlete is lactose-intolerant. Some athletes complain that milk makes their mouths feel like cotton, but there is no scientific proof that milk creates any unusual condition in the mouth.

"MAKING WEIGHT"

Wrestling and some other sports require that competitors weigh in to qualify for the weight category in which they will compete. This can create tremendous pressures on athletes to manipulate their weights to meet the desired weight class. Attempts to increase muscle mass significantly in athletes before sexual maturation has been completed may be detrimental. A good training program for adolescents will provide sufficient exercise to develop the muscles and skills needed for effective competition with other teenagers. A well-balanced diet, often consisting of four meals a day, is the best means of insuring that teenagers who are competing in sports are well nourished.

EDUCATIONAL IMPLICATIONS

Generally athletes are quite concerned about their nutrition, for they recognize that nutrition plays a key role in their performance. However, it is imperative that they receive accurate and useful information. Cho and Fryer (1974) studied the nutrition knowledge of physical education majors at the university level. As a part of the study, the sources of the students' nutrition knowledge were explored. If students rated coaches as being the primary or secondary source of nutrition information, scores for the nutrition knowledge test were lower than for students who ranked their coaches' information as of lesser importance to them. On the test of nutrition knowledge, physical education majors scored significantly lower than students from a basic nutrition class. Because coaches are viewed as an important source of nutrition information by many athletes, and because lower scores in nutrition knowledge were found for students who were relying on coaches for information, there is a compelling argument for including at least a basic nutrition course in the curriculum of physical education majors at the university level; these college graduates would then provide high school athletes better information on dietary needs of an athlete than is currently available. This approach to education for coaches would be most helpful in avoiding the propagation of nutrition fallacies about the need for honey, protein supplements, vitamin supplements, and on ad infinitum!

CASE STUDIES

These two case studies have been selected to illustrate the types of problems that may exist in the diets of some teenagers. They reflect the freedom many teenagers have in the selection of food during the day. In addition, these cases emphasize the importance of developing an appreciation of the value of good nutrition before the individual reaches this independent state.

DAVID

This particular case is of interest because it provides actual proof that children from upper-middle and upperclass families do not automatically have adequate diets. Certainly, a high income combined with the educational achievement of the parents in these social classes may influence the nutritional status of the children, but these factors do not guarantee adequacy. The boy in this study is proof of this; he is the son of a physician.

David, a senior in high school, is 6 ft tall and weighs 152 lb. He is slightly thin and is troubled with acne. As can be observed in the five days of menus listed in Tables 9.7 and 9.8, several changes should be made in his diet to meet David's dietary needs. Intake reflects the common problems of this age group: a hurried breakfast and a snack-type dinner, often eaten hastily with friends rather than family at an organized and well-planned family meal. David needs to change his habits to include a bigger breakfast consisting of juice, a glass of milk, cereal, meat or eggs, and toast. He would probably eat a better breakfast and dinner if the family arranged to eat these meals together. Regular meals in an organized setting would promote increased consumption of milk, fruit, and vegetables. It is interesting to note that his dietary pattern, which included foods often selected by adolescents, provided approximately the recommended level of protein. His vitamin C intake was also adequate. Gross inadequacies were found in the levels of calcium, iron, vitamin A, and the B vitamins. These values were calculated for one day, but a review of total intake for the week shows a continuing pattern of very low consumption of milk, very restricted choices of fruits, and distinctly limited use of vegetables. The narrowness of the diet choices provides potential for inadequate intake of trace minerals in addition to the noted deficiencies.

TABLE 9.7 David's Dietary Record for Five Days

Day	Breakfast	Lunch	Dinner	Snack
Monday	Oatmeal Orange juice	Roast beef sandwich Apple Potato chips	Hamburger in bun Soft drink	Chocolate ice cream
Tuesday	Oatmeal Tomato juice	Ham sandwich Apple Orange	Toasted cheese sandwich Milk	

Wednesday	Scrambled eggs
	Milk
		Beef sandwich
		Apple
			Hot roast beef
			  w/ gravy
			Mashed potatoes
			  w/ gravy
			Soft drink	

Thursday	Oatmeal Orange juice	Roast beef sandwich Apple Potato chips	Hamburger in bun French fries Black coffee	
Friday	Cold cereal w/ milk Orange Juice	Tuna sandwich Apple	Hamburger in bun Soft drink	

LIFELONG NUTRITION

TABLE 9.8   Analysis of David's Nutrient Intake for a Day

Food	Kcal	Protein (g)	Calcium (mg)	Iron (mg)	Vitamin A (IU)	Thiamin (mg)	Riboflavin (mg)	Niacin (mg)	Ascorbic Acid (mg)
Oatmeal (1 c)	230	5	21	1.4	0	0.19	0.05	0.3	0
Orange juice (1 c)	110	2	22	0.2	500	0.21	0.03	0.8	112
Roast beef sandwich (1)	250	88	32	2.2	10	0.08	0.15	3.2	Tr
Apple (1)	70	Tr	8	0.4	50	0.04	0.02	0.1	3
Potato chips (10)	115	1	8	0.4	Tr	0.04	0.01	1.0	3
Hamburger (1)	310	27	42	3.4	26	0.12	0.24	5.7	—
Soft drink (1 1/2 c0	115	0	0	0	0	0	0	0	0
Ice cream (3 fl oz)	100	2	66	Tr	200	0.02	0.12	0.1	Tr
Day's total	*1200*	*53*	*199*	*8,0*	*786*	*0.70*	*0.62*	*11.2*	*118*
RDA	*2800*	*59*	*1300*	*12*	*5000*	*1.2*	*1.3*	*16*	*60*

To make adequate modifications in David's food patterns, it would be wise to determine the reasons for this narrow approach toward food selection. The impediments to eating a broader range of foods and larger amounts should be identified, and ways of modifying the situation should be sought. However, improvement in acne as a result of dietary changes is not anticipated; acne has not responded to treatment through diet.

ROSA

Rosa presents an interesting contrast to David because she is from a family with limited income and many children (twelve, to be exact). The diet at home reflects both the Spanish-American heritage and the food patterns that are common among families of limited incomes. This case emphasizes the value of a good school nutrition program at lunchtime. Rosa works in the school cafeteria and is able to have all the fruit juice and other food that she wishes at the noon meal. It is apparent that this opportunity is invaluable in helping to improve her food intake, although she does not adequately avail herself of the opportunity to obtain free milk. Her menus for three days are given in Table 9.9. Rosa's diet, when analyzed by use of the Food Guide, Pyramid still reveals some shortcomings in her food selections. For example, on Tuesday she had no milk, and on Wednesday she had only one serving. This pattern resulted in an adequate intake of calcium despite her consumption of corn tortillas, either as the tortilla alone or in tacos and enchiladas. If wheat flour tortillas were used rather than limed corn tortillas, her calcium intake would be alarmingly low. In the fruit and vegetable category, she easily met the requirement for a source of vitamin C each day. However, a source of vitamin A was lacking, and her total intake of fruits and vegetables was too restricted. The meat and meat substitute category was satisfied, as was the bread and cereal group.

Although Rosa has economic limitations in modifying her food intake at home, she could be encouraged to promote a few changes that would fit the family food budget. The most obvious change to be suggested is the elimination of soft drinks and the substitution of nonfat milk, preferably with the use of nonfat dried milk solids. This change alone would improve the nutritional intake significantly and would also save the family money. The economy of this substitution might permit the family to purchase some vegetables. For example, carrots could be purchased at a relatively low cost to aid in meeting vitamin A needs. Other seasonal choices could be made frequently, too.

TABLE 9.9   Rosa's Dietary Record for Three Days

Day	Breakfast	Lunch	Dinner	Snack
Monday	Oatmeal Orange juice	Hamburger in bun Potato chips Orange juice Strawberry ice cream	1 piece fried chicken Refried beans Tortillas w/ butter Milk	Apple Vanilla ice cream
Tuesday	No breakfast	2 fish sticks 2 slices bread w/butter Orange juice Lemon pie	3 tacos Soft drink	Apple
Wednesday	Doughnut Cocoa	Tamale Orange juice 2 slices bread w/butter Fruit jello	2 enchiladas Soft drink	Apple Potato chips

Rosa could make wiser choices at school by being sure to eat the fruits and vegetables available in the Type A lunch being served.

FACTORS IN IMPROVING DIETS OF ADOLESCENTS

It is important not only to identify the nutrition problems of teenagers, but also to consider ways to improve the situation. A multifaceted approach toward overcoming nutritional problems in teenagers seems to be the only way to achieve any observable, lasting changes. Behavioral changes in eating habits of adolescents require an approach based on education and strong personal interests.

EDUCATION

Nutrition for the teenager is probably most effective when education is begun in the elementary grades and continues throughout junior and senior high school programs. Unfortunately, such a solution is difficult to implement effectively on a large scale. Elementary schools usually allot time for the study of nutrition, but many teachers have never had an opportunity to take a college nutrition course that would provide the background necessary to teach accurately and effectively. It is imperative that teachers in the elementary grades have at least one good nutrition course in their college program. It must be recognized that many elementary school children are teaching their parents nutrition as they learn it in school. Therefore, misinformation or inadequate information about nutrition from teachers confuses parents as well as children and greatly hinders an effective nutrition program.

Although home economic teachers in junior and senior high school are the persons officially designated to present factual and stimulating nutrition information, the importance of nutrition should not be stressed only in these classes. All high school students, regardless of their sex or curriculum objectives, need to have a working knowledge of nutrition, and not all students are enrolled in high school home economics classes. The role of nutrition can also be emphasized in biology classes by pointing out the needs of various animals and by doing feeding experiments in these classes. Social studies teachers can add considerable interest to their subject by examining some of the nutrition problems found in other countries and determining the impact that nutritional patterns have had on the country's history and development. Physical education teachers are often in a unique position to make a significant contribution toward improved nutrition for the teenager. Certainly, any coach should be concerned about his team's diet, and the close relationship that the girls' physical education teacher may have with her students can also be an effective avenue for introducing sound ideas regarding nutrition.

If this many-pronged approach to nutrition education is to be effective, it is imperative that the teachers in the program have an adequate understanding of basic nutrition themselves. Such an understanding is possible through a carefully conceived college nutrition course taught to all teachers in the aforementioned areas. State credential requirements for all elementary teachers, and for secondary school teachers in the fields of physical education and the biological and social sciences, should specifically include a basic nutrition course. In most states, this course is now required only of home economics majors. This program needs to be extended.

The per-student fiscal allocation for nutrition education that is now a part of the Federal school lunch program adds considerable potential for increasing nutrition education efforts in the schools. Through funded programs to develop nutrition education materials and to train school lunch personnel and others related to the nutrition program, improved knowledge of nutrition and modification of dietary habits can be the result.

EMPHASIZING APPEARANCE

An important reason for unhappiness in the teens is the failure to be accepted by the group, and appearance is one major criterion for acceptance. The extremely thin or heavy individual is automatically subject to rejection by the group. Not only are their bodies less attractive, but their clothing looks less stylish. The problem of weight alone may be sufficient reason for the group to refuse admittance to a particular boy or girl.

Concern with personal appearance may frequently motivate the adolescent boy to consume large amounts of food to fill out his frame. The larger growth spurt that usually begins for boys between the ages of 11 and 13 requires considerable quantities of wholesome food to meet the nutritional demands of such rapid growth. During this period, a boy's body may become lanky and lean. To the adolescent boy, such an appearance is not pleasing, and he will attempt to eat more food to fill out his body. To satisfy appetites and achieve the desired weight gain, boys usually eat a large quantity of food and frequently drink large amounts of milk; as a result, they are likely to be eating adequately. Even with high-calorie, relatively non-nourishing snacks, it is possible for a teenage boy to meet his recommended allowances each day. This should not be construed to mean that teenage boys are never malnourished — it is certainly possible to find adolescent boys who are poorly fed. The point is that boys are less likely to be poorly nourished than girls.

Teenage girls need to focus their attention on the total picture they present rather than concentrating their nutritional objectives exclusively on their figures. They need to recognize the importance of regulating their choice of foods so that their entire appearance is at its best. With adequate nutrition education, they can learn how to budget their calories to consume the nutrients needed for healthy skin, clear eyes, shiny hair, and a general sense of physical well-being without indulging in the excess calories that lead to overweight.

If girls can be encouraged to use raw vegetables and fruits as snack foods, they can participate in the sociability of snacks with their friends without consuming high-calorie foods with low nutrient value. Another practice to be emphasized among teenage girls is the use of skim milk if they are worried about their weight.

The selection of foods lower in sugar as snacks not only has the advantage of aiding the general appearance, but is also valuable in avoiding dental health problems. The presence of carbohydrate materials in the mouth provides an excellent medium for tooth-decaying bacteria, and few people in the United States are able to brush their teeth directly after snacking. The selection of nourishing, relatively low-calorie snacks, such as fruits or raw vegetables, helps the figure as well as the smile.

DIETARY PATTERNS OF PARENTS

Bruch (1957) emphasized the influence of parents on overweight in children; the tendency to imitate one's parents may also cause poor nutrition habits in the children of normal weight who have a poor example to copy. Some parents urge children toward obesity because they view fat as a symbol of financial success.

Mothers in particular may need to examine their own dietary habits before expecting any drastic changes in their children's diets. Although mothers are usually the persons responsible for planning and preparing family meals, they are frequently poorly nourished themselves. Their example is adopted by many teenagers, especially girls. Mothers should be careful to eat a good breakfast, a practice that is healthful for them and sets a desirable example for their children to follow.

The father's example, as well as the mother's, should not be underestimated. Over a period of years, children will acquire many of their parents' and siblings' habits.

FAMILY ADJUSTMENTS

An understanding family can be helpful in continuing good dietary patterns or in establishing good nutritional habits where poor ones existed. When problems of overweight exist, a reducing regimen is more easily followed by most people if someone else is genuinely interested in the progress being made. A member of the family may well serve as the interested bystander during a period of weight reduction, but this person must be careful to avoid nagging.

Families sometimes may be able to improve the nutrition of their teenagers by adjusting the meal schedule to a more convenient time. If this is not possible, a hot dinner might be kept warm in the oven until the tardy teen arrives.

One means of improving diets may be, surprisingly enough, through snacks. This may appear to contradict the critical comments previously made about snacks, but a nutritious snack can help meet the body's daily need for nutrients. For example, a protein food (such as milk) at snack time may be used very efficiently by the body. Raw fruits and vegetables, when washed and ready to eat directly from the refrigerator, may be tempting snack items.

SUMMARY

The nutritional requirements of teenagers are high because of the large growth spurt characteristic of both adolescent boys and girls. Studies have shown that the dietary habits of adolescent boys are more nearly adequate than those of girls, but it is apparent that much work remains to be done to improve the nutrient intake of both adolescent boys and girls. Particular efforts are required to increase the intake of iron, calcium and vitamin A during this critical decade of life.

Adolescents are particularly concerned about developing a satisfactory self-image, and this priority influences their dietary patterns. Their need to strengthen their confidence and establish a degree of independence are two other priorities in the teens that also shape dietary patterns. Peer influences promote some shifts in food patterns and choices, such as increased consumption of snacks in social situations, meal skipping, adoption of vegetarian food practices, and testing of fad reducing diets.

Athletes require additional food to supply the energy required for sports. The needs can be supplied by increasing the size of servings provided in the Daily Food Guide. It is not necessary to provide protein or vitamin supplements. A pregame meal high in carbohydrate and low in fat, with two to three glasses of liquid, is recommended for athletes participating in a sport which extends over a period of time, such as a basketball game. This meal should be consumed about three hours before the event.

Improvements in the nutritional practices of teenagers may be fostered through nutrition education programs, through illustration of the relationship between a pleasing physical appearance and good nutrition, and through family cooperation. Another means of improving teenagers' nutrition knowledge in school is through nutrition education for coaches and others who teach subjects where nutrition education may be incorporated into the high school curriculum.

BIBLIOGRAPHY

ABDULLA, M., ET AL   Nutrient intake and health status of lactovegetarians: Chemical analyses of diets using duplicate portion sampling technique. *Am. J. Clin. Nutr. 40:* 325. 1984.

AMERICAN ASSOCIATION FOR HEALTH, PHYSICAL EDUCATION, AND RECREATION *Nutrition for Athletes — Handbook for Coaches.* Amer. Assoc. Health, Physical Education, and Recreation. 1201 16th St., Washington, D.C. 1971.

BAKER, L. AND K.R. LYEN   Anorexia Nervosa. In *Adolescent Nutrition.* Ed. M. Winick. Wiley. New York. p. 13. 1982.

BAYER, A.E.   Eating out of control: Anorexia and bulimia in adolescents. *Child. Today 13(6):* 7. 1984.

BRASSEL, J.A.   Changes in body composition during adolescence. In *Adolescent Nutrition.* Ed. M. Winick. Wiley. New York. p. 13. 1982.

BRUCH, H.   *Importance of Overweight.* Norton. New York. 1957.

CHO, M. AND B.A. FRYER   Nutritional knowledge of collegiate physical education majors. *J. Am. Diet. Assoc. 65:* 30. 1974.

DAHLQUIST, A.   Lactose intolerance. *Nutr. Abst. Rev. 54:* 649. 1984.

DANIEL, W.A., JR.   Nutritional requirements of adolescents. In *Adolescent Nutrition.* Ed. M. Winick. Wiley. New York. p. 19. 1982.

ERHARD, D.   New vegetarians. *Nutr. Today 8(5):* 4. 1973.

FRISCH, R.E. AND J.S. NAGEL   Prediction of adult height of girls from age of menarche and height at menarche. *J. Pediat. 85:* 838. 1974.

GARN, S.M. AND D.C. CLARK   Nutrition, growth, development, and maturation: Findings from the Ten-State Nutrition Survey of 1968-1970. *Pediat. 56:* 306. 1975.

HAGER, T.   High-risk "heart" families: A genealogical look. *J. Am. Med. Assoc. 250:* 1663. 1983.

HASKELL, W., ET AL   *Nutrition and Athletic Performance.* Bull Publishing. Palo Alto, CA. 1982.

HEALD, F.P.   New concepts in atherosclerosis as it applies to adolescents. In *Adolescent Nutrition.* Ed. M. Winick. Wiley. New York. p. 175. 1982.

HERBERT, P.N., ET AL   High-density lipoprotein metabolism in runners and sedentary men. *J. Am. Med. Assoc. 252:* 1034. 1984.

HODGES, R.E.   Vitamin and mineral requirements in adolescence. In McKigney, J.I. and H.N. Munro. *Nutrition Requirements in Adolescence.* MIT Press. Cambridge, MA. p. 127. 1976.

KALCH, F.I. AND W.D. MCARDLE   *Nutrition, Weight Control, and Exercise.* Lea and Febiger. Philadelphia. 2nd ed. 1983.

KEYS, A.   Serum cholesterol response to dietary cholesterol. *Am. J. Clin. Nutr. 40:* 351. 1984.

KNITTLE, J.L., ET AL   Adolescent obesity. In *Adolescent Nutrition.* Ed. M. Winick. Wiley. New York. p. 151. 1982.

LANZKOWSKY, P.   Iron deficiency in adolescents. In *Adolescent Nutrition.* Ed. M. Winick. Wiley. New York. p. 73. 1982.

McCoy, H., ET AL   Nutrient intakes of female adolescents from 8 southern states. *J. Am. Diet. Assoc. 84:* 1453. 1984.

McGILL, H.C., ET AL   *Developmental Nutrition: Atherosclerosis.* Ross Laboratories. Columbus, OH. 1974.

McKIGNEY, J.I. AND H.N. MUNRO   *Nutrition Requirements in Adolescence.* MIT Press. Cambridge, MA. 1976.

NELSON, M.   Dietary practices of adolescents. In *Adolescent Nutrition.* Ed. M. Winick. Wiley. New York. p. 35. 1982.

PENNER, K.P. AND K.M. KOLASA   Secondary teachers' nutrition knowledge, attitudes, and practices. *J. Nutr. Ed. 15:* 141. 1983.

PERRON, M. AND J. ENDRES   Knowledge, attitudes, and dietary practices of female athletes. *J. Am. Diet. Assoc. 85:* 573. 1985.

PUGLIESE, M.T., ET AL   Fear of obesity: Cause of short stature and delayed puberty. *New Eng. J. Med. 309:* 513. 1983.

ROSSO, P. AND S.A. LEDERMAN   Nutrition in pregnant adolescents. In *Adolescent Nutrition.* Ed. M. Winick. Wiley. New York. p. 47. 1982.

ROUSE, I.L., ET AL   Vegetarian diet and blood pressure. *Lancet 2:* 742. 1983.

ROWE, N.H., ET AL   Effects of ready-to-eat breakfast cereals on dental caries experience in adolescent children: A three-year study. *J. Dent. Reserach 53(1):* 33. 1974.

RUSH, D.   Symposium on national evaluation of school nutrition program. *Am. J. Clin. Nutr. (Suppl.):* 363. 1984.

SHARMAN, I.M., ET AL   Effects of vitamin E and training on physiological function and athletic performance in adolescent swimmers. *Brit. J. Nutr. 25:* 265. 1971.

SINGLETON, N. AND D.S. RHOADS   Assessment of nutrition education of students in grades 3 to 12. *J. Am. Diet. Assoc. 84:* 59. 1984.

SMITH, N.   *Food for Sport.* Bull Publishing. Palo Alto, CA 1976.

SMITH, N.   Nutrition and the adolescent athlete. In *Adolescent Nutrition.* Ed. M. Winick. Wiley. New York. p. 63. 1982.

TANNER, J.M., ET AL   Standards from birth to maturity for height, weight, height velocity, and weight velocity: British children. *Arch. Dis. Child. 4:* 455. 1966.

TRUESDELL, D.D., ET AL   Nutrients in vegetarian foods. *J. Am. Diet. Assoc. 84:* 38. 1984.

U.S. DEPARTMENT OF AGRICULTURE   *Nationwide Food Consumption Survey, 48 States, 1977–78.* Preliminary Report No. 2. Washington, D.C. 1980.

WHARTON, R. AND R.W. CROCKER   Adolescent obesity. *Child. Today 13(6):* 12. 1984.

WILLIAMS, M.   *Nutrition for Fitness and Sport.* Wm. C. Brown. Dubuque, IA. 1983.

WINICK, M., ED.   *Adolescent Nutrition.* Wiley. New York. 1982.

CHAPTER TEN

Managing Weight

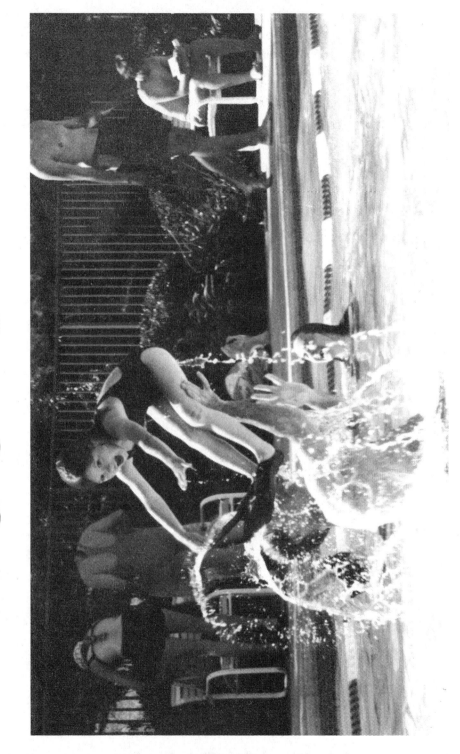

DIMENSIONS OF THE ENERGY CRISIS

Energy is a word of crisis proportions in the personal lives of many people whose weights are at either extreme of the weight spectrum. Anorexia nervosa and bulimia entered the public vocabulary in the 1980s. Obesity has long been a familiar word, and it is a growing concern to an unfortunately large segment of the population. Although overweight and obesity are much more common problems demographically than anorexia nervosa and bulimia, the latter two are increasingly being diagnosed, particularly among adolescents. All is not wonderful in the land of food abundance. This chapter deals with these two ends of the weight control energy crisis in childhood and its importance in achieving and maintaining a healthful weight in adulthood.

In our nation, where food is so abundant, nutritionists are coping with overweight and obesity as troublesome and dangerous health outcomes of our naturally bountiful food supply. This development in the science of nutrition represents a complete about-face from the original studies of deficiency conditions. However, health implications and the negative physical image of overweight have been instrumental in focusing public attemtion on weight control. The general acceptance that "thin is beautiful" has led to the emerging problem of extreme thinness, a nutritional problem that can be every bit as life-threatening as obesity. Approaches to weight management control deserve special consideration in this book because of the significant roles parents play as models for their children and gatekeepers of the family's food supply.

Obesity originating in childhood is more difficult to control in adulthood than is adult-onset obesity. Clearly, the original avoidance of obesity is more desirable than weight reduction programs. Children can be taught about weight control as they proceed through school, but it is the parents' responsibility to help develop suitable attitudes toward food and exercise during the early, formative years. Parents need basic nutrition knowledge if they are to guide their children success-fully.

This chapter provides information about achieving and maintaining weight control. Extensive research is being conducted on the causes and treatment of deviations from normal weight in children and adults; as these findings become available, modification in diet therapy may evolve.

Weight control is important both for the development of a satisfactory self-image in childhood and adolescence and for maintenance of optimal physical health. Activity levels may be reduced due to overweight. Children who are excessively heavy may relate to others in a different manner and others may, in turn, respond differently if body weight is not within a normal range.

Children who grow up to be obese adults may find that employment and promotion can be influenced negatively by the burden of obesity. Mortality statistics add another dimension of concern; although obesity is not cited as the cause of death, the mortality rate for overweight patients with diabetes, cirrhosis of the liver, appendicitis, and cardiovascular disorders is signifi-cantly higher than for those within the recommended weight range.

Weight management to achieve optimal growth and body size is a goal that is easier to state than it may be to achieve in practice. The fact is that abundant and healthful food is readily available for the majority of children in this country. The complications that may interfere with achieving a desirable weight include social interactions within the family and at school, innumerable food messages in the environment, and lack of physical activity as well as other influences on lifestyles. However, the overall tendency among American adults is an increase in weight — despite the development of various fat and sugar substitutes, which were intended to help reduce the incidence of obesity.

DEFINING WEIGHT PROBLEMS

BMI
Body mass index; expression of weight in relation to height.

The standards used to define overweight and obesity are the subject of considerable debate. The preferred method of defining obesity is by the use of the body mass index (BMI). This value is obtained by the formula:

$$BMI = \frac{\text{weight (in pounds)}}{\text{height}^2 \text{ (in inches)}} \quad x \quad 704.5$$

Adults with a BMI greater than 27 are considered obese, which indicates possible health risks. Meisler and St. Jeor (1996) found that the range of a BMI between 19 and 25 had the lowest health risks. The BMI of parents may foreshadow the weight management needs of children.

BMI can be approximated using the coordinates in Fig. 10.1 and also by using the metric formula:

$$BMI = \frac{\text{weight (in kg)}}{\text{height}^2 \text{ (in meters)}}$$

Another measure of importance is the waist-to-hip ratio. Increased health risks are associated with men who have a waist-to-hip ratio greater than 1.0 and with women with a value of 0.8 or more. Additionally, men with a waist measuring more than 40 inches or women with waists greater than 35 inches have increased health risks.

Overweight among America's children is a growing concern, as can be seen from Fig. 10.2, which summarizes trends revealed in the National Health Examination Survey (NHES), and the three subsequent National Health and Nutrition Examination Surveys (NHANES I, II, and III). The incidence of obesity is somewhat greater in children than in adolescents (Table 10.1),

Weight (pounds)

	100	105	110	115	120	125	130	135	140	145	150	155	160	165	170	175	180	185	190	195	200	205
5'0"	20	21	21	22	23	24	25	26	27	28	29	30	31	32	33	34	35	36	37	38	39	40
5'1"	19	20	21	22	23	24	25	26	26	27	28	29	30	31	32	33	34	35	36	37	38	39
5'2"	18	19	20	21	22	23	24	25	26	27	27	28	29	30	31	32	33	34	35	36	37	37
5'3"	18	19	19	20	21	22	23	24	25	26	27	27	28	29	30	31	32	33	34	35	35	36
5'4"	17	18	19	20	21	21	22	23	24	25	26	27	27	28	29	30	31	32	33	33	34	35
5'5"	17	17	18	19	20	21	22	22	23	24	25	26	27	27	28	29	30	31	32	32	33	34
5'6"	16	17	18	19	19	20	21	22	23	23	24	25	26	27	27	28	29	30	31	31	32	33
5'7"	16	16	17	18	19	20	20	21	22	23	23	24	25	26	27	27	28	29	30	31	31	32
5'8"	15	16	17	17	18	19	20	21	21	22	23	24	24	25	26	27	27	28	29	30	30	31
5'9"	15	16	16	17	18	18	19	20	21	21	22	23	24	24	25	26	27	27	28	29	30	30
5'10"	14	15	16	17	17	18	19	19	20	21	22	22	23	24	24	25	26	27	27	28	29	29
5'11"	14	15	15	16	17	17	18	19	20	20	21	22	22	23	24	24	25	26	26	27	28	29
6'0"	14	14	15	16	16	17	18	18	19	20	20	21	22	22	23	24	24	25	26	26	27	28
6'1"	13	14	15	15	16	16	17	18	18	19	20	20	21	22	22	23	24	24	25	26	26	27
6'2"	13	13	14	15	15	16	17	17	18	19	19	20	21	21	22	22	23	24	24	25	26	26
6'3"	12	13	14	14	15	16	16	17	17	18	19	19	20	21	21	22	22	23	24	24	25	26
6'4"	12	13	13	14	15	15	16	16	17	18	18	19	19	20	21	21	22	23	23	24	24	25

Height (inches)

Fig. 10.1   Body Mass Index Chart.

TABLE 10.1   Percentage of Overweight Children and Adolescents by Gender and Race/Ethnicity[a]

Ethnic Background	Children (%)		Adolescents (%)	
	Boys	Girls	Boys	Girls
White, Non-Hispanic	13.2	11.9	11.6	9.6
Black, Non-Hispanic	14.7	17.9	12.5	16.3
Mexican-American	18.8	12.5	15.0	14.0
Overall	14.7	13.7	12.3	10.7

[a]Overweight is defined as BMI at or above gender and age-specific 95th percentile (NHANES III, 1988–1994).

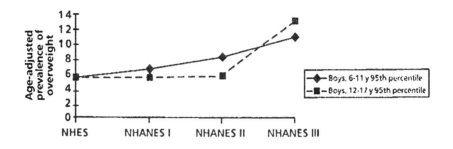

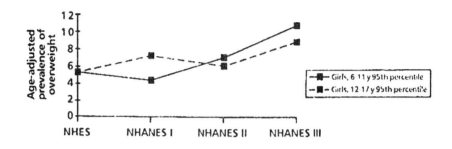

Fig. 10.2   Age-adjusted prevalence of overweight in boys and girls ages 6–11
and 12–17 (from NHES and NHANES I, II, and III). From Rolls, B.J.
and J.O. Hill, *Carbohydrates and weight management*. ILSI Press.
Washington, D.C. 1998.

with males having slightly greater incidence than females. On
the basis of race/ethnicity, Mexican-American males and Black
(non-Hispanic) females exhibited the highest incidence of obesity.

Another way to determine overweight, but perhaps the
simplest and most convenient is to compare body weight with
recommended desirable weights (see weight tables in Appendix A
and Table 4.1).

ENERGY BALANCE

When a person consumes the same amount of energy in
food that is expended for basal metabolism, activity, and thermic
effect of food, a constant body weight is the result. When more
kilocalories are consumed than are expended, the individual is in
positive caloric balance, and weight gain occurs. Conversely,

weight is lost when energy intake is less than energy expenditure. Thus, weight control can be considered in practical mathematical terms. Growing children and pregnant women should be in slightly positive caloric balance. Persons who wish to lose weight will need to be in negative caloric balance.

Each pound of body weight gain due to deposition of fat represents 3500 cal in excess of the energy needed for maintaining the body and its activities. This surplus of calories need not occur in just one day, but ordinarily represents a gradual accumulation that becomes evident as fatty deposits. For example, eating a piece of cake with icing on it each day could provide sufficient calories in a week to add 1 pound of fatty deposits.

When weight loss is the goal, food intake needs to be modified from the individual's usual dietary pattern so that caloric intake is somewhat less than that needed for body maintenance. If intake is reduced by approximately 500 calories per day, weight loss in a week should be approximately 1 pound. Such precise correlation of weight loss with energy intake may not show up immediately because of the weight of water in body tissues and other physical adjustments. However, about 1 pound is the average loss for each 3500 cal decrement. This formula sounds simple, but these calories should be eliminated without reducing the nutritional adequacy of the diet.

The other part of the energy equation is the calories used in physical activity. People seeking to lose weight need to focus their efforts on increasing their level of exercise while also decreasing caloric intake. The combination of an increased need for calories and a decreased intake enhances the likelihood of achieving a caloric deficit of 3500 calories weekly.

CONCERN FOR WEIGHT CONTROL

INFANCY

There has been considerable debate over the influence of genetic disposition toward obesity versus environmental factors in some infants and children. Although causative influences are not yet fully defined, the facts regarding incidence of obesity in families are available. When both parents are obese, children in the family have an 80 percent chance of also being obese. The likelihood of a child being obese when only one parent is obese

Obesity that begins in early years may continue to be a problem later in life unless dietary changes and increased activity are encouraged.

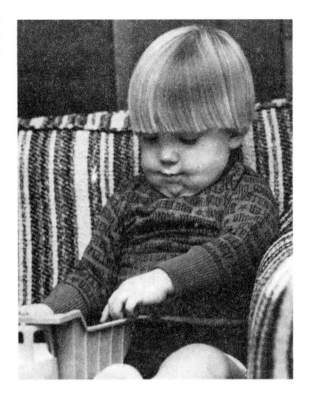

drops by half, to 40 percent. With both parents of normal weight, the likelihood of overweight children drops to slightly more than one chance in twenty or about 7 percent. Such figures clearly indicate the advantage of being born to parents who wisely stay within the desirable weight range.

One intriguing area of research into obesity was that in which the development of fat cells was studied. Hirsch and Knittle (1970) reported on cellularity in adipose tissue, noting that the number of fat cells was greater in obese than in nonobese infants. The formation of adipose cells appears to be particularly great during the latter part of gestation and the early period of infancy, and these cells continue to form until about the age of 4, and then again between the ages of 7 and 11. Weight gain during these critical periods presumably is the result both of new cells and of increase in the size of existing cells. At other periods, weight gain apparently is due primarily to an increase in the size of the cells rather than to the creation of new cells.

The theory of critical periods for forming new fat cells suggests that weight control is particularly significant at these times so that excessive numbers of cells will not be created. The extension of this approach is that a person with fewer fat cells is less likely to become obese than the individual who has a large number of fat cells, which were created in infancy as a consequence of the feeding regimen or inactivity in early life. However, research has not verified this interpretation.

Approaches to dealing with obesity are varied, but the preventive perspective is of considerable importance today. Since approximately 80 percent of children who are overweight will carry this pattern into their adult years, the need to avoid overweight in childhood is apparent.

If an infant is being bottle fed, parents should be encouraged to avoid the urge to force-feed the last portion of the

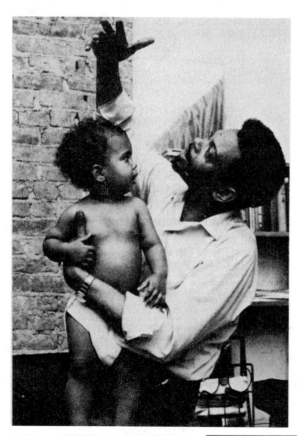

This interested baby is likely to remain a desirable weight because of the activity and eating patterns of the father.

bottle, a practice that often occurs because of the visible supply of milk remaining in the bottle. Whole milk should still remain the basis of the formula for the bottle-fed infant. Low-fat and skim milk have too high an electrolyte content in relation to water and place a strain on the kidneys.

The addition of solid foods, as noted in Chapter 6, now is suggested at approximately six months of age. Children who are gaining very rapidly and who are approaching the 85th percentile of weight for length certainly should not be receiving solid foods at an early age; many solid foods for babies have a higher caloric density than either human milk or cow's milk formulas. For example, high-meat dinner infant foods as well as fruits, meats, egg yolks, and puddings and desserts prepared for infants all contribute significantly more calories per 100 grams than are provided by either human or cow's milk. Pureed vegetables, however, are lower in caloric density than milk. Extensive use of zwieback and crackers as pacifiers may also lead to excessive caloric intake. Infant foods should be fed in modest amounts rather than encouraging the infant to finish the jar. Pureed vegetables and soups are relatively low in energy value and can be used when feeding overweight infants. Cereals, egg yolk, and strained meats make important contributions to the diet, but can be fed in modest amounts. Overfeeding should clearly be avoided during infancy.

Another dimension to weight control during the early period of life is activity level. Once a baby begins to crawl, exercise can be encouraged by permitting free movement rather than confining the would-be explorer to the playpen or a chair. Incidentally, this approach has the side benefit of providing more exercise for parents, too.

Parents who are alert to the need for weight control can promote optimal growth by using correct feeding practices and allowing an environment for activity. However, it is important that this concern not reach the point where parents become anxious and neurotic about dietary practices and activity.

CHILDHOOD

In most cases, children's appetites closely parallel their need for food, so weight control may largely be a self-regulating mechanism. When children tend to be sedentary or when adults attempt to force them to eat, however, some change in dietary habits is usually necessary. Weight control is safest and most effective when undertaken with profesional supervision, possibly including medical surveillance. Often weight control can be achieved by letting a child grow into the weight, i.e., avoiding weight gain while height catches up.

INDIVIDUAL PERCEPTIONS Weight control throughout childhood is important for both psychological and physiological reasons. Even before adolescence is reached, boys and girls are generally concerned about their appearance and aware of the importance of appropriate weight. Interpretations of the appropriateness of a teenager's weight may be quite different from the viewpoint of the adolescent and from that of a dietitian. Height-weight tables serve as a useful guide to interpretation of weight versus height data, but the teenagers may have quite a different perception of desirable weight.

In 1970, the National Center for Health Statistics reported that 31 percent of the boys studied were concerned about being underweight and 22 percent were concerned about being overweight. Girls in the same age bracket showed approximately a reverse of these statistics — 24 percent of the girls were concerned about being underweight, and 34 percent were worried about being overweight. These concerns were expressed in spite of the fact that 40 percent of the boys and girls had weighed themselves within the week prior to the interview, and 70 percent had weighed themselves within the preceding month. Clearly, weight control is a constant concern for many teenagers. This may lead to fad diets rather than appropriate and healthful dietary measures.

PROFESSIONAL GUIDANCE Particularly for teenagers, a strong word of caution is needed in the field of weight control, because there are so many self-styled experts and fad diets that appear in popular literature and the media. Well-meaning friends and acquaintances will gladly share their "authoritative knowledge" of ways to lose weight. Beware not only of this personal advice, but also of weight reduction suggestions in "diet" books and popular magazines.

The appearance of a diet in print is no guarantee of its efficacy or its safety. Insist on knowing the qualifications of the person who is recommending a diet. Being a published writer is simply not sufficient to make a nutrition expert of a layman. Qualified nutritionists and dietitians shoul have a sound academic background in organic chemistry, biochemistry, physiology, psychology, and nutrition, and at least a B.S. or B.A. degree from an accredited university with a major in dietetics or nutrition. Many also have earned their M.S. or Ph.D. degrees in nutrition or dietetics, adding greater depth to their understanding of weight control and other nutritional problems. Another criterion for judging the qualifications of nutrition professionals is by determining whether they are members of The American Dietetic Association. Membership in this professional association is available only to persons with the academic background described. In addition, some professionals are Registered Dietitians, a designation often indicated by the letters R.D. following the name. This is additional proof of the professional qualifications of the individual.

UNDERWEIGHT

Because the more common dietary problem in the United States today is that of overweight, less attention often is given to the problems of the underweight individual. A thin child, however, usually has lowered resistance to infection, reduced physical energy, diminished alertness, and a less attractive appearance.

Personal tastes in physical proportions may vary, but evidence indicates that health will be optimal when weight is within the normal range (see Appendix A). One of the problems associated with severe underweight is the increased incidence of tuberculosis. Because underweight is usually caused by small food intake, it is likely that the thin person is receiving inadequate amounts of essential nutrients needed by the body, not simply inadequate calories. These deficiences can create health problems at any age, but they are particularly important to remedy in growing children. Therefore, when a child is underweight, it is essential to examine the dietary pattern and develop an appropriate plan for overcoming the shortages.

CAUSES

When a physical examination fails to reveal any physical cause for underweight, it is necessary to assess both the diet and the mealtime environment. The caloric content of the meals served each day may be increased, but major changes usually need to be made in the home environment. Parents can play an important part in helping a child gain weight when they understand the specific problems that have caused their child to be too thin. Often, the doctor or nutritionist will be able to detect an underlying problem that needs to be corrected. Common focal points to consider are: the mother's and father's attitudes toward food, the emotional climate at the table and in the home, feelings of sibling rivalry, the mealtime schedule, and the child's activity pattern.

Frequently, dietary problems encountered in underweight children have been of long duration and may be traced back to the first few months of life. Some mothers or fathers are almost professional worriers when it comes to feeding their children, and they communicate this concern about appetite to their babies. When parents regularly coax their children to eat, it is not surprising that some children acquire poor appetites and resist almost anything that is fed to them. Still other children discover early in life that they can control their parents by refusing to eat the food that parents urge on them.

Some family tables resemble a battleground, at least in an emotional sense. Sensitive children may become so tense at the table, as a result of family arguments, that eating becomes a difficult task.

Sometimes adults have unrealistic ideas of the amount of food a child needs to eat. Such adults may try to force children to eat more food than they need or want. One common technique employed by the adult to achieve a greater food intake is to insist that the child remain at the table until the food is gone. This grandstand play usually creates strong hostility between the two participants and makes the likelihood of a good appetite at the next meal more remote. Sometimes parents thoughtlessly discuss their children's eating habits where the children can hear them. If a child overhears himself characterized as a picky, fussy eater, he will begin to feel that this is indeed just what he is going to be.

Another example of parents' influence on their children's dietary patterns was provided by a distinctly thin and rather anxious preschool child who cautiously checked with her mother about any unfamiliar food that was served. She would ask her mother whether she would like the new food before tasting the item. The mother took this responsibility very seriously, weighing her knowledge of the food and her child before responding. If she thought the new food might not be acceptable to the child, she would tell her daughter that she might not like it. Needless to say, the new food, if sampled, was not accepted. The result of this continuing interaction was a preschooler who was underweight and who ate a very narrow spectrum of food with little enthusiasm. Although this story seems unlikely, it is true. It illustrates the fact that parents are often so close to feeding situations that they are unaware of how they are interacting with their children.

In some instances, food problems are directly attributable to problems rooted in sibling rivalry. A child who feels he is not getting his fair share of attention may decide that refusal to eat at meals is a good way to gain family attention. True, it may not be expressions of approval that are received, but at least some recognition as an individual is gained. Fussy eating habits at the table may gradually become this child's trademark.

Most children have better appetites for meals when they play actively and eat at regular intervals each day. A few children may become poor eaters simply because they are too tired and too hungry to eat well at the table. Children who are very tired rarely are able to eat much food. This generalization is as applicable at breakfast as it is at dinner. Some children are fed too little or too infrequently. These conditions, leading to underweight and malnutrition, have been observed in this country in families where parents have little concern for their children.

TREATMENT

ENVIRONMENTAL CHANGES   The adjustments necessary in an environment to promote better appetite will vary with the situation. Parents who are too concerned about the child's dietary needs will find that Johnny eats more food when they concentrate on preparing appetizing, tempting meals and refrain from reminding him that he should eat more.

It may be difficult to change a tense atmosphere at the table to one of congeniality, but change will occur if everyone in the family makes an effort. Subtle aids in the form of soft background music, an attractive centerpiece, and special preplanned topics of conversation can be used to initiate this difficult transition. Considerable effort over a long period of time is necessary to achieve a permanent change in group behavior at the table. This change in mood, however, can be accomplished to the benefit of the entire family.

Sibling rivalry can be alleviated by conscious effort to give recognition and approval to all the children equally, or as needed, throughout the day. Genuine expressions of approval at the table may improve the appetite when a child feels neglected or rejected, but such comments should not be centered exclusively around approval of greater food intake.

Scheduling of meals and bedtime may require special effort if parents' work schedules require a late dinner. It is usually possible, however, to arrange the daytime schedule to include a nap if children need to stay up late to have some time with their parents. The children's dinner could be served early and a light dessert served when their parents have dinner. Other adjustments may need to be implemented to meet specific family scheduling problems. The important thing is to be sure that adequate rest is provided and that food intake is spaced appropriately to ensure a hungry, interested child at meals.

DIETARY MODIFICATION Some general suggestions can be made to modify the caloric intake of thin children, but usually the most satisfactory adjustments can be made when a dietitian has the opportunity to examine the typical food pattern of the family and then make specific suggestions. The meal plan for thin children should still include a well-balanced diet rather than concentrating on a narrow selection of high-calorie foods. Whole milk is preferable to skim milk or buttermilk for these children. The use of milk in soups and puddings is also recommended. Small increases in serving sizes, particularly in the servings of meats and bread and cereal products, are frequently effective in causing modest weight gains. Snacks may be increased to provide more calories, but quantity and timing should be planned to avoid interfering with mealtime appetites.

Parents may find special ways of increasing their children's food intake if they view the problem objectively. It is most important to avoid making a big production of dietary changes to increase a child's weight. Subtle changes from the kitchen are more effective than long lectures on the need for change.

ANOREXIA NERVOSA

Some persons, notably adolescent girls, develop a seriously distorted body image of perceived overweight and follow a diet they feel will bring about enough weight loss to achieve desired thinness. A typical profile shows these people to be: female; adolescent; high academic achievers; somewhat isolated socially; from affluent families with other high achievers; from families with friction between father and mother, psychological problems in the family, and either obesity or excessive thinness

ANOREXIA NERVOSA Extreme thinness, possibly life-threatening, resulting from dietary modifications pursued to achieve a thin body image.

in family members. Obviously, not everyone who fits this profile will become totally absorbed in an intense desire to achieve an extremely thin body. On the other hand, some boys and older females who do not match all the descriptive elements in the profile also may be obsessed with the need to achieve a thin physique.

The condition resulting when motivation to be thin causes people to follow dietary practices that result in serious weight loss and even in death is called anorexia nervosa, a name that literally translates as "loss of appetite due to nerves." Although anorexia nervosa has been recognized for many years, public attention was not focused on this problem until the 1980s. With greater media attention, the incidence of anorexia nervosa being reported has increased sharply. However, undiagnosed cases and lack of awareness of its existence probably caused anorexia nervosa to be unreported in the past. There is no way to determine if the problem is actually increasing, but this may be the case. The bright side is that the increasing recognition of anorexia nervosa may lead to improved diagnosis and treatment, which could save lives in the future.

The diagnosis of anorexia nervosa is difficult, because people who have the problem may not go for a physician's examination. In fact, people with anorexia nervosa may not even be recognized as having a problem for quite a long time, even within their own families; the onset may be gradual, and proximity makes recognition difficult. Outsiders may be able to recognize the overt indications of excessive activity and gradual weight loss witithout a diagnosed illness, two indications of a possible case of anorexia nervosa.

HYPOTHERMIA
Abnormally low body temperature of 95°F or lower.

Even when the person is examined by a physician, diagnosis may be difficult; there is no clear-cut group of symptoms exhibited by anorexics. Physicians use such information as: present weight in comparison with highest preceding weight and recommended weight for height; total body potassium; body temperature (hypothermia); hypotension (low blood pressure); psychological assessment; use of diuretics and laxatives; and activity patterns. Death can result when the body becomes seriously underweight. Cases have been reported where patients' body weights were only about 50 percent of the recommended weight. A body temperature of less than 95°F (hypothermia) is another serious indication of possible death. Serum potassium levels about 50 percent the normal level have also been observed as dangerous in cases of anorexia nervosa.

Development of anorexia nervosa with its dangerously low weight is seen as an attempt by the patient to lose enough weight to meet the desired physical image; this is done by sharply limiting food intake and following an active physical program to burn up calories from the food that is consumed. Excessive activity and limited food intake result in weight loss despite the body's ability to make certain physiological adjustments, such as the onset of amenorrhea, to reduce the amount of energy needed to maintain the body. In fact, it appears that the delay in sexual maturation that accompanies anorexia nervosa may be one of the goals of some adolescents pursuing this destructive dietary course.

Whether or not sexual motivations are underlying causes of anorexia nervosa, the condition usually has psychological factors, as well as dietary restrictions; these need to be identified and resolved if the patient is to be helped back toward a normal life. Often, patients with anorexia nervosa do not perceive their physiques as others do; they are frequently convinced that they still need to lose weight when their appearance is alarmingly gaunt to others. The patient's perspective cannot be understood until the psychological factors complicating individual cases are identified and studied; intervention strategies can then be developed.

Treatment of a person with anorexia nervosa should be the joint effort of a physician and either a psychologist or psychiatrist. Sometimes, nutritional intervention may be necessary with intravenous or nasogastric tube feedings, but food through the mouth is desirable as soon as possible. Fortunately, the gastrointestinal tract in anorexia nervosa is usually quite capable of good digestion and absorption of nutrients when the patient is willing to eat. Attempts at psychiatric rehabilitation should be avoided until sufficient weight has been gained to be certain that the patient is out of physical danger. When psychiatric intervention occurs, the family should usually be included in the rehabilitation efforts so that the patient can receive appropriate support in the family setting.

The nutritional therapy appropriate for treating anorexics is still a matter of some debate. Often, there is not very much interest in food; in fact, the urge to avoid eating may remain quite intense during the recovery phase. Around 35 calories per pound of body weight is a suggested goal for refeeding anorexics. Careful and frequent physician involvement is essential to achieving a safe regimen of weight gain. A team approach by the physician and psychiatrist or psychologist is important to recovery from anorexia nervosa.

BULIMIA

Bulimia is a condition characterized by periodic episodes of gorging on food, followed by self-induced vomiting to avoid the weight gain that normally results from excessive eating. The profile of individuals who have bulimia is comparable to that for anorexia nervosa. In fact, some anorexics have bulimia. Bulimia can be particularly hard to detect, because some people use self-induced vomiting as a means of maintaining an ideal weight; not everyone with bulimia is excessively thin. Because both the gorging and the vomiting episodes can be done in complete secrecy, even family members may not be aware of this dietary behavior. A dentist, however, may be painfully aware of the problem because of the erosive damage resulting from the acidic environment in the mouth when gastric juice and its hydrochloric acid are vomited repeatedly. The esophagus may also reveal damaged caused by hydrochloric acid from the stomach.

If patients with bulimia are also anorectic and have lost a considerable amount of weight, they will require the type of treatment described in the preceding section. However, if the present weight is normal, behavioral modification and psychological counseling may be the way to correct the problem. This condition must be corrected, even though the patient's weight is under control, because repeated vomiting is physically damaging to the body, particularly to the teeth and esophagus.

OVERWEIGHT

Overweight affects the very rich and the very poor, adults and children. It is the most common nutrition problem throughout the United States today. This condition in children is of particular concern because overeating is likely to become a way of life that carries on into adulthood. Cases of long duration are very difficult to treat successfully even when they represent a distinct health hazard. It is far easier to treat the problem when it begins than to wait until adulthood and try to change the habits of a lifetime.

Overweight Children and Future Health Prospects

To assess the health hazards associated with overweight in children, we must look into the future; these overweight children, in all probability, may become overweight adults. Overweight is generally detrimental to the health of adults. It should be pointed out, however, that the suicide rate in overweight individuals is lower than in persons of normal weight, a finding that has more significance in the teenage group than in the population as a whole. Eating apparently provides a solution of sorts for some individuals with emotional problems.

Some of the common health problems in the adult American population are conditions frequently associated with overweight. It has been shown conclusively that blood pressure increases with increasing weight and decreases with weight reduction. Hypertension is two and one-half times more likely to occur in an overweight individual than in a person of normal weight. Tendency toward atherosclerosis is twice as common in the overweight as in the underweight. with the normal individual being somewhere in between these two extremes. Nine out of ten diabetics over 40 are overweight.

Studies of Norwegians during World War II, when diets were highly restricted, revealed some indisputable facts. A distinct drop in circulatory diseases accompanied the restriction in diet, and hospital patients showed less clotting in the veins following surgery. These trends were reversed as food once again became readily available after the war.

Insurance statistics indicate that permanent loss of excess weight can definitely improve the chance of survival of a formerly overweight person, but the person in the best position is the one who has never been too heavy. The percentage mortality of overweight men is 142 percent (normal weight equals 100 percent) and drops to 113 percent if the excess weight is lost permanently. Volatile weight control, or frequent reduction and gain, is more dangerous than maintenance of a constant high weight.

With such overwhelming evidence regarding the health hazards of overweight, it is an important parental responsibility to help children avoid excessive weight gain during childhood.

CAUSES OF OVERWEIGHT

Numerous specific causes of overweight may be cited, but they are due ultimately to an excess of caloric intake in relation to the body's energy expenditure, a case of too much food in relation to exercise. Children who have weight problems resulting from improper diet are of paramount interest in this chapter. Cases of overweight caused by a physical malfunction require medical treatment. Actually, only a small percentage of persons weigh too much because of physical abnormalitites like metabolic disorders or glandular malfunctions.

It is easy to say that a person is overweight because of eating too much, but permanent desirable weight control can rarely be accomplished unless the reasons behind excessive intake are understood and corrected.

DEVELOPMENTAL OBESITY   Some children exhibit progressive, excessive weight gain from infancy throughout childhood. One possible explanation for this developmental overweight is that the typical activity patterns of an individual may be inborn. Because a less active individual requires fewer calories daily than a normally active person, the less active child will gradually become overweight while eating a diet that is average for children the same age.

Some parents use food as a reward for their children. Parents may give children dessert for cleaning their plates or ice cream or candy for good behavior. These extras not only add calories, but also build in a strong psychological support from food, thus promoting inappropriate weight gain in children.

Perhaps a significant factor in the incidence of developmental overweight is the mother who measures her maternal prowess by the plumpness of her child. It is far more important to have a child within the normal weight range for height than it is to have the fattest baby in the neighborhood.

Food may become a comfortable form of security for some children. This attitude toward food, when maintained a long time, is likely to result in excessive weight gain. Sometimes this pattern may be instituted as a result of propping an infant's evening bottle so that milk is continually available while the child drifts off to sleep. This practice not only has the potential for creating a strong tie between the bottle and a sense of security, but is also poor because the teeth are bathed in the sugar-containing liquid, promoting caries. Bottle propping may also lead to the development of otitis (inflammation of the ear) because spilled milk is a fine medium for microorganismal growth.

REACTIVE OVERWEIGHT This type of weight gain may result from an adjustment to a crisis, such as loss of a loved one. Some children and adults, too, seem to derive psychological comfort from food in times of stress.

Sexual adjustment may be an underlying reason for some teenagers being overweight; theoretically, a fat figure may be a defense for individuals wishing to avoid contacts with the opposite sex or secretly desiring to have physical attributes of the other sex.

Disturbance in the home as a cause of overweight is a difficult one to resolve. Bulleen et al (1963), studying adolescent girls at two summer camps, found that overweight girls more frequently came from less happy family situations than did girls of normal weight. It appeared that the insecurity felt by the overweight girls from the disturbed families was related to their fear of leaving their families.

Other less dramatic factors such as a genuine fondness for food and our society's sedentary way of life could be mentioned here also. Certainly, there are many reasons for overweight children.

INFLUENCE OF OVERWEIGHT ON ADOLESCENTS

Studies to gain greater understanding of the causes of excess weight have given some insights into the problems associated with adolescent obesity. Bulleen et al (1963) interviewed two groups of girls, one overweight and the other of normal weight, to determine the reasons for the difference in the size of the individuals. This study revealed that overweight girls dated less, were less vigorous in their actions, participated in fewer activities, and indulged in more eating sprees than girls of normal weight. The overweight girls recognized their lack of activity, but seemed to be unaware that this inactivity contributed to their overweight condition.

PREVENTION OF OVERWEIGHT

At any age level, but particularly with children, the need for weight control before extra weight becomes a problem should be emphasized. It is far easier to maintain a normal weight than to try to remove unnecessary pounds that have earned a child the nickname of 'Fatty.' By the time this point is reached, the child is faced with the dual problem of a psychological need to change the self-image as well as the physical problem of shedding the excess weight. This is a large order for anyone, and it is a task that frequently could have been avoided.

Education to reduce the problem of overweight in American children is not a simple matter; the roots of overeating underlie much of our society, from the influences of family income and cultural background to the impact of technology on our physical activity patterns. Obviously, there is no single solution to overcome a problem of such complexity. A multi-faceted educational approach, however, can help people achieve a better understanding of the underlying causes, and, with increased understanding, perhaps progress will be achieved.

One effective way to help prevent overweight in children is to encourage active play, plenty of walking and sports, and to minimize the time spent viewing television. The current popularity of jogging, roller skating, soccer, basketball, and other team sports suggests that some progress is being made toward eliminating public lethargy and enhancing physical status.

Perhaps the most significant and long-lasting effects in nutrition education can be accomplished by the obstetrician. A pregnant woman is usually anxious to do whatever her doctor recommends to promote development of a healthy baby. Obstetricians can conduct classes for groups of expectant women or they can talk to them individually about the need for proper nutrition (including weight control) during pregnancy. These sessions should also include the nutritional needs of the young, and special emphasis should be given to developing attitudes within the family that will help all members achieve and maintain an appropriate weight.

Other physicians can also play important roles in nutrition education geared toward prevention of undesirable weight gain. Usually, doctors have sufficient contact with preschool children and parents to permit assessment and appropriate intervention when overweight begins to develop. Early intervention enables small changes to be made in the diet so that the child grows into the weight gain instead of becoming so heavy that an actual loss is required. Essentially, the best strategy when a child is gaining too much weight is to provide a diet that maintains weight, but does not cause weight gain, until the child's height catches up with weight. Advice from doctors may be very effective with some parents because of the high esteem in which they hold their child's pediatrician.

Physicians who have little or no education in nutrition can help their overweight patients by referring them to a nutritionist or dietitian, preferably an R.D. (Registered Dietitian) for nutrition counseling and assistance with weight control problems. Increasingly, an R.D. is included in the health team in clinics. Others operate private practices to counsel people with a variety of nutrition-related problems, including overweight and underweight.

The role of the physician and R.D. in nutrition education need not, indeed should not, be limited to advice regarding the preschooler. Some children experience weight control problems that appear to be related to their entry into school (at the age of 5 or 6). Other developmental crises, experienced near the beginning of puberty and again in the middle teens as emphasis begins to be placed on heterosexual acceptance, may trigger weight problems. Although the doctor probably will see these children less frequently than the preschooler, it still is possible to provide appropriate guidance when needed.

Educators can play an important part in nutrition education within the school program. Home economics teachers and school nurses are in particularly favorable positions to emphasize the value of good nutrition and weight control. Other teachers, including biology and physical education instructors, can also help develop an interest in nutrition. It is important, however, that teachers refer students in need of special weight control assistance to appropriate medical or dietetic personnel rather than undertake the project themselves.

TREATMENT OF OVERWEIGHT AND OBESITY

GUIDELINES FOR DIETING   If a child is overweight in relation to height (see Figs. 10.3 and 10.4), supervision of dietary modification should be done jointly by a physician and dietitian. A physician can monitor health aspects and a dietitian can provide nutrition counseling to the child and parents. They will be able to analyze the problems and work out an appropriate dietary plan to curb any weight increases while the child is growing into the existing weight. Small dietary changes can then be implemented to maintain consistent weight in relation to increasing height. It is important to avoid jeopardizing potential gains in height by excessive dietary restrictions. The concept of growing into

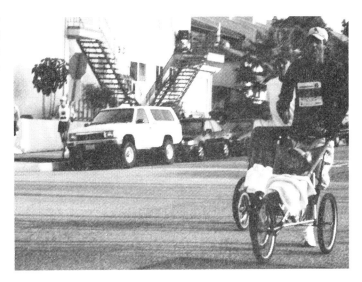

Active parents with good dietary and exercise patterns set a good example to help their children maintain an appropriate weight.

existing weight is the preferred approach to correcting problems of overweight in childhood.

A dietitian can plan and implement an appropriate weight control diet while encouraging the child to follow the diet plan and increase exercise. Children, like older dieters, often appreciate having someone around who is genuinely interested in their progress. This is undoubtedly one of the reasons doctors and dietitians are effective in treating weight control cases. However, they can be successful only if the overweight child really wants to modify weight. A child entering puberty is likely to be receptive to a weight control program because of peer group pressure to be normal.

A key part of weight control for children is to increase activity levels. Fortunately, the current physical fitness craze provides considerable reinforcement of this principle. Emphasis among many children today is focused on some favorite activity, whether it be racquetball, swimming, jogging, aerobics, or any other active sport. Fashion designers have added significantly to this lifestyle by creating jogging suits, stretch tights and other attire for athletes and active children. The fact that jogging suits are even available for babies is further evidence of the importance youngsters and young adults place on fitness. Sensible levels of activity comparable to jogging about 12 miles weekly are suggested; excessive exercise can create health problems by

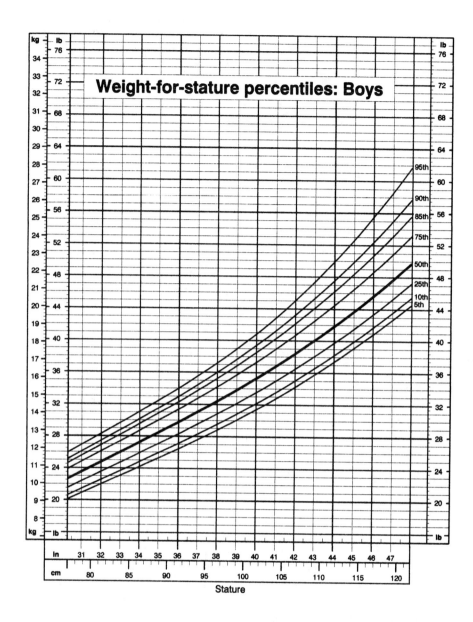

Fig. 10.3   Weight-for-stature percentiles (5th, 10th, 25th, 50th, 75th, 90th, and 95th) for boys (National Center for Health Statistics in collaboration with the National Center for Chronic Disease Prevention and Health Promotion). 2000.

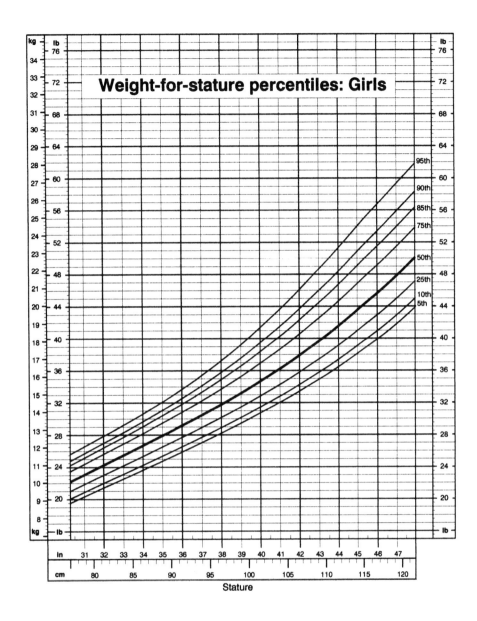

Fig. 10.4   Weight-for-stature percentiles (5th, 10th, 25th, 50th, 75th, 90th, and 95th) for girls (National Center for Health Statistics in collaboration with the National Center for Chronic Disease Prevention and Health Promotion). 2000.

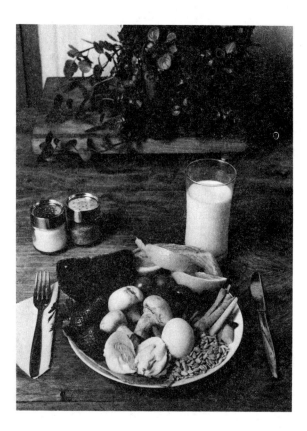

Menus for losing weight can be both tempting and satisfying.

reducing fat stores below desirable levels and are not recommended.

A boon to dieting is the development of new interests during the adolescent years. When a person is busy with other matters, food becomes secondary and less tempting. Parents can help younger children with weight problems by providing new and interesting ideas for play when food seems to be troubling them. Walks together or short trips are also helpful.

There are two purposes of any good diet designed for weight control: 1) to adjust weight in relation to height at a reasonable rate, and 2) to retrain the appetite so that the lost weight will not be regained. To lose weight, it is necessary to eat fewer calories than when the extra weight was gained and/or burn up more calories. Most children and adults are successful in keeping off the weight if the diet is similar to what is ordinarily eaten in the home.

Young et al (1971) explored the merits of various frequencies of feeding in relation to weight reduction and body composition. These researchers, using a carefully constructed experimental design, tested the effect of dividing the day's intake into six meals, three meals, and one meal daily. Results indicated that frequency of eating had no significant effect on weight loss or on fat losses (skinfold thickness or body circumference). Reaction to the various frequencies of feeding favored three meals. Some subjects felt that six meals daily were a nuisance, while only one meal created a strain.

The following suggestions are appropriate guidelines for any weight reduction program:

1. Weight reduction is best undertaken when the patient first begins to gain too much weight.

2. The decision to reduce must be internalized within the patient; another person cannot provide the primary motivating force for reduction.

3. Moderate activity will help modify the normal physical activity pattern and assist in developing actual physical need for more calories. Walking, bicycling, or similar activities are suggested.

4. Acquisition of new hobbies or interests will help prevent the boredom that often leads to overeating.

5. An attempt should be made to understand and modify the psychological factors that may have caused the weight problem.

6. The assistance of an interested person — layman, dietitian, or physician — can provide the extra boost needed to persist in the reduction program.

7. The diet plan itself should provide sufficient satiety value to keep the patient from feeling like a martyr, but it must still reduce the caloric intake sufficiently to provide the necessary relative weight loss.

8. The dieter should be prepared to expect slow weight loss, but it must not be so slow that interest and motivation are lost.

9. Emphasis must be constantly placed on the importance of keeping the weight off once it is lost. Volatile weight losses and gains are harmful to health.

10. The diet should be patterned as closely as is practical on the customary diet of the individual. This makes it easier to follow the diet. It also makes retraining of diet habits to maintain lower weight a simple process, because retraining occurs during the diet period itself.

11. A good weight reduction diet will provide necessary nutrients, but restrict calories. Particular attention should be given to including the nutrients needed by children for growth.

12. For the person with a modest weight problem, weight control can probably be achieved by reducing the size of servings and avoiding second helpings.

13. Parents can help children with weight control by not giving undue emphasis to food. Food should not be used as a threat or as a reward.

14. Simple changes in the diets of children can be very effective in avoiding excess pounds. After age 2, skim milk can be substituted very satisfactorily for whole milk, and it provides far fewer calories. Raw fruits, carrots, celery sticks, and other raw vegetables provide the desired crunchiness and bulk children often seek in a snack. If these items are available, and if ice cream, cookies, and crackers vanish from the kitchen, weight control problems often depart, too. Table 10.2 provides some comparative figures

FAD DIETS AND THEIR RISKS

Particular problems in reduction diets come to the fore in the adolescent period. Girls are particularly susceptible to the siren song of fad diets, but boys are not immune to the appeal of diets that make impressive claims for effortless weight loss. There is no way to predict what weird diets will assault the overweight consumer in the next several years, but there are ways to evaluate the wisdom and safety of diets as they come along. The one predictable fact is that "easy" diets with undocumented claims of great success will continue to multiply.

Any diet that is proposed as a reducing diet should include the range of foods in the quantities suggested in the Food Guide Pyramid. Portion control and appropriate selection of foods with little or no fat are the keys to a lifetime of success in

TABLE 10.2   Caloric Values of Some Selected Snack Foods[a]

Food	Cal	Food	Cal
Milk, whole (1 c)	160	Milk, skim (1 c)	90
Tomato juice (1 c)	45	Apple juice (1 c)	120
Apple (1 medium)	70	Cabbage, raw (1 c)	25
Cake, chocolate w/icing (1/16 of 10" cake)	445	Cantaloupe (1/2 of 5" dia.)	60
		Carrot, grated (1 c)	45
Cheese, cheddar (1"-cube)	70	Celery, diced (1 c)	15
Doughnut, cake (1)	125	Orange, medium (1)	60
Potato chips (10 chips)	115	Tomato, medium (1)	35
Radishes (4 small)	5		

[a]Data from Nutritive value of foods, *Home and Garden Bulletin 72*, revised US Department of Agriculture, Washington, D.C. 1978.

weight control at recommended levels. Any diet being considered for weight reduction should be measured against the Food Guide Pyramid.

Be wary of diets making any of the following claims:

1. Eat all you want and lose weight.

2. Watch the pounds melt away.

3. This is the "easy way" to lose weight.

4. Bread is fattening.

5. A single food or a very limited menu is the best way to lose weight, because it helps fat melt away.

6. A diet pill causes effortless weight loss.

Remember, some diets and diet products can be dangerous, even life-threatening. Liquid protein diets and related diet products that result in intake of only about 300 calories daily have greatly restricted energy available from the dietary formula. Considerable breakdown of tissue protein is ultimately used to maintain the body, which is almost in a state of fasting. These types of products have been the cause of death for some dieters.

Some liquid diet products are available for persons who are seeking a diet that requires little effort on their part. Unfortunately, no retraining of dietary habits occurs in such a diet, and lost weight is usually regained quickly. Another disadvantage is the lack of dietary fiber in such products.

Diet "candies" and various other products are marketed as appetite suppressants. Some drugs are touted by their manufacturers as easy ways to lose weight; their action may be due to a diuretic effect or other physiological action. The use of catecholaminergic drugs (e.g., phentermine) and/or serotoninergic drugs (e.g., d, l-fenfluramine) to reduce appetite and increase levels of norepinephrine and serotonin in the brain has proven to be effective in short-term weight loss programs for some people. Medical supervision and lifestyle changes to increase activity and modify dietary habits are essential to avoid regaining weight after the drugs are stopped.

Non-nutritive and low-calories sweeteners are used widely in products varying from diet colas to ice cream. Ingredient labels must list all ingredients, which makes it possible to identify the presence of such sweeteners as aspartame and

Fad diet aids constantly bombard consumers in the marketplace. Unfortunately, many dangerous recommendations and products are marketed side-by-side with correct information. Consumers need to be particularly wary and well-informed when they are seeking a means of losing weight.

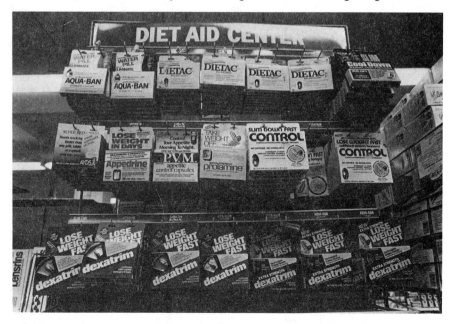

saccharin, as well as the many forms of sugars that can be used. The nutrition label lists calories and carbohydrate in a defined serving size of the food. Fat replacements such as Olestra and Caprenin, are being incorporated in an array of foods to help consumers reduce fat and calorie intake. Food labels carry this information. Consumption of foods containing these reduced calorie alternatives rather than their regular counterparts can be helpful in reducing calorie consumption. However, it is necessary to try to retrain eating habits to reduce the quantity of food eaten even though these alternatives are available. Control is an important facet of reducing regimens because of the need to establish eating patterns that assure an appropriate level of food intake and adequate nutrient content.

SUMMARY

Weight control is a component of good nutrition that needs to be monitored and corrected as necessary. When the body's need for energy (calories for basal metabolism, physical activity, and thermic effect of food) is in concert with calories in the food consumed, a person will not gain weight. However, if one is eating a diet providing more energy than needed, weight will be gained. Conversely, weight is lost when the body's energy needs exceed the energy provided in the diet.

Even in childhood, weight control is a matter of importance. During adolescence, awareness of and dissatisfaction with body size can create an intense drive to reduce weight. In some cases, the drive to reduce far below recommended weight results in such serious weight loss that physical consequences may include death. Anorexia nervosa, a condition found most commonly in teenage girls, results in excessive thinness to the point of emaciation; it is an attempt by some teenagers to fulfill the urgent desire to be very thin. Bulimia may accompany anorexia nervosa or may be found in some teenagers who have not undergone any serious weight loss. Both problems have psychological dimensions to them and require dietary modifications augmented with psychiatric counseling.

Obesity and overweight are problems that occur more frequently than underweight. Alteration of eating patterns (sometimes accomplished by behavior modification techniques) is needed if weight control is to be established and maintained after completing a diet. Overweight children need diets with enough calories to maintain existing weight until their growth in height is consistent with their weight.

Diets that maintain good nutrition while establishing weight control should be based on the food groups (milk, meat and meat alternatives, fruits, vegetables, breads and cereals). Portion control is vital to achieving desired weight loss. Establishment of healthful dietary habits for a lifetime should be the goal of any weight control diet.

Fad diets, diet devices, and medications are potentially harmful and often ineffective. Any weight control plan should be evaluated to be sure that a broad diet is included and that there are sufficient sources of energy available to prevent burning body tissues for energy. Diets that promise effortless success in weight reduction or make similar claims are often ineffective and dangerous.

BIBLIOGRAPHY

ANDING, J.D., ET AL   Blood lipids, cardiovascular fitness, obesity, and blood pressure: presence of potential coronary heart disease risk factors in adolescents. *J. Am. Diet. Assoc. 96(3):* 238. 1996.

ANONYMOUS   Position of the American Dietetic Association: weight management. *J. Am. Diet. Assoc. 97(1):* 71. 1997.

ANONYMOUS   Unwarranted dieting retards growth and delays puberty. *Nutr. Rev. 41:* 14. 1983.

ASHWELL, M.   Brown adipose tissue — relevant to obesity? *Human Nutr.: Appl. Nutr. 37A:* 232. 1983.

BROWN, M.R., ET AL   High protein, low calorie liquid diet in treatment of very obese adolescents: Long-term effect on lean body mass. *Am. J. Clin. Nutr. 38(7):* 20. 1983.

BRYCE-SMITH, D. AND R.I.D. SIMPSON   Case of anorexia nervosa responding to zinc sulphate. *Lancet 11:* 350. 1984.

BULLEEN, B.A., ET AL   Attitudes towards physical activity, food, and family in obese and nonobese adolescent girls. *Am. J. Clin. Nutr. 12:* 1. 1963.

GARFINKEL, P.E. AND D.M. GARNER   *Anorexia Nervosa: Multidimensional Perspective.* Brunner/Mazel. New York. 1982.

GOODSTEIN, R.K.   *Eating and Weight Disorders: Advances in Treatment and Research.* Springer Publishing. New York. 1983.

GUO, S.S., ET AL   Predictive value of childhood body mass index values for overweight at age 35 years. *Am. J. Clin. Nutr. 59:* 547. 1994.

HAFEN, B.Q.   *Nutrition, Food, and Weight Control.* Allyn and Bacon. Boston. 1981.

HEALD, F.P.   Nutrition in adolescence. *Clin. Nutr. 2(5):* 19. 1983.

HIMES, J.H.   Infant feeding practices and obesity. *J. Am. Diet. Assoc. 75:* 122. 1979.

HIMMS-HAGEN, J.   Brown adipose tissue thermogenesis in obese animals. *Nutr. Rev. 41:* 261. 1983.

HIRSCH, J. AND J.L. KNITTLE   Cellularity of obese and nonobese human adipose tissue. *Fed. Proc. 29:* 1516. 1970.

HUSE, D.M. AND A.R. LUCAS   Dietary patterns in anorexia nervosa. *Am. J. Clin. Nutr. 40:* 251. 1984.

JAMES, W.P.T.   Energy requirements and obesity. *Lancet 2:* 386. 1983.

KATCH, F.I. AND W.D. MCARDLE   *Nutrition, Weight Control, and Exercise.* Lea & Febiger. Philadelphia. 2nd ed. 1983.

KORCOK, M.   Those who 'eat and run' may lead healthier lives. *J. Am. Med. Assoc. 250:* 2589. 1983.

MCSHERRY, J.A.   Diagnostic challenge of anorexia nervosa. *Am. Fam. Phys. 29:* 141. 1984.

MEYER, E.E. AND C.G. NEUMANN   Management of obese adolescents. *Ped. Clin. N. Am. 24(1):* 123. 1977.

NEUMAN, P. AND P. HALVORSON   *Anorexia Nervosa and Bulimia: Handbook for Counselors and Therapists.* Van Nostrand Reinhold. New York. 1983.

NEUMANN, C.G.   Obesity in pediatric practice: obesity in preschool and schoolage child. *Ped. Clin. N. Am. 24(1):* 117. 1977.

NEWMARK, S.R. AND B. WILLIAMSON   Survey of very-low calorie weight reduction diets. *Arch. Int. Med. 143:* 1195. 1983.

POLIVY, J.   Psychological consequences of food restriction. *J. Am. Diet. Assoc. 96(6):* 589. 1996.

POWER, C., ET AL   Body mass index and height from childhood to adulthood in the 1958 British birth cohort. *Am. J. Clin. Nutr. 66:* 1094. 1997.

PUGLIESE, M.T., ET AL   Fear of obesity: Cause of short stature and delayed puberty. *New Eng. J. Med. 309:* 513. 1983.

REES, J.M.   Eating disorders in adolescents: a model for broadening our perspective. *J. Am. Diet. Assoc. 96(1):* 22. 1996.

ROLLAND-CACHERA, M.R., ET AL   Adiposity rebound in children: Simple indicator for predicting obesity. *Am. J. Clin. Nutr. 39:* 129. 1984.

ROLLS, B.J. AND J.O. HILL   *Carbohydrates and Weight Management. ILSI Press.* Washington, D.C. 1998.

SATTER, E.M.   Internal regulation and evolution of normal growth as the basis for prevention of obesity in children. *J. Am. Diet. Assoc. 96(9):* 860. 1996.

SORENSEN, T.I.A. AND S. SONNE-HOLM   Risk in childhood of development of severe adult obesity: retrospective, population-based case-cohort study. *Am. J. Epidemiol. 127:* 104. 1988.

STUNKARD, A., ET AL   Influences of social class on obesity and thinness in children. *J. Am. Med. Assoc. 221:* 579. 1972.

TAITZ, L.S.   Obesity in pediatric practice: infantile obesity. *Ped. Clin. N. Am. 24(1):* 107. 1977.

Van Itallie, T.B. and M.R. Yang   Cardiac dysfunction in obese dieters: Potentially lethal complication of rapid, massive weight loss. *Am. J. Clin. Nutr. 39:* 695. 1984.

Vasselli, J.R., et al   Modern concepts of obesity. *Nutr. Rev. 41:* 361. 1983.

Webb, P. and T. Abrams   Loss of fat stores and reduction in sedentary energy expenditure from undereating. *Human Nutr.,: Clin. Nutr. 37C:* 271. 1983.

Whisenant, S.L. and B.A. Smith   Eating disorders: current nutrition therapy and perceived needs in dietetics education and research. *J. Am. Diet. Assoc. 95(10):* 1109. 1995.

White, P.O. and T. Mondeika   *Diet and Exercise: Synergisms in Health Maintenance.* Am. Med. Assn. Chicago. 1982.

Worthington, B.S. and L.E. Taylor   Balanced low-calorie vs. high-protein-low-carbohydrate reducing diets. *J. Am. Diet. Assoc. 64:* 47. 1974.

Wurtman, J.J.   Involvement of brain serotonin in excessive carbohydrate snacking by obese carbohydrate cravers. *J. Am. Diet. Assoc. 84:* 1004. 1984.

Young, C.M., et al   Frequency of feeding, weight reduction, and body composition. *J. Am. Diet. Assoc. 59:* 466. 1971.

SECTION FOUR

The Adult Years

CHAPTER ELEVEN

Adults

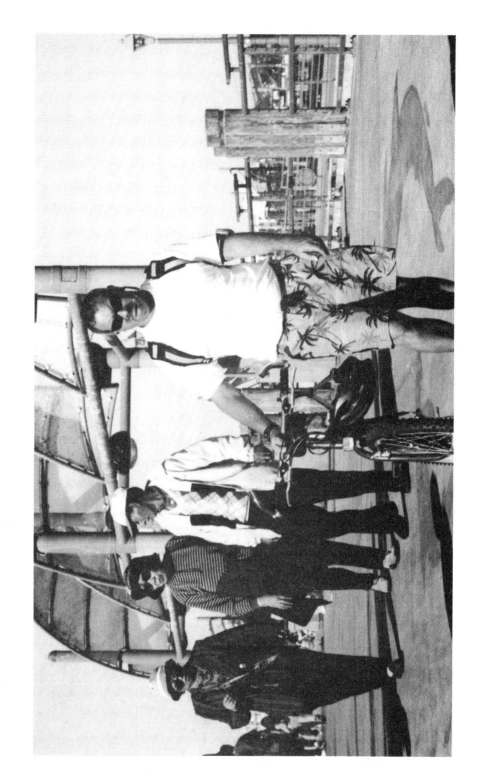

OVERVIEW

Adults are really "walking histories" bearing the imprint of nutritional status throughout life — the prenatal period, infancy, childhood, adolescence, and adulthood right up to today. Such visual evidence as height and incidence of decayed, missing, or filled teeth is noticed rather easily. However, many other effects of long-term nutritional status are present, but may not be readily apparent. A prime example is the integrity of bones, for nutrition over the years plays a vital role in maintaining bone density.

The familiar expression, "You are what you eat," certainly summarizes the importance of nutrition in our daily lives. For adults, a minor change to say, "You are what you eat and have eaten," is a particularly accurate way of pointing out the significance of dietary patterns throughout life. Health, vigor, work capacity, and happiness are key components of life, and nutrition is a vital foundation for achieving them. The food habits of adults determine, at least in part, the rate at which the physical, emotional, and mental changes of aging are evidenced.

Some people reach adulthood with vigorous, normally functioning bodies and minds. Others permanently carry many nutritional scars. The scars may not be detectable immediately, but animal experiments have shown that faulty nutrition in early life may induce physical problems in later life. The nutritional needs of the adult must, therefore, be considered both from the standpoint of those who have been well

409

*nourished as children and those whose diets were inade-
quate in the early years or teens.*

SOCIOPSYCHOLOGICAL
INFLUENCES ON DIET

You might be tempted to assume that a person who is well nourished throughout childhood has established the dietary patterns needed for a lifetime of good nutrition. Certainly this would be helpful if it were true, but many physiological, psychological, and sociological changes occur that influence dietary patterns during the remaining stages of the life cycle. When people live together, there is usually at least a small change in dietary patterns as people blend their tastes into a single menu, and if there is an intermixture of cultures, the dietary alterations may be significant. And the social makeup of the people living together may change over time so that the dietary adjustments may very well be made more than once in a lifetime.

The occupation of an adult may be responsible for other dietary shifts a person makes. Corporate personnel in the sales division and other professional people are confronted with the prospect of many meals away from home when they entertain clients or travel on business. Heavy schedule pressures may interfere so that some professional people do not have time to eat lunch at all. Still others may have jobs with heavy responsibilities and considerable tension, which culminate in physical problems such as hypertension, thus necessitating dietary changes not necessarily of the person's choosing. Some women who have been calorically indiscreet during pregnancy may also join the ranks of those who are modifying their diets. People working at home continually are confronted with ready access to food and the problems of excess weight if they yield to the urge to snack frequently. Food provides a strong temptation for people who like to sample frequently while cooking. Those who find working at home lonely or frustrating may use food as a means of escape.

Two-income households are very common today, a fact which has created some significant changes in family meal patterns. The problem of having time to prepare meals at home is further compounded by the long commutes that many workers must make. The bottom line for such families is often a dinner bought on the way home, eaten at a restaurant, or prepared from convenience items (frozen meals and/or mixes). The actual nutritional merits of such dinners will vary widely, depending on the choices that are made.

Regardless of the specific meal situations in a household there is a basic need for all people in the family to be fed, and some patterns to accomplish this task will evolve for each household. For some people, the pattern may involve breakfast eaten while driving to work, lunch at the desk, and a microwaved frozen dinner. Another household may have an organized family breakfast, lunches purchased away from home, and a nourishing, tempting dinner eaten together at the family dining table. Countless other variations can be observed all around you, and you may follow yet a different pattern. The point is that there are many ways in which people eat, but the long-term impact of these daily decisions can greatly influence your health as you proceed through life. Good nutrition can be viewed as a form of health insurance to minimize physical problems in the future.

Young adults are faced with many opportunities and challenges as they proceed to complete their education, enter the work world, and establish their own households. This is a period involving a real juggling act, one in which the challenges of earning a good income in an interesting job, maintaining a pleasing and healthy lifestyle, and often managing the intricacies of parenting all must be met satisfactorily! No wonder today's young adults seem to be perenially on the move and running from behind. The good news is that you can juggle these tasks with some careful planning — planning that includes setting some priorities and making some educated choices — and then following up on your plans. Even good nutrition and exercise can become regular parts of your days. Remember that a goal of young adults is to help assure optimal health through good nutrition (and even to try to correct physical problems that may be developing due to previous poor nutrition habits).

A TIME FOR AN OUNCE OF PREVENTION

Early adulthood is a pivotal time for people to take stock of their nutritional status and to honestly assess their eating patterns. Necessary modifications can still be made that can have critical influences on their health as they grow into their senior years. The old saying that "An ounce of prevention is worth a pound of cure" surely applies to health. However, continuing efforts to monitor eating patterns and nutritional status are required. Small changes continued over a long period of time can have either beneficial or detrimental effects, depending on the changes. Smart food choices are basically what is needed to derive the benefits of good nutrition to help promote optimal health. A row of bottles with fancy supplements is not appropriate.

Just what are the particular health conditions that are of special concern when considering how you are eating? For both men and women, overweight and obesity provide a primary focus because of the significance of excess weight in some other health problems. Coronary heart disease, hypertension, type 2 diabetes, stroke, gallbladder disease, osteoarthritis, sleep apnea, respiratory problems, and certain cancers appear at a higher rate among overweight and obese people than among the population as a whole.

Research is continuing at a furious pace to investigate the impact of various food choices on heart disease and on various cancers. The importance of dietary patterns throughout the adult years in helping to avoid not only these health problems, but also osteoporosis is emerging. Doubtless there will be much more information available to help consumers within the next 10 years.

The various conditions that can be influenced by dietary choices are examined in the following sections. Recognition of the importance of diet in relation to these common health problems is vital to helping adults practice healthy nutrition habits, beginning right now!

OVERWEIGHT AND OBESITY

Not only is excess weight a growing problem in the United States, but it also is projected to grow still larger. The National Nutrition and Health Examination Survey conducted between 1960 and 1962 found the prevalence of overweight and obesity in persons 20 and older was over 43% of the population (Table 11.1). That number ballooned to almost 55% between 1988 and 1994, the period measured in the National Health and Nutition Examination Survey (NHANES III). Of particular concern is the rapid increase in obesity (BMI of 30.0 or greater kg/m^2) from 14.4% of women and men in NHANES II (1976–80) to 22.3% of women and men in NHANES III (1988–1994) (see Table 11.2).

NHANES I, II, AND III National Health and Nutrition Examination Survey I (1971–74), II (1976–80), III (1988–94); federal studies to assess health and nutritional status of a representative sample of Americans.

TABLE 11.1   Prevalence (%) of Overweight and Obesity (BMI $\geq$ 25.0 kg/m^2) Among Adults 20 and Older in the United States, 1960–1994[a]

Population Group	NHES I 1960–62 (age 20–74)	NHANES I 1971–74 (age 20–74)	NHANES II 1976–80 (age 20–74)	NHANES III 1988–94 (age $\geq$ 20)
Men				
(20–29)	39.9	38.6	37.0	43.1
(30–39)	49.6	58.1	52.6	58.1
(40–49)	53.6	63.6	60.3	65.5
(50–59)	54.1	58.4	60.8	73.0
(60–69)	52.9	55.6	57.4	70.3
(70–79)	36.0[b]	52.7[b]	53.3[b]	63.1
(all ages)	48.2	52.9	51.4	59.4
Women				
(20–29)	17.0	23.2	25.0	33.1
(30–39)	32.8	35.0	36.8	47.0
(40–49)	42.3	44.6	44.4	52.7
(50–59)	55.0	52.2	52.8	64.4
(60–69)	63.1	56.2	56.5	64.0
(70–79)	57.4	55.9[b]	58.2[b]	57.9
(all ages)	38.7	39.7	40.8	50.7
Both Sexes (all ages)	*43.3*	*46.1*	*46.0*	*54.9*

[a]Adapted from Flegal, K.M., et al. Overweight and obesity in the United States: prevalence and trends, 1960–1994. *Int. J. Obes. 22:* 39. 1998.
[b]Ages (70–74)

At all ages, obesity occurs at a greater rate in women than in men, a pattern that has held true in all the surveys included in Table 11.2 except in NHES I (ages 20–29). The pattern of incidence of obesity with regard to age is the same in men as in women. Among adults, the lowest incidence of obesity is when they are between age 20 and 29. There is an increase in the decades of the 30s and 40s, but the highest incidence of obesity is found in the 50s for both men and women. After the 50s, there is a gradual reduction in the percentage of the population that is obese, but the numbers are still very sobering, especially when the trend seems to be ever increasing numbers.

TABLE 11.2   Prevalence (%) of Overweight and Obesity (BMI ≥ 30.0 kg/m^2) Among Adults 20 and Older in the United States, 1960–1994[a]

Population Group	NHES I 1960–62 (age 20–74)	NHANES I 1971–74 (age 20–74)	NHANES II 1976–80 (age 20–74)	NHANES III 1988–94 (age ≥ 20)
Men				
(20–29)	9.0	8.0	8.1	12.5
(30–39)	10.4	13.3	12.1	17.2
(40–49)	11.9	14.2	16.4	23.1
(50–59)	13.4	15.3	14.3	28.9
(60–69)	7.7	10.3	13.5	24.8
(70–79)	8.6[b]	11.1[b]	13.6[b]	20.0
(all ages)	10.4	11.8	12.2	19.5
Women				
(20–29)	6.1	8.2	9.0	14.6
(30–39)	12.1	15.1	16.8	25.8
(40–49)	17.1	17.6	18.1	26.9
(50–59)	20.4	22.0	22.6	35.6
(60–69)	27.2	24.0	22.0	29.8
(70–79)	21.9	21.0[b]	19.4[b]	25.0
(all ages)	15.1	16.1	16.3	25.0
Both Sexes (all ages)	*12.8*	*14.1*	*14.4*	*22.3*

[a]Adapted from Flegal, K.M., et al. Overweight and obesity in the United States: prevalence and trens, 1960–1994. *Int. J. Obes. 22:* 39. 1998.
[b]Ages (70–74)

Some interesting differences can be noted in Table 11.3, which presents data on overweight and obesity in different racial groups in the United States, as measured in NHANES III (1988–94). Among Whites and non-Hispanic Whites, the incidence of overweight was greater than obesity for both men and women. This was also true for Black, non-Hispanic Black, and Mexican-American men, but the reverse was true for these groups of women. Black and non-Hispanic Black women had the highest incidence of obesity, followed fairly closely by Mexican-American women.

Obesity and overweight are a rapidly growing nutritional concern among the whole population.

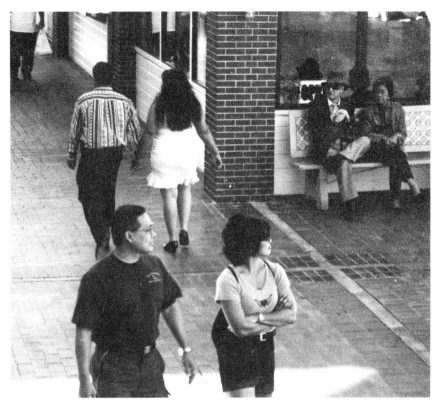

Just over $51.6 billion was spent in medical and disability costs in 1995 for conditions resulting from or aggravated by obesity, and indirect costs for this problem were estimated to be about $47.6 billion in 1995. Clearly, obesity is both an expensive problem, as well as a personal health hazard.

Extensive coordinated efforts have been made to identify health achievements and problems on a national level in the United States. At the present time, work is in progress to draft the document "Healthy People 2010 Objectives," which is being developed under the Assistant Secretary for Health in the Department of Health and Human Services. This developing document will be based on assessment of progress toward the goals that were set forth in "Healthy People 2000" and new projections for achievement by 2010.

Work on the nutrition section is divided into 20 objectives, three of which address weight control: healthy weight, obesity in

TABLE 11.3 Prevalence (%) of Overweight (BMI ≥ 25.0 kg/m²) and Obesity (BMI ≥ 30.0 kg/m²) by Race/Ethnicity in the United States, as Determined in NHANES III (1988–1994)[a]

Race/Sex	Overweight	Obese	Total overweight and Obese
White			
Men	41.0	20.0	61.0
Women	25.7	23.5	49.2
Black			
Men	35.9	20.6	56.5
Women	29.3	36.5	65.8
White, non-Hispanic			
Men	40.7	19.9	60.6
Women	24.7	22.7	47.4
Black, non-Hispanic			
Men	36.0	20.7	56.7
Women	29.3	36.7	66.0
Mexican-American			
Men	43.3	20.6	63.9
Women	32.6	33.3	65.9

[a]Adapted from Flegal, K.M., et al. Overweight and obesity in the United States: prevalence and trends, 1960–1994. *Int. J. Obes. 22:* 39. 1998.

adults, and overweight and obesity in children/adolescents. The proposed objectives directed toward the adult population are:

1. Increase to at least 60% the prevalence of healthy weight (defined as a BMI equal to or greater than 19.0 and less than 25.0) among all people aged 20 and older. (Baseline: from 1988 to 1994, 41% of all people aged 20 years and older were at a healthy weight, 39% of males and 44% of females).

2. Reduce to less than 15% the prevalence of BMI at or above 30.0 among people aged 20 and older. (Baseline: from 1988 to 1994, 22% of people aged 20

and older had BMIs ≥ 30.0 (20% of males and 25% of females).

3. Reduce to 5% or less the prevalence of overweight and obesity (at or above the sex- and age-specific 95th percentile of BMI from the revised NCHS/CDC growth charts) in children (aged 6–11) and adolescents (aged 12–19). (Baseline: in 1988–1994, 11% of all children and 10% of all adolescents were overweight or obese.)

CARDIOVASCULAR DISEASE

CARDIOVASCULAR DISEASE (CVD) General term covering various abnormalities and dysfunctions of the heart and blood vessels.

Cardiovascular disease (CVD) is a broad term that covers dysfunction of both the heart and blood vessels. Included conditions are atherosclerosis (e.g., coronary heart disease leading to heart attacks), cerebrovascular disease (e.g., stroke), and hypertension (high blood pressure). The risk of developing cardiovascular disease (including hypertension) as well as Type 2 diabetes, is increased with increasing overweight and obesity (Table 11.4).

Ideally, coronary arteries are capable of delivering adequate oxygenated blood to the heart to meet its need for oxygen and other nutrients. However, the ideal situation is often compromised gradually as people age, and they begin to deposit

TABLE 11.4   **Risk of Cardiovascular Disease, Hypertension, and Type 2 Diabetes Among Overweight and Obese people Compared with Normal Weight Persons[a]**

Category (BMI)	Disease Risk and Waist Circumference	
	Men (≤ 40") Women (≤ 35")	Men (≥ 40") Women (≥ 35")
Overweight (25.0–29.9)	Increased	High
Obese (30.0–34.9)	High	Very high
(35.0–39.9)	Very high	Very high
Extremely obese (≥ 40)	Extremely high	Extremely high

[a]Adapted from *Preventing and Managing the Global Epidemic of Obesity.* Report of the World Health Organization Consultation of Obesity. WHO. Geneva. June, 1997.

fatty streaks in arteries and the eventual buildup of fibrous plaque. Atherosclerosis is the condition characterized by the formation and buildup of these deposits. As these deposits increase, blood flow in the arteries may become somewhat obstructed, a situation termed ischemia. Coronary heart disease (CHD) is characterized by atherosclerotic lesions in the coronary arteries.

Hypertension is abnormally high blood pressure. This condition is dubbed "the silent killer" because it can strike people who have no idea that they have this condition. Blood pressure tends to rise as the arteries lose some elasticity due to aging. The diagnosis of hypertension is made when systolic blood pressure is 140 mm Hg or greater and diastolic blood pressure is 90 mm Hg or greater.

In addition to overweight, obesity, and hypertension, there are other risk factors associated with coronary heart disease. Among these factors, the levels of the various blood lipids are of significance. Total serum cholesterol, low-density lipoprotein-cholesterol (LDL), high-density lipoprotein-choles-

ATHEROSCLEROSIS
Condition in which fatty streaks and fibrous plaque are deposited in the arteries.

ISCHEMIA
Obstruction of arterial blood flow due to buildup of fatty streaks and fibrous plaque in the arteries.

CORONARY HEART DISEASE (CHD)
Condition in which oxygen supply to the heart is reduced by atherosclerotic lesions.

HYPERTENSION
Systolic blood pressure of at least 140 mm Hg and a diastolic blood pressure of at least 90 mm Hg.

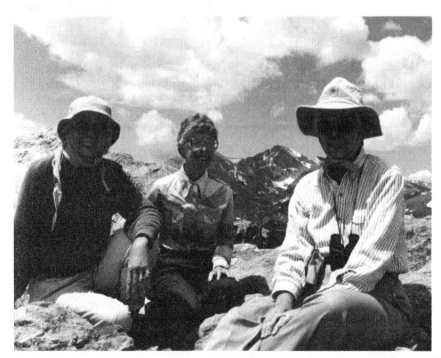

Hiking provides excellent aerobic exercise as well as some spectacular vistas for these middle-aged ladies.

TABLE 11.5   Blood Lipid Values as Risk Factors in CHD[a]

Compound	Relative risk of CHD			
	Normal (mg/dL)	Borderline-high (mg/dL)	High (mg/dL)	Very high (mg/dL)
Total cholesterol	<200	200–239	>240	
LDL-cholesterol	<130	130–159	≥160	
HDL-cholesterol	>35		<35	
Triglycerides	<200	200–400	400–1,000	>1,000

[a]Adapted from *Clinical Guidelines on the Identification, Evaluation, and Treatment of Overweight and Obesity in Adults.* National Institutes of Health, National Heart, Lung, and Blood Institute. Department of Health and Human Services. Washington, D.C. 1998. p. 64–65.

terol (HDL), and triglyceride levels are rated in relation to their influence on the risk of coronary heart disease (Table 11.5).

Cholesterol is transported in the blood to all body tissues combined with fat and protein in compounds called lipoproteins. These lipoproteins have different densities, and, in general, are referred to as high density lipoproteins (HDL) and low density lipoproteins (LDL). It has been found that the cholesterol in HDL is less likely to be deposited in arterial walls than that in LDL. Thus, the former is popularly referred to as "good" cholesterol and the latter as "bad" cholesterol. Moderate, frequent physical activity (exercise) favors the formation of HDL and decreases LDL, as does a small amount of alcohol in the diet, for example, a glass or two or wine.

It should be pointed out that cholesterol is present in all animal tissues, that it is an essential substance, and among other things, that it serves as the starting material for the body to synthesize vitamin D and some of the sex hormones.

The dietary intake of fats has an influence on blood lipid levels and, therefore, is an important topic in the development of the "Healthy People: 2010 Objectives." The U.S. Dietary Guidelines recommend that no more than 30% of the day's calories come from fat. Furthermore, less than 10% of the day's calories should be from saturated fats. These recommendations have been heeded by enough people to have caused a noticeable drop in fat consumption (33% calories from fat and 11% calories from saturated fat in 1994–1996). Despite these averages, many people in 1994–1996 were not reducing their fat intake to the recommended levels (Table 11.6).

TABLE 11.6 Percent of Various American Populations Meeting Goal of ≤30% Total Fat and <10% Saturated Fat, 1994–1996[a]

Population Group	% Meeting Dietary Guideline[b]	
	Total Fat	Saturated Fat
Male		
(20–39)	29	32
(40–59)	28	33
(≥60)	34	42
Female		
(20–39)	38	41
(40–59)	33	42
(≥60)	40	47
African American, *non-Hispanic*	25	29
Hispanic	33	35
White, non-Hispanic	34	35

[a]Adapted from *Continuing Survey of Food Intakes by Individuals (CSFII)*, US Department of Agriculture (2-day average).
[b]US Dietary Guidelines goal of no more than 30% calories from fat and less than 10% calories from saturated fat.

The fact that far less than half the population was meeting the guidelines for fat and saturated fat intake in 1994–1996 does not appear to daunt the optimists who are shaping the 2010 Objectives. Instead, they are proposing that the target objective be that at least 75% of the population age 2 and older meet both the maximum intake of 30% fat and less than 10% saturated fat. Such a strong recommendation is based on the recognized importance of controlling fat intake as a measure toward helping to minimize the risk of cardiovascular health problems.

Dietary patterns are a factor in the development of cardiovascular problems, but other factors also are involved. Smoking has been identified as a risk factor, and that (like diet and exercise) can be controlled by the individual. Men in their middle years are more likely to have a heart attack than are women, although women exhibit an increased risk after menopause. Other potential risk factors are diabetes, high homocysteine levels, and the incidence of heart attacks (particularly early in life) in the family lineage. Ancestors and sex are inherent in each individual, but lifestyle choices can be made to optimize cardio-vascular health throughout life.

RESEARCH INSIGHTS

Stampfer, M.J., et al., Primary prevention of coronary heart disease in women through diet and lifestyle. *N. Engl. J. Med. 343:* 16. 2000.

Stampfer, et al. (2000) noted that pharmacologic approaches to managing hypertension and blood lipid levels, as well as therapy in treating cases of acute myocardial infarction and congestive heart failure, have helped to reduce coronary heart disease, but present possible side effects and expense. These authors undertook this study to determine the impact of combining compliance with behavioral and dietary guidelines on preventing coronary problems and strokes.

This longitudinal study tracked 84,129 female Registered Nurses 14 years, beginning in 1980. Questionnaires at 2-year intervals provided the data analyzed in this project. Items included height, weight, smoking (current and past practices), occurrence of myocardial infarction in a parent before age 60, menopausal status and hormone use, physician-diagnosed hypertension and high cholesterol levels, physical activity (time and type), and a food-frequency and portion-size questionnaire (beginning in 1980 with 61 items and expanding to 116 items in 1984) which also included use of vitamin supplements (multi-and single vitamins). Women were classified regarding their risk level in 5 categories. Low risk was defined as never smoked or had not smoked within the past 10–14 years, moderate alcohol (5 g/day), at least 30 minutes of moderate or vigorous activity daily, body mass index of less than 25, and diet low in trans fat and glycemic load and high cereal fiber and omega-3 fatty acids and folate, and finally, a high ratio of polyunsaturated to saturated fat. Incidence of myocardial infarction or death due to coronary problems and also stroke incidence or stroke-related deaths were tracked throughout the 14 years of the study. Coronary heart disease was the cause of 296 deaths and 832 nonfatal coronary heart disease events. There also were 705 strokes. Smoking more than 14 cigarettes daily increased heart risks more than 5 times compared with non-smokers, while smoking between 1 and 14 tripled the risk. Women in the top 40% for diet scores were at less risk than those with poorer diets, but the influence was appreciably less than that for smoking. Those exercising more than 5.5 hours/week also reduced their risk compared with less active nurses. A BMI of 30 or more increased risk more than 50% above those with a BMI of less than 23.0. Consuming alcohol at a level approximately equal to a glass of wine daily reduced risk compared with no alcohol. Women in the low-risk category for all 5 factors had 5 coronary heart disease incidents compared with 62 for women who were in the low-risk category for 3 factors. The risk of a coronary event for the women at low risk in all 5 categories was estimated to be 80% lower than the rest of the population. The data from this study clearly support the benefits of optimizing behaviors and lifestyle, as defined by the factors considered in this research.

CANCER

Cancers of various types represent a major health problem in the United States, particularly among adults. Considerable public attention has been drawn to lung cancer and the major role that smoking plays in the incidence of this type of cancer. In the past few years there also has been considerable focus on the relationships between various environmental contaminants and cancers. More recently, various foods in the diet have been pin-pointed for their possible contributions toward promoting cancer and especially toward protecting against cancers. Research around diet and food is extensive, and some information is beginning to emerge that is shaping dietary recommendations.

The carcinogenic effects of charcoal-broiled meats, particularly when the surface is charred, have been noted and publicized for many years. The link noted between nitrates used at high levels for preserving bacon and some other meats led to studies that resulted in reduced levels of nitrate (but still protective against harmful microorganisms) in today's bacon, weiners, and other preserved meats. On-going efforts are directed toward noting and studying other potentially carcinogenic factors in foods.

Today much of the research relating to food and cancers is centered around the potential protective effects that certain foods and/or their components may have in relation to the development of cancer. Phytochemicals are receiving headlines as their potential for protecting against cancer is being studied. Literally, phytochemicals are chemicals from plants. Actually, there are various types of chemical compounds in certain plants that may provide various unique functions in the body without serving as nutrients. The mechanisms of some of these phytochemicals are not well understood at the present time, but there is some evidence accumulating that the compounds may be effective in protecting against certain physical problems.

PHYTOCHEMICAL
Compound found in a plant that may perform a protective role (non-nutritive) against certain physical problems.

Phytoestrogens are phytochemicals that are chemically somewhat similar to estrogens produced by the body. The structural similarity appears to allow phytoestrogens to occupy some reactive sites in the body that otherwise would be receptive to natural estrogens, which may be a factor in protecting against breast cancer. This type of reaction is an example of an antiestrogen action. Other times phytoestrogens are weakly estrogenic in their behavior, thus promoting bone density to aid in protecting against osteoporosis. Soybeans are rich in isoflavones, which are valued as phytoestrogens.

FUNCTIONAL FOOD
Foods observed to have some health benefits beyond just their nutritive content.

Although phytochemicals are gaining considerable recognition and the study that is needed to clarify their possible roles and benefits in human health, it is important to remember that these compounds occur in nature as just part of the complex components of the foods we eat. Observations regarding the possible beneficial effects of phytochemicals actually are usually the result of consumption of specific foods or groups of foods, followed by efforts to identify the specific components in the foods that may account for the health influences of these foods in the diet. These foods considered to have protective functions against various health problems are termed "functional foods."

Among the plant foods identified as functional foods are grains (particularly oats), legumes (especially soybeans), and fruits and vegetables (notably tomatoes, citrus, cranberries, crucifers, tea, dark green and leafy vegetables, garlic, and onions). Some of the phytochemicals thought to be responsible for the perceived functional properties of these and other functional foods are presented in Table 11.7.

OMEGA-6 FATTY ACIDS
Fatty acid family in which the first double bond is at the sixth carbon atom from the methyl group at the end of the molecule.

OMEGA-3 FATTY ACIDS
Fatty acid family in which the first double bond is at the third carbon atom from the methyl group at the end of the molecule.

Recognition of the significant roles these and other functional foods play in promoting human health underscores the importance of eating a wide array of foods as major components of the diet. The U.S. Dietary Guidelines and the Food Guide Pyramid have been developed as the major vehicles for emphasizing the importance of eating fruits, vegetables, and cereal products in abundance each day. The slogan "5 a Day" has been publicized extensively to highlight the need for at least 5 servings of fruits and vegetables each day.

The possible role of fatty acids in cancer also has been the subject of considerable study. Attention has been directed toward the polyunsaturated fatty acids (PUFA), with particular efforts being made to understand the significance of the omega-6 (ω-6) and omega-3 (ω-3) fatty acids. This designation means that the first double bond in these families is located 6 or 3 carbon

TABLE 11.7   Selected Phytochemicals, Their Sources, and Possible Protective Role

Compound	Source	Possible Role
Isoflavones Genistein	Soybeans (tofu, tempeh, soy flour, TVP, soy protein isolate, soy milk)	Antiestrogenic to help protect against breast cancer; weak estrogenic effect to promote bone density and protect against osteoporosis; perhaps useful in reducing symptoms of menopause; lower serum cholesterol
Carotenoids Lycopene	Tomatoes	Antioxidant action suppresses growth of cells in prostate, stomach, colon, and rectal cancers
β-carotene	Carrots; winter squash; dark green, leafy vegetables	Antioxidant action may protect against some cancers and myocardial infarction
β-glucan	Oat bran, oatmeal	Reduction of cholesterol (total and low-density lipoprotein)
Allium	Garlic, onions	Possible reduction of cancers of gastrointestinal tract
Glucosinolates Indoles Isothiocyanates	Cruciferous vegetables (broccoli, cabbage, Brussels sprouts, cauliflower)	Protection against breast cancer
Limonoids Limonene	Citrus fruits	Possible protection against cancer
Polyphenols Catechins	Tea	Some evidence of protection against breast cancer
Flavonoids	Tea	May reduce risk of cardiovascular disease
Phenols	Red wine	May have antioxidant effect to prevent oxidation of LDLs to impede atherogenesis
Plant lignans	Flaxseed	May possibly reduce risk of breast cancer; may aid in lowering LDL- and total cholesterol

atoms from the methyl (non-working) end of the fatty acid, respectively. Sometimes these are designated as N-6 and N-3 rather than as omega because of the recognition of the location of the first double bond from the non-working end of the molecule.

The ω-6 family is represented by an essential polyunsaturated fatty acid — linoleic acid, which has 18 carbon atoms and 2 double bonds. Among the plant sources of linoleic acid are the oils extracted from soybeans, safflower, corn, and canola. All of

LINOLEIC ACID
Polyunsaturated 18-carbon fatty acid with the first of its 2 double bonds occurring at the omega-6 carbon.

α-LINOLENIC ACID

Polyunsaturated 18-carbon fatty acid with the first of its 3 double bonds at the omega-3 carbon.

EICOSAPENTANOIC ACID

Omega-3 fatty acid with 20 carbon atoms and 5 double bonds; abbreviated EPA.

DOCOSAHEXANOIC ACID

Omega-3 fatty acid with 22 carbon atoms and 6 double bonds; abbreviated DHA.

these oils are commonly used in the diet as oils and/or margarines. The ω-3 family includes α-linolenic acid, an essential fatty acid which also is an 18-carbon polyunsaturated fatty acid. However, the first of its 3 double bonds occurs at the third carbon from the methyl end. Soybean, flax seed, and canola oils are excellent sources of ω-3 fatty acids.

In the body, metabolism of the ω-6 polyunsaturated fatty acids results in the formation of arachidonic acid, which has 20 carbon atoms and 4 double bonds, with the first double bond occurring at the ω-6 carbon atom. Metabolism of the ω-3 polyunsaturated fatty acids leads to a formation of eicosapentanoic acid (fortunately abbreviated EPA) and docosahexanoic acid (DHA). Eicosapentanoic acid has a structure of 20 carbon atoms and 5 double bonds, beginning with the ω-3 carbon atom. Docosahexanoic acid (DHA) has 22 carbon atoms and 6 double bonds, beginning at the third carbon from the methyl end (Fig. 11.1) The ω-3 fatty acids are found in fish oils. Tuna, salmon, sardines, and anchovies are especially good sources of ω-3 fatty acids, but other fish also are of merit.

The fact that the ω-6 and ω-3 polyunsaturated fatty acids are metabolized differently in the body is of apparently some significance in influencing production of prostaglandins in the body. Prostaglandins are hormone-like regulatory eicosanoids that help regulate blood pressure and other actions in the body which are important to help avoid heart attacks and strokes. This role has been the foundation for the recommendation of increased fish consumption and reduced beef and other red meats to help promote heart health.

More recently, the possible link between reduced intake of ω-6 polyunsaturated fatty acids and somewhat greater intake of ω-3 polyunsaturated fatty acids and reduced incidence of intestinal cancers was noted. Results of extensive studies are not yet available, but there appears to be wisdom in eating fish, particularly those that are excellent sources of ω-3 polyunsaturated fatty acids. However, consumption of fish liver oil supplements is not suggested, but rather consumption through dietary sources is suggested. Emphasis on use of canola and soybean oils and limiting polyunsaturated fat intake to no more than 10% are recommended.

OSTEOPOROSIS

Osteoporosis can be translated literally as "porous bones," for it is a condition characterized by reduced bone mass.

ω-6 Acids

$$CH_3(CH_2)_4CH=CHCH_2CH=CH(CH_2)_7COOH$$
Linoleic Acid

$$CH_3(CH_2)_4(CH=CHCH_2)_4(CH_2)_2COOH$$
Arachidonic Acid

ω-3 Acids

$$CH_3(CH_2CH=CH)_3(CH_2)_7COOH$$
α-Linolenic Acid

$$CH_3(CH_2CH=CH)_5(CH_2)_3COOH$$
Eicosapentanoic Acid

$$CH_3(CH_2CH=CH)_6(CH_2)_2C00H$$
Docosahexanoic Acid

Fig. 11.1 Selected omega-6 and omega-3 fatty acids and their metabolic products.

This situation becomes evident among older people when they begin to show evidence of a widow's hump or suffer broken bones that may result from a fall or perhaps simply from structurally faulty bones. The genesis of osteoporosis actually is based in childhood and the early adult years, for these are the years when storage of calcium is occurring in the bones to form structurally sound bones throughout the body. Deposition can occur into the decade of the 30s, but then withdrawal of calcium from the skeleton begins to dominate over deposition, the result being a gradual diminishment of bone mass or bone density. In women, demineralization is accelerated following menopause, apparently due to reduced levels of estrogens.

OSTEOPOROSIS Condition characterized by reduced bone mass.

Several risk factors have been identified for developing osteoporosis. Females are more susceptible to developing osteoporosis than are males; Whites and Asians are at greater risk than Blacks or Hispanics, although anybody can develop osteoporosis. Other uncontrollable risk factors include family history, unusually short or tall physique, diabetes mellitus, hyperparathyroidism, hyperthyroidism, early menopause, low testosterone (in men), and advancing age. Risk factors that can and should be avoided include low calcium intake, limited physical actvity, smoking, and excessive alcohol consumption.

Although some demineralization of the skeleton is a consequence of aging, the extent of physical disability related to this process can be minimized through long-term dietary efforts. In particular, calcium intake from dietary sources needs to be a focus of everybody's eating patterns throughout life. Milk needs to be a pillar of meal and snack planning for children of all ages. Unfortunately, the widespread pattern of using sodas as the beverage rather than milk has resulted in a smaller consumption of calcium among today's children. This is setting them up for a future that includes osteoporosis unless milk becomes a corner-stone of their diets long before they enter the 30s. Clearly, young adults need to be aware of the importance of building stores of calcium in their bones to maximize the amount of calcium deposited before they enter the withdrawal phase that occurs after the late 30s.

LACTOSE
INTOLERANCE
Discomfort following ingestion of milk due to inadequate lactase, the enzyme needed to digest lactose (the sugar in milk).

The easiest way to obtain adequate calcium at any age is to drink milk (whole, lowfat, or fat free). However, some people avoid milk because of allergies or because of lactose intolerance. Unfortunately, apparently far more people think they have lactose intolerance than actually do have this problem of digesting lactose (McBean and Miller, 1998). Many people also do not understand that lactose intolerance is not the same problem as an allergy to milk (allergic response to proteins in milk).

The actual extent of lactose intolerance is hard to assess because of the possibility of individuals misinterpreting symptoms following ingestion of milk. Rosado, J. et al, (1987) found that many people avoided milk and milk products or used lactose digestive aids because they thought they might possibly have a problem if they consumed milk. This avoidance occurred despite the lack of proof that they were lactose intolerant. It is true that many of the world's population groups may have some lactose intolerance. These groups include a high proportion of adult Asians, many Hispanics and Blacks, and some Caucasians. However, a review of research on the ability of lactose-intolerant individuals to tolerate varying levels of milk in the diet (McBean and Miller, 1998) found that many of the subjects could consume 1 or 2 glasses of milk daily without discomfort, particularly if they consumed the milk at breakfast and dinner rather than all at one time and if they also ate some solid food along with the milk. This conclusion suggests that milk need not be avoided in the diets of most people who think they have lactose intolerance, but that they should consume no more than a cup at a time and that the milk should be accompanied by solid food.

DIABETES MELLITUS

Diabetes mellitus is a group of conditions characterized by glucose intolerance. Type II (noninsulin-dependent) diabetes may occur in adults, particularly among those who are obese. People who have a family history of diabetes mellitus should be checked periodically to determine their fasting blood glucose levels and their levels following administration of a glucose "load." If their fasting blood glucose level is above 140 at different testings, their level at random testings is 200 or more, and the glucose tolerance test shows a level above 200 after 2 hours, the diagnosis may be diabetes mellitus. Diet modifications likely will be necessary to manage the course of the disease. Often the most important aspect of dietary management is to effect some weight loss. This change alone can often ameliorate the problems of diabetes, Clearly, in diabetes (as in some other adult health conditions) overweight and obesity are central to the occurrence of the problem.

NUTRITIONAL NEEDS

ENERGY REQUIREMENTS

The crisis that is building in America regarding unhealthful weights of people of all ages requires that careful thought be given to finding solutions to alleviate the situation throughout the nation. Adults, as a group, show a pattern of increasing weight during the early and middle adult years, usually followed by some leveling off or declining weight in the golden years. It is particularly important to focus on this problem in the early adult years, not only because of the importance of controlling weight gain before it begins to be an imposing problem, but also because this is a time when parents set a very important example for their children. This example will subtly influence what happens to these children as they reach adulthood, too.

Among the reasons that adults tend to gain weight even though they are no longer growing is that their metabolism gradually is slowing throughout adult life. The consequence of this gradual and subtle change in the need for energy for metabolic

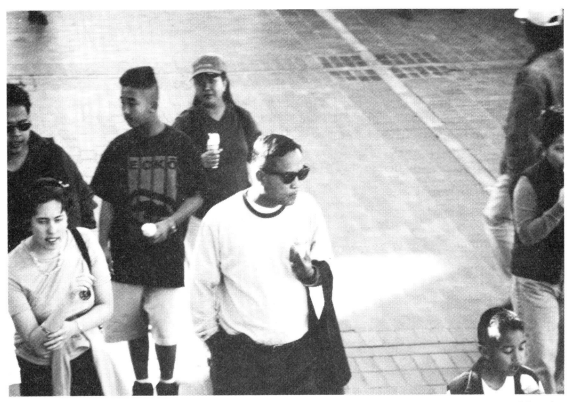

Snacking adds extra calories for these strollers, a pattern that contributes to the weight problem in the United States.

demands is that weight is gained even though caloric intake may remain unchanged. The reduced need for calories for basal metabolism means that fewer calories need to be available to keep the body operating. Any excess calories are manifested ultimately as increased fatty deposits, a sight all too familiar to many adults.

Reduced activity frequently is a part of the lifestyle changes that develop in the transition from the teens to being an adult. The demands of jobs and families tend to place severe limits on the time and energy adults may have for exercise. Sedentary lifestyles require fewer calories than do physically active patterns. Again, this can evolve into a routine that requires very limited energy from food. The net result of reduced activity and gradually slowing metabolism is a need to limit caloric intake during the adult years. The limitations that are necessary are dependent on the physical activities that define the lifestyle of each person. The energy levels recommended for reference adults in 1989 are presented in Table 11.8.

A pound of weight gain represents an intake of approximately 3,500 kilocalories more than are expended. The usual pattern of weight gain in the adult years is a gradual, rather than a sudden, weight gain. This subtle change might be about 5 pounds annually, which translates to consuming only about 50 calories per day more than are expended. The voracious appetite and growth demands of the teens are likely to have resulted in eating patterns that arc firmly established at a higher level than is needed in adulthood. A minor decrease in the size of servings will be enough to avoid the typical weight gains of adulthood. The important thing is to check weight on a weekly basis at the same time of day to detect weight gain when it starts rather than when 10 extra pounds are already accumulated. Avoidance of excess weight is far easier than weight loss.

The keys to weight control include:

1. Limiting fat intake to no more than 30% of calories (by such measures as using nonfat dairy products, trimming fat from meats, keeping meat portions to

TABLE 11.8   Recommended Energy Intakes[a]

Age	Weight		Height		REE[b]	Average energy allowance (cal)[c]		
	(kg)	(lb)	(cm)	(in)	(cal/day)	Multiples	(/kg)	(/day)[d]
Males								
(20–24)	72	160	177	70	1780	1.67	40	2900
(25–50)	79	174	176	70	1800	1.60	37	2900
(≥51)	77	170	173	68	1530	1.5	30	2300
Females								
(20–24)	58	128	164	65	1350	1.60	38	2200
(25–50)	63	138	163	64	1380	1.55	36	2200
(≥51)	65	143	160	63	1280	1.50	30	1900

[a]Adapted from Recommended Dietary Allowances, revised 1989 (abridged) by the National Academy of Sciences. National Academy Press. Washington, D.C.
[b]Calculation based on FAO equation, then rounded. REE = resting energy expenditure.
[c]Range of light to moderate activity (variation is ±20%).
[d]Figure is rounded.

about 4 ounces maximum; and using limited amounts of butter, margarine, and salad dressings).

2. Monitoring portion sizes (Table 11.9).

3. Eating an abundance of vegetables and fruits.

4. Generally avoiding snacking, particularly avoiding chips, dips, and other high-calorie snack foods; finding something else to do rather than reaching for a snack.

5. Exercising at least 3 times a week (weight bearing and aerobic).

You will hear countless suggestions for controlling weight. Some border on the bizarre and totally incredible, while others may provide practical help. The important thing is to be aware of your weight and to make minor adjustments in your eating pattern if you see your weight beginning to increase.

Weight reduction diets ultimately have to provide fewer calories than are being expended by the body. Those that emphasize only a few foods and that deviate from the recommendations in the Daily Food Guide do not provide the basis for a lifetime of healthful eating. A good weight reduction diet builds good dietary patterns and habits for healthy eating the rest of your life. Dietary habits that provide the variety and quantity of food needed for good health should be established during the time a weight correction plan is being followed. At the time that the desired weight goal is reached, the habits that have been developed will enable you to maintain a healthful weight.

One of the particularly important habits that should be developed and maintained is regular exercise, preferably aerobic and weight bearing. Three or more times a week for at least 30 minutes is a useful recommendation, but people who find it easy to say that tomorrow is going to be the day for exercise may be wise to make exercise a daily event. Walking is an inexpensive and effective activity; swimming is a vigorous means of exercising without causing stress on joints in the legs and ankles. The important point is that exercise needs to be done regularly and with enthusiasm. It should be an activity that is enjoyable for the person and convenient to do. Excuses to avoid exercising need to be eliminated as much as possible.

TABLE 11.9   Recommended Servings and Serving Sizes[a]

Food Group	Suggested Servings	Serving Size
Vegetables	3–5 Include dark-green leafy and deep-yellow often	1 c raw leafy 1/2 c any other kind
Fruits	2–4 Include citrus, melon, or berries daily Choose as desserts Use juices as beverages in place of sodas	1 med. apple, orange, banana 1/2 c small, diced fruit 3/4 c juice

Breads, cereals,
  rice, pasta
	6–11
	Include variety of grains
	Eat several servings of whole grains daily
		1 slice bread
		1/2 bun, bagel, or English
		  muffin
		1 oz dry, ready-to-eat
		  cereal
		1/2 c cooked rice, cereal,
		  or pasta

Milk, yogurt,
  and cheese
	2–3
	Choose fat free or light (lowfat) milks most
	  of the time
	Choose lowfat yogurt and lowfat cheese most
	  of the time
	Use regular cheeses in smaller servings and
	  less often
		1 c milk or yogurt
		1 1/2 oz cheese

Meats, poultry,
  fish, dry beans
  and peas, eggs,
  and nuts
	2–3
	Total daily of 6 oz cooked flesh foods
	Trim fat
	Remove skin from poultry
		3 oz cooked lean red meat,
		  skinless poultry, or fish
		1 c cooked dried beans or
		  peas
		2 eggs

[a]Adapted from *Dietary Guidelines for Americans*. Human Nutrition Service, US Department of Agriculture. Hyattsville, MD. 1990.

NUTRIENT RECOMMENDATIONS

The Recommended Dietary Allowances (RDA) generally are lower for women than for men, and they are the same or even a bit higher than earlier in life despite the fact that the actual need for calories is slightly reduced in adulthood (Table 11.10). Note that the iron recommendation is higher for women than for men until women reach menopause, at which time the RDA for iron is dropped to the same level as for men. This adjustment recognizes the need for iron to compensate for the loss of iron during menstruation.

TABLE 11.10   Recommended Dietary Allowances for Men and Women[a]

Nutrient	Men			Women[b]		
	(19–24)	(25–50)	(≥50)	(19–24)	(25–50)	(≥50)
Protein (g)	58	63	63	46	50	50
Vit. A (μg RE)[c]	1,000	1,000	1,000	800	800	800
Vit. K (μg)	70	80	80	60	60	60
Iron (mg)	10	10	10	15	15	10
Zinc (mg)	15	15	15	15	15	10
Iodine (μg)	150	150	150	150	150	150

[a]Adapted from Recommended Dietary Allowances, Revised 1989 (abridged). Food and Nutrition Board, National Academy of Sciences — National Research Council. Washington, D.C. 1989.
[b]The recommendations for pregnancy are in Table 4.6.
[c]Retinol equivalents. 1 retinol equivalent = 1 μg retinol or 6 μg β-carotene.
[d]α-Tocopherol equivalents. 1 mg d-α-tocopherol = 1 α-TE.

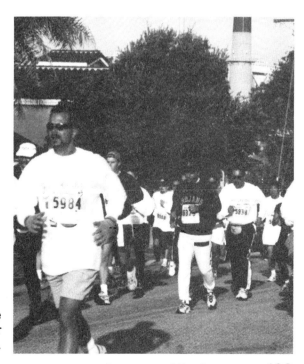

Jogathons and marathons inspire some adults to work at keeping fit with regular aerobic exercise.

Table 11.11 presents the Recommended Intakes for Individuals that were published in 2000. The nutrients for which Adequate Intakes (AI) had been established at that time were calcium, phosphorus, magnesium, vitamin D, fluoride, thiamin, riboflavin, niacin, vitamin B₆, folate, vitamin B₁₂, panthothenic acid, biotin, choline, vitamins C and E, and selenium. The recommendations reflect a somewhat greater need by men than by women for some of these nutrients.

TABLE 11.11   Recommended Intakes for Adults[a]

Nutrient (daily amounts)	Men				Women			
	(19–30)	(31–50)	(51–70)	(>70)	(19–30)	(31–50)	(51–70)	(>70)
Calcium (mg)	1,000	1,000	1,200	1,200	1,000	1,000	1,200	1,200
Phosphorus (mg)	700	700	700	700	700	700	700	700
Magnesium (mg)	420	420	420	420	310	320	320	320
Vitamin D (μg)[b,c]	5	5	10	15	5	5	10	15
Fluoride (mg)	4	4	4	4	3	3	3	3
Thiamin (mg)	1.2	1.2	1.2	1.2	1.1	1.1	1.1	1.1
Riboflavin (mg)	1.3	1.3	1.3	1.3	1.1	1.1	1.1	1.1
Niacin (mg equiv.)[d]	16	16	16	16	14	14	14	14
Vitamin B₆ (mg)	1.3	1.3	1.7	1.7	1.3	1.3	1.5	1.5
Folate (μg)[e]	400	400	400	400	400	400	400	400
Vitamin B₁₂ (μg)[f]	2.4	2.4	2.4	2.4	2.4	2.4	2.4	2.4
Pantothenic acid (mg)	5	5	5	5	5	5	5	5
Biotin (μg)	30	30	30	30	30	30	30	30
Choline (mg)[g]	550	550	550	550	425	425	425	425
Vitamin C (mg)	90	90	90	90	75	75	75	75
Vitamin E (mg)	15	15	15	15	15	15	15	15
Selenium (μg)	55	55	55	55	55	55	55	55

[a]Adapted from Dietary Reference Intakes: Recommended Intakes for Individuals. Food and Nutrition Board, Institute of Medicine, National Academy of Sciences. Washington, D.C. 2000.
[b]In the absence of adequate exposure to sunlight.
[c]As cholecalciferol. 1 μg = 40 IU Vitamin D.
[d]As niacin equivalents (NE). 1 mg niacin = 60 mg tryptophan.
[e]1 μg food folate = 0.6 μg folic acid from fortified food or supllement.
[f]Because 10–30% of people older than 50 may malabsorb food-bound Vitamin B₁₂, it is advisable for older people to consume foods fortified with Vitamin B₁₂ or take a supplement containing Vitamin B₁₂.
[g]Although AIs have been set for choline, there are few data to assess whether a dietary supply of choline is needed at all stages of the life cycle, and it may be the requirement can be met by endogenous synthesis at some of these stages.

TABLE 11.12   Fatty Acid Content in Selected Foods (100 g quantities)[a]

Food	Total fat (g)	Cholesterol (mg)	Fatty Acids			
			Saturated (g)	Mono-saturated (g)	Poly-saturated (g)	18:3 (g)
Butter	81.1	219	50.5	23.4	3.0	1.2
Margarine, regular stick						
Corn	80.5	0	13.2	45.8	18.0	N/A
Soybean	80.5	0	16.7	39.3	20.9	1.5
Oil						
Corn	100.0	0	12.7	24.2	58.7	
Cottonseed	100.0	0	25.9	17.8	51.9	
Olive	100.0	0	13.5	73.7	8.4	
Peanut	100.0	0	16.9	46.2	32.0	
Rapeseed (canola)	100.0	0	6.8	55.5	33.3	11.1
Safflower	100.0	0	9.1	12.1	74.5	
Soybean	100.0	0	14.4	23.3	57.9	6.8
Sunflower	100.0	0	10.1	45.4	40.1	

[a]Adapted from *Composition of Foods: Fats and Oils (Raw, Processed, Prepared)* Agriculture Handbook No. 8–4. US Department of Agriculture. Science and Education Administration. Washington, D.C. Rev. 1979.

EATING FOR OPTIMAL HEALTH

From the foregoing examination of many aspects of health and its interrelationships with dietary practices in adulthood, you can appreciate the importance of putting this knowledge into practice for the rest of your life. Clearly, what people eat can have a tremendous influence on them throughout their adult years. Food preferences, cultural food patterns, lifestyles, and income are among the major factors that determine what and how much people eat. Because of this individuality, specific menus are of limited use. However, some general guidelines can serve as guideposts in eating for good health.

1. Include 2 and preferably more glasses of fat free or low fat milk plus calcium-fortified orange juice or

other rich sources of calcium every day to provide at least 1000 mg calcium daily.

2. Select foods low in fat to limit the calories from fat to 30% of the day's calories, with no more than 10% of the day's calories coming from saturated fats, 10% from polyunsaturated fats (preferably omega-3 sources), and 10% from monounsaturated fatty acids (Tables 11.12 and 11.13). This guideline can be met by such practices as:

—Trimming fat from all meats
—Eating fish at least 3 meals per week
—Limiting serving sizes and frequency of eating red meats
—Including poultry frequently
—Choosing soybean and canola oils and using them sparingly
—Incorporating olive oil in salads and some other preparations because of its content of monounsaturates.

3. Eat at least 2 servings of fruit and 3 servings of vegetables daily. Include:

—Citrus or other good source of vitamin C daily
—Dark green, leafy or yellow vegetables at least every other day
—Frequent servings of foods rich in phytochemicals (Table 11.7).

4. Include plenty of fiber (at least 20 grams) daily by selecting (Table 11.14):

—Whole grain breads and cereal products
—Eating edible peels of fruits and vegetables
—Choosing whole fruits and vegetables rather than juices most of the time.

5. Eat a good breakfast and 2 other meals daily, but eliminate or keep snacks to a minimum

—Eat nutrient-rich breakfast, including citrus or other rich source of vitamin C, fat free milk, and whole-grain cereal or bread product (or other comparable nutrient-loaded, fairly low calorie menu).

Food	Total fat (g)	Chol-esterol (mg)	Saturated (g)	Mono-unsaturated (g)	Poly-unsaturated (g)	18:3[b] (g)	20:5[c] (g)	22:6[d] (g)
Bass, Freshwater	2.0	59	0.4	0.7	0.7	Tr	0.1	0.2
Catfish, Channel	4.3	58	1.0	1.6	1.0	Tr	0.1	0.2
Cod, Pacific	0.6	37	0.1	0.1	0.2	Tr	0.1	0.1
Flounder, Yellowtail	1.2	—	0.3	0.2	0.3	Tr	0.1	0.1
Haddock	0.7	63	0.1	0.1	0.3	Tr	0.1	0.1
Halibut, Pacific	2.3	32	0.3	0.8	0.7	0.1	0.1	0.3
Ocean Perch	1.6	42	0.3	0.6	0.5	Tr	0.1	0.1
Pike, Walleye	1.2	86	0.2	0.3	0.4	Tr	0.1	0.2
Salmon								
Atlantic	5.4	–	0.8	1.8	2.1	0.2	0.3	0.9
Coho	6.0	—	1.1	2.1	1.7	0.2	0.3	0.5
Snapper, Red	1.2	—	0.2	0.2	0.4	Tr	Tr	0.2
Swordfish	2.1	39	0.6	0.8	0.2	—	0.1	0.1
Trout, Brook	2.7	68	0.7	0.8	0.9	0.2	0.2	0.2
Tuna, Albacore	4.9	54	1.2	1.2	1.8	0.2	0.3	1.0
Crab, Alaska								
King	0.8	—	0.1	0.1	0.3	Tr	0.2	0.1
Blue	1.3	78	0.2	0.2	0.5	Tr	0.2	0.2
Dungeness	1.0	59	0.1	0.2	0.3	—	0.2	0.1
Lobster, Northern	0.9	95	0.2	0.2	0.2	—	0.1	0.1
Shrimp, Northern	1.25	125	0.2	0.3	0.6	Tr	0.3	0.2
Scallop. Atlantic	0.8	37	0.1	0.1	0.3	Tr	0.1	0.1

[a]Adapted from *Provisional Table on the Content of Omega-3 Fatty Acids and Other Fat-Components in Selected Foods*. US Department of Agriculture. Human Nutrition Information Service. Nutrient Data Research Branch. Nutrition Monitoring Division. Washington, D.C. 1988.
[b]Linolenic acid.
[c]Eicosapentaenoic acid (EPA).
[d]Docosahexenoic acid (DHA).

TABLE 11.14   Selected Sources of Dietary Fiber (100 g quantities)[a]

Food	Total Dietary Fiber (AOAC)	Food	Total Dietary Fiber (AOAC)
Bread		Banana	1.6
Cornbread	2.6	Blueberries	2.3
Cracked wheat	5.3	Grapes, Thompson, raw	0.7
French	2.3	Kiwifruit, raw	3.4
Mixed grain	6.3	Nectarines, raw	1.6
Oatmeal	3.9	Orange	
Pita, white	1.6	Raw	2.4
Pita, whole wheat	7.4	Juice	0.2
Pumpernickel	5.9	Peach, raw	1.6
Rye	6.2	Pineapple, raw	1.2
Whole wheat	7.4	Strawberries	2.6
White	1.9	Baked beans, canned	7.7
Tortilla		Beans, Great Northern, cooked	5.4
Corn	5.2	Tofu	1.2
Wheat flour	2.9	Spaghetti, cooked	1.6
Bran flakes	18.8	Broccoli, cooked	2.6
Corn flakes	2.0	Carrots, raw	3.2
Rice		Peas, cooked	2.8
Brown, cooked	3.5	Potatoes, baked w/ skin	4.0
Parboiled, cooked	0.5		
Apples			
Raw, w/ skin	2.2		
Raw, w/o skin	1.9		
Juice	0.1		
Sauce, sweetened	1.2		

[a]Adapted from *Provisional Table on the Content of Fiber in Selected Foods*. US Department of Agriculture. Human Nutrition Information Service. Nutrient Data Research Branch. Nutrition Monitoring Division. Washington, D.C. 1988.

—Watch portion sizes and fat content of the menus chosen.

—Drink water or fat free milk or pasteurized fruit juice (not sweetened fruit drink) or nibble on a raw vegetable if snacking is needed.

—Avoid snacking while watching television or doing other sedentary activities.

6. Eliminate most desserts except on special occasions.

—Healthful choices include baked custard, rice pudding, and fresh fruits.

—Very small portions provide the pleasure, without adding huge amounts of calories. (Serve only 2 or 3 bites rather than requiring will power to halt the fork or spoon.)

—Avoid candy almost all of the time by saying "no" when it is offered and by not keeping any at home or at work.

7. Reward yourself for practicing these and other healthy eating habits by going on a walk or other fun physical activity with family and/or friends.

SUMMARY

Adulthood is a critical time for eating well; your future health can be influenced significantly by how you choose to eat now. For parents, the healthful example they are setting for their children will help assure that good food habits are established before the adolescent years — a truly wonderful gift they can give to their children!

Particular attention needs to be directed toward eating a varied, adequate diet that provides all of the nutrients needed by the body without eating foods high in fat and empty calories that can promote unhealthful weight gain. When weight is managed for maintenance at the recommended weight (BMI between 19.0 and 25.0), serious health risks may be decreased. Inclusion of functional foods that provide phytochemicals, fiber, omega-3 fatty acids, and perhaps other health benefits beyond the defined roles of the nutrients can also contribute to maintenance of optimal health. The risk of developing osteoporosis can be reduced by consuming plenty of milk and other food sources of calcium. Exercise (load-bearing and aerobic) helps to protect against osteoporosis while also helping to combat weight gain and maintaining good muscle tone throughout the body.

Strategies to eat for good nutrition and health need to be developed individually to meet lifestyle and food preferences. However, a wide variety of foods emphasizing intake of milk, fruits, vegetables, and breads and cereal can be entwined with modest intake of protein foods (frequently fish and poultry) and a small amount of fat (a maximum of a third of the fat being from saturated fat, and the other two-thirds of the fat being split about equally between monounsaturated and omega-3 or other polyunsaturated fatty acids).

BIBLIOGRAPHY

ANDERSON, J.J.B. AND S.C. GARNER Phytoestrogens and human function. *Nutr. Today 32 (6):* 232. 1997.

ANONYMOUS Ω-3 fatty acids: review of role and benefits. *J. Am. Diet. Assoc. 98(9):* 963. 1998.

CAMERON, K.E., ET AL Prescription appetite suppressants in weight management. *Nutr. Today 32(5):* 202. 1997.

CONNOR, W.E. Do the ω-3 fatty acids from fish prevent deaths from cardiovascular disease? *Am. J. Clin. Nutr. 66:* 188. 1997.

CROSS, A.T., ET AL Snacking patterns among 1,800 adults and children. *J. Am. Diet. Asoc. 94(12):* 1398. 1994.

CULLINEN, K. AND M. CALDWELL. Weight training increases fat-free mass and strength in untrained young women. *J. Am. Diet. Assoc. 98 (4):* 414. 1998.

DJURIC, Z., ET AL Oxidative DNA damage levels in blood from women at high risk for breast cancer are associated with dietary intakes of meats, vegetables, and fruits. *J. Am. Diet. Assoc. 98(5):* 524. 1998.

DREVON, C.A. Marine oils and their effects. *Nutr. Rev. 50(4):* 38. 1992.

EXPERT PANEL ON FOOD SAFETY AND NUTRITION. Functional foods: role in disease prevention and health promotion. *Food Tech. 52(11):* 63. 1998.

GLANZ, K., ET AL Why Americans eat what they do: taste, nutrition, cost, convenience, and weight control concerns as influences of food consumption. *J. Am. Diet. Assoc. 98(10):* 1118. 1998.

GREEN, G.W. AND S.R. ROSSI States of change for reducing dietary fat intake over 18 months. *J. Am. Diet. Assoc. 98(5):* 529. 1998.

GREENE, G.W., ET AL   State of change for reducing dietary fat to 30% of energy or less. *J. Am. Diet. Assoc. 94(10):* 1105. 1994.

HARNACK, L.M., ET AL   Guess who's cooking? Role of men in meal planning, shopping, and preparation in U.S. families. *J. Am. Diet. Assoc. 98(9):* 995. 1998.

HARRIS, W.S.   Ω-3 fatty acids and serum lipoproteins: human studies. *Am. J. Clin. Nutr. 65 (suppl.):* 16455. 1997.

HEANEY, R.P.   Bone mass, nutrition, and other lifestyle factors. *Nutr. Rev. 54:* S3. 1996.

HERTZLER, S.R., ET AL   How much lactose is low lactose? *J. Am. Diet. Assoc. 96(3):* 243. 1994.

HOLMAN, R.T.   Slow discovery of the importance of ω-3 essential fatty acids in human health. *J. Nutr. 128:* 427S. 1998.

KATZ, F.   USDA surveys show what Americans eat. *Food Tech. 52(11):* 50, 1998.

KENNEDY, E.   1995 Dietary Guidelines for Americans: an overview. *J. Am. Diet. Assoc. 96(3):* 234. 1994.

KURTZWEIL, P.   Staking a claim to good health. *FDA Consumer 32(6):* 16. 1998.

LI, B.Y., ET AL   Antithetic relationship of dietary arachidonic acid and eicosapentaenoic acid on eicosanoid production in vivo. *J. Lipid Res. 35:* 1869. 1994.

MCBEAN, L.D. AND G.D. MILLER   Allaying fears and fallacies about lactose intolerance. *J. Am. Diet. Assoc. 98(6):* 671. 1998.

NATIONAL HEART, LUNG, AND BLOOD INSTITUTE EXPERT PANEL ON IDENTIFICATION AND TREATMENT OF OVERWEIGHT AND OBESITY IN ADULTS. Executive summary of the clinical guidelines on the identification, evaluation, and treatment of overweight and obesity in adults. *J. Am. Diet. Assoc. 98(10):* 1178. 1998.

NATIONAL INSTITUTES OF HEALTH.   National Heart, Lung, and Blood Institute. Clinical Guidelines on the Identification, Evaluation, and Treatment of Overweight and Obesity in Adults. *U.S. Depart. of Health and Human Services.* Washington, D.C. 1998.

NICKLAS, T.A., ET AL   Impact of breakfast consumption on nutritional adequacy of diets of young adults in Bogalusa, Louisiana: ethnic and gender contrasts. *J. Am. Diet. Assoc. 98(12):* 1432. 1998.

Packard, P.T. and R.P. Heaney   Medical nutrition therapy for patients with osteoporosis. *J. Am. Diet. Assoc. 97(4):* 414. 1997.

PETERSON, J. AND J. DWYER   Taxonomic classification helps identify flavonol-containing foods as a semiquantitative food frequency questionnaire. *J. Am. Diet. Assoc. 98(6):* 677. 1998.

PRINCE, D.M. AND M.A. WELSCHENBACH   Olestra: a new food additive. *J. Am. Diet. Assoc. 98(5):* 565. 1998.

RIPPE, J.M.   Obesity epidemic: challenges and opportunities. *J. Am. Diet. Assoc. 98(10 suppl.):* S5. 1998.

RIPPE, J.M.   Role of physical activity in the prevention and management of obesity. *J. Am. Diet. Assoc. 98(10 supp):* S31. 1998.

ROCK, C.L.   Dietary Reference Intakes, antioxidants, and beta carotene. *J. Am. Diet. Assoc. 98(12):* 1412. 1998.

ROLLS, B.J. AND J.O. HILL   *Carbohydrates and Weight Management.* ILSI Press. Washington, D.C. 1998.

ROSADO, J.L., ET AL   Milk consumption, symptom response, and lactose digestion in milk intolerance. *Am. J. Clin. Nutr. 45:* 1457. 1987.

SCHWARTZ, M.W. AND R.J. SEELEY   New biology of body weight regulation. *J. Am. Diet. Assoc. 97(1):* 54. 1997.

SHEARD, N.F.   Fish consumption and risk of sudden cardiac death. *Nutr. Rev. 58(6):* 177. 1998.

SHICK, S.M., ET AL   Persons successful at long-term weight loss and maintenance continue to consume a low-energy, low-fat diet. *J. Am. Diet. Assoc. 98(4):* 408. 1998.

SUBAR, A.F., ET AL   Dietary sources of nutrients among U.S. adults, 1989 to 1991. *J. Am. Diet. Assoc. 98(5):* 537. 1998.

TOWERS, P.A., ET AL   Role of milk in human health. *Nutr. Today 32(5):* 219. 1997.

VAN HORN, L., ET AL   Dietitian's role in developing and implementing the first federal obesity guidelines. *J. Am. Diet. Assoc. 98(10):* 1115. 1998.

WELLAND, D.   Fighting phytos. *Health (Nutrition Magazine from U.S. Foodservice) 1:* 1. 1998.

WHELAN, J.   Polyunsaturated fatty acids: signaling agents for intestinal cancer? *Nutr. Today 32(5):* 213. 1997.

YOUNG, L.R. AND M. NESTLE   Variation in perceptions of a "medium" food portion: implications for dietary guidance. *J. Am. Diet. Assoc. 98(4):* 458. 1998.

CHAPTER TWELVE

Seniors

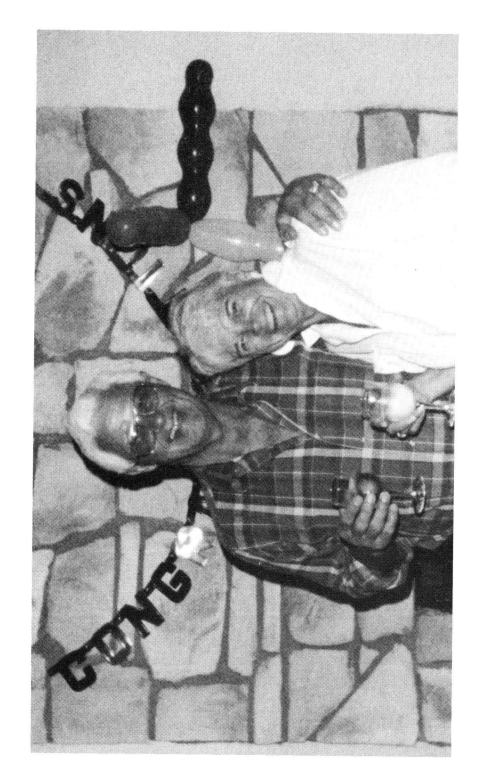

OVERVIEW

Regardless of whether they are called "the elderly," "senior citizens," "golden agers," or "retirees," the reality is that there are such wide differences in the health status, lifestyles, and attitudes that it is impossible to lump people 60 and above into any single category. In fact, there is little agreement even on the age at which individuals are classified as old. Social Security will begin paying full benefits to eligible, non-working people at age 65 and pays all eligible people at age 70 even if they are still working. Proposed changes in Social Security probably will raise the age requirements, a move that is perhaps consistent with the fact that life expectancy for people being born now in the United States have a life expectancy of about 75 years. This figure is well above the expectation of 47 years at the beginning of the 20th century. In the mid-90s, 13% of the U.S. population were 65 or older; the fastest growing population group is 85 or older.

The fact that people are living longer is only part of the picture — there is far more to life than simply breathing. Attention increasingly is being directed toward the quality of life in the later years. Active lifestyles relatively free of pain and other physical limitations are the goal of the majority of today's older generation. Good dietary patterns and optimal nutrition are keys to helping to extend the active, participatory dimension of life. This chapter focuses on the

445

subtle and sometimes profound changes that affect the elderly and their nutritional needs.

PHYSICAL CHANGES

Although physical changes happen at varying rates in individuals, certain changes are inevitable during the course of a very long life. For example, basal metabolic rate declines by about 5% between the ages of 40 and 50 and about 7.5% between 50 and 60, but the rate declines by 10% between 60 and 70. After 70, the rate of decline is about 12.5%!

Other significant changes also are occurring. Loss of muscle mass and strength and decreasing bone density accompany aging, although appropriate exercises and nutrition can be used to minimize the changes. The senses may become less acute; decreased ability to smell and taste food may interfere with the pleasure of eating. Reduced secretions are noted throughout the body. For instance, saliva, hydrochloric acid in the stomach, and sebaceous gland secretions are gradually diminished in the later years of life. Absorption of calcium and vitamin B_{12} is less efficient. The skin becomes more wrinkled, less resilient, and may reveal some pigmented or "age" spots. Gastric motility is slowed, leading to constipation. In addition to graying and/or loss of hair, nails tend to grow slower and to be a bit thicker. Reduced output of such body compounds as hormones and enzymes can be noted throughout the body as aging progresses.

Obviously, the entire body is involved in the aging process, but evidence of these changes may be obvious in some people by the time they are in their 50s, while others are quite sprightly and active into their 80s and even beyond. Many factors contribute to the physical state of an elderly person. The results of genetics, illnesses and injuries, stresses throughout life, eating habits, and activity patterns all come together in the later years to impact significantly on the quality of life for seniors.

NUTRITIONAL REQUIREMENTS

Nutritional requirements for seniors are similar to those for younger adults. However, the physical changes associated with aging may affect the foods an older person eats and may

TABLE 12.1   Recommended Dietary Allowances for Men and Women >50 Years Old[a]

Nutrient	Men	Women
Protein (g)	63	50
Vit. A (μg RE)[b]	1,000	800
Vit. K (μg)	80	65
Iron (mg)	10	10
Zinc (mg)	15	12
Iodine (μg)	150	150

[a]Adapted from Recommended Dietary Allowances, Revised 1989 (abridged). Food and Nutrition Board, National Academy of Sciences — National Research Council. Washington, D.C. 1989.
[b]Retinol equivalents. 1 retinol equivalent = 1 μg retinol or 6 μg β-carotene.
[c]α-Tocopherol equivalents. 1 mg d-α-tocopherol = 1 α-TE.

alter the efficiency of absorption and utilization in the body. The Recommended Dietary Allowances for men and women 51 and older are presented in Tables 12.1 and 12.2.

In his 1997 review article, Blumberg (1997) explored the issue of whether recommended nutritional intakes for seniors needed to be raised beyond the levels identified to be adequate to avoid frank nutritional deficiencies. Particularly in the case of seniors who may have physical limitations in optimum use of nutrients, he suggested that modest increases in certain nutrients might improve the quality of life. Decreased bone density and decreased calcium bioavailability in seniors increase their need for calcium. Related to these problems are the decreased ability to synthesize cholecalciferol in the skin and the increased production of parathyroid hormone in the winter, both of which underline the significance of vitamin D and its close relationship to calcium utilization.

The decreased immune function in seniors increases the need for zinc and both vitamins A and E. The increase in pH in the stomach raises the requirements for both folic acid and vitamin B_{12}, as well as for calcium, zinc, and iron. Higher levels of the antioxidant vitamins C and E and also β-carotene can help to counter the increased oxidative stress in aging. To help

TABLE 12.2   Recommended Intakes for Men and Women >50 Years Old[a]

Nutrient (daily amounts)	Men		Women	
	(51–70)	(>70)	(51–70)	(>70)
Calcium (mg)	1,200	1,200	1,200	1,200
Phosphorus (mg)	700	700	700	700
Magnesium (mg)	420	420	320	320
Vitamin D (μg)[b]	10	15	10	15
Fluoride (mg)	4	4	3	3
Thiamin (mg)	1.2	1.2	1.1	1.1
Riboflavin (mg)	1.3	1.3	1.1	1.1
Niacin (mg equiv.)[c]	16	16	14	14
Vitamin B_6 (mg)	1.7	1.7	1.5	1.5
Folate (μg)[d]	400	400	400	400
Vitamin B_{12} (μg)[e]	2.4	2.4	2.4	2.4
Pantothenic acid (mg)	5	5	5	5
Biotin (μg)	30	30	30	30
Choline (mg)[f]	550	550	425	425
Vitamin C (mg)	90	90	75	75
Vitamin E (mg)	15	15	15	15
Selenium (μg)	55	55	55	55

[a]Adapted from Dietary Reference Intakes: Recommended Intakes for Individuals. Food and Nutrition Board, Institute of Medicine, National Academy of Sciences. Washington, D.C. 2000.
[b]As cholecalciferol. 1 μg = 40 IU Vitamin D.
[c]As niacin equivalents (NE). 1 mg niacin = 60 mg tryptophan.
[d]As dietary folate equivalents (DFE). 1 μg food folate = 0.6 μg folic acid from fortified food or supplement consumed with food = 0.5 μg of synthetic (supplemental) folic acid taken on an empty stomach.
[e]Because 10–30% of people older than 50 may malabsorb food-bound Vitamin B_{12}, it is advisable for older people to consume foods fortified with Vitamin B_{12} or take a supplement containing Vitamin B_{12}.
[f]Although AIs have been set for choline, there are few data to assess whether a dietary supply of choline is needed at all stages of the life cycle, and it may be the requirement can be met by endogenous synthesis at some of these stages.

counter the tendency for increased homocysteine levels, more folate, vitamin B_6, and vitamin B_{12} may be effective. Also, reduced efficiency in utilizing pyridoxal means an increased need for vitamin B_6 in the diet.

Campbell et al (1994) did nitrogen balance studies in older, healthy women and men, which resulted in their estimate of an adequate dietary protein intake of 0.91 + 0.043 g/kg/day for this group. Their recommendation for protein intake for seniors is 1.0 to 1.25 g/kg/day. This is significantly higher than the 0.8 g/kg/day RDA. The incidence of protein-calorie malnutrition that has been noted among home-bound and institutionalized elderly helps to underline the possible significance of increasing the recommended intake of protein.

*HYPERHOMO-
CYSTEINEMIA
Elevated level of
homocysteine; may be
a risk factor for
vascular problems.*

Hyperhomocysteinemia has been found in several studies (Perry, et al, 1995: Clark, et al, 1992; Stampfer, et al, 1992) to be associated with increased risk of cardiovascular and stroke episodes. Folate and/or vitamin B_{12} are effective agents in reducing homocysteine levels. The levels of these vitamins needed to reduce homocysteine in those with hyperhomocysteinemia are markedly greater than the amounts required to avoid anemia.

THE WORLD OF THE ELDERLY

Although much already is known regarding the nutritional needs of the elderly, nutritional status among seniors all too often leaves room for considerable improvement in diets. The dietary habits of a lifetime exist in each individual, which makes changes difficult. However, there are many other aspects of senior life that combine to influence just what food actually is eaten.

INFLUENCE OF HEALTH CONDITIONS

Seniors with serious health problems face challenges to their normal dietary patterns. In some cases, they may be taking medication(s) that have profound influences on their appetites, taste perceptions, and even tolerance of foods. Changes in diet for people with cardiovascular problems are likely to include dietary changes, particularly reduction in fat. Weight loss also is likely to be an objective in the dietary treatment of cardiovascular patients.

Even among the elderly, overweight and obesity are all too common. The NHANES III results from the study conducted from 1988 to 1994 showed that 63.1% of men between ages of 70 and 79 were classified as obese or overweight. The incidence at 80 and older for men dropped to 50.6, which still is an alarming figure considering the impact of excess weight on health and the quality of life. Somewhat fewer women (57.9%) in the same study between the ages of 70 and 79 were overweight and obese, and the number dropped to 50.1% at age 80 and above. These figures

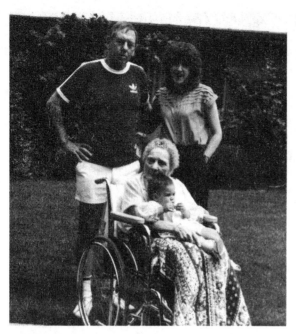

Health problems often complicate the problem of providing adequate nutrition for the elderly, but family support can help to stimulate appetite and interest in eating.

highlight the need for improved dietary patterns to help seniors achieve a healthier weight.

Adequate nutrition for seniors is an achievable goal if social, psychological, environmental, and economic factors do not interfere. These influences need to be understood and appreciated when considering ways of assuring that seniors are well nourished. Obviously, there are innumerable variations in individual situations.

SOCIO-PSYCHOLOGICAL INFLUENCES

Although there is variation among individuals, problems that are common to a large fraction of mature adults exist. In the United States, with its youth-oriented culture, there is an emphasis on the relationship of social status to job status. A person who occupies a position of authority in the business world is treated with dignity and respect. However, with retirement, one may find the social status that was inherently attached to the position is gone. One then may join the ranks of the elderly who have the task of searching once again for the tangible and satisfactory identity that gives status in the eyes of the world. The dignity accorded the elderly in cultures that embrace the aged within the family circle is denied a distressing fraction of people in the United States following their retirement.

Some retired people find new recognition and status through volunteer work. Others tend to brood over their totally different way of life, finding little reason for existing, and simply waiting for death.

Many older citizens have made virtually no preparation for the ever-lengthening years of retirement. People who have worked long hours for many years may not have developed hobbies that are of value when the pressures of work have been left behind. Their lives may become filled only with boredom. Senior Citizen Centers are available in many cities and towns to combat the empty hours. There are even whole towns dedicated to the retired citizen. These retirement villages specialize in providing the practical and human needs that are difficult to manage in the workaday world. Recreation facilities are geared toward the capabilitities of the older citizen, and the emphasis is on compatible companionship. For the person in good health who chooses to gravitate toward these clubs and communities, the empty hours of the day become very full.

ECONOMIC FACTORS

The void created by lack of employment during the retirement years is but one of the adjustments frequently required. The loss of one's mate requires considerable adaptation on the part of the bereaved at any point in life, but in later years, there is less activity to direct the mind away from the immediate problems one faces. Adjustments during the time of bereavement may mean giving up the home that has been the family gathering place for many years; feelings of depression may be very intense, and life may seem overwhelmingly empty. For a woman, widowhood may impose financial responsibilities she has never had to understand and handle before. For a widower, the problems of managing home and meals become immediately pressing. Previously shared responsibilities become the sole burden of the survivor, and the golden years may abruptly lose their burnish.

Some people have sufficient funds to make these remaining years comfortable and free of financial worry, but the large majority of elderly citizens are tightly caught in the press created by the economy and the very limited income available under most retirement plans. The picture is complicated still further by the prolonged period of retirement that must be financed. More than 5 million people over age 65 have to live on fixed incomes that are too little to enable them to live in the manner that they did when they were still working. This obvious deterioration in standard of living is degrading to anyone and is no more acceptable to the aged than to younger people. In some instances, this shortage of funds freezes older people into life in a portion of town where life is changing. More affluent residents may have moved away, to be replaced by people who cannot or do not maintain the area. There is less pleasure to be drawn from the immediate environment, and the rate of crime in the area may rise. Cramped budgets of the elderly require skillful management if they are to cover the bare necessities. A move to a more pleasant area is not a financial possibility for them.

Social occasions sharpen appetites and add sparkle to the daily routine of retirees.

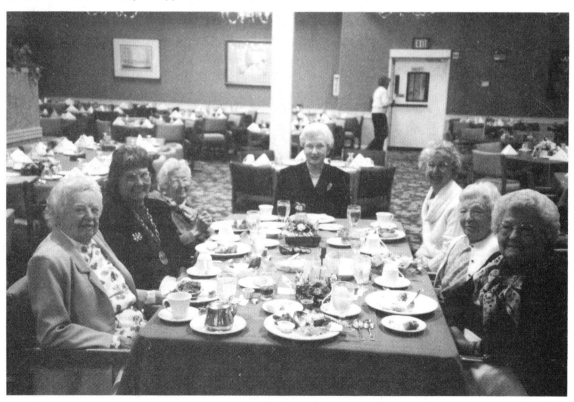

NARROWING HORIZONS

As if these problems are not sufficient, general health deteriorates eventually. Concern with health is very real to the aged. Some of the problems can be treated very well; others are costly and threatening to life itself; others are merely imagined. In the desire to avoid possible ailments or to improve ailments resulting from hypochondriacal musing, older people are easy prey for the hawker of patent medicines and "health foods." Today's older generation grew up when the general pattern was to see a doctor only when virtually on one's deathbed. To them it may seem less ominous (and less costly) to try the wares of the "health-peddling" entrepreneur in preference to visiting the physician, a choice that may be injurious to the health of the individual.

In today's mobile society, the ability to drive a car is seemingly as important as eating and breathing. Unfortunately, many seniors have deteriorating vision, which makes driving (especially at night) a problem for them. Eventually, they may even have to quit driving. This seriously restricts mobility and independence, particularly if public transportation is not readily available. A walk to the bus may be more than some seniors can manage, and then there also is the problem of walking at the other end of the ride, plus returning home again on the bus. This is such a daunting prospect that the elderly may become virtually homebound. Yet a further dimension of the inability to continue driving is the problem of carrying groceries and other purchases. Loss of strength makes such tasks beyond the realm of reality for many.

Isolation leads to depression among some seniors. When seniors live alone, they may long for opportunities to talk to somebody. The stimulation of conversation and social interactions can greatly improve the quality of life for seniors who feel isolated. Without such stimuli, interest in eating healthily simply may evaporate.

ADAPTING TO CHANGE

This overview of the realities of being a part of this somewhat isolated generation, of course, is not complete in all aspects, nor is it all true for any one individual. However, this provides the background needed to view the nutritional needs and problems of the elderly in the perspective of today's world. This population group, perhaps more than any other, can only be

RESEARCH INSIGHTS

Marcus, E.L. and E.M. Berry, Refusal to eat in the elderly. *Nutr. Rev. 56(6):* 163. 1998.

This review article by Marcus and Berry (1998) examines problems of weight loss and anorexia among elderly people; interdisciplinary approaches to alleviating these problems are also considered. Among the physiologic changes during aging that can lead to gradual weight loss are reduced energy intake, slowing basal metabolic rate, decreased lean body mass, reduced appetite, reduced satiety, and reduced senses of taste and olfaction. In addition to physiologic changes due to aging, older patients with anorexia (sometimes termed tardive anorexia because of its delayed onset in life) may have other health conditions, feelings, and attitudes that are influencing their willingness to eat. Among the reasons underlying this behavior in patients in institutional settings may be the wish to die, dislike of the food offered, distractions from eating, or a protest against a caregiver. Patients who are cognitively impaired (e.g., Alzheimer's patients) may have reduced appetite underlying refusal to eat because of mental difficulties. Depression is the leading cause of inadequate food intake in the elderly, whether they are living at home or in an institution. Refusal to eat may be linked in some cases to suicide, either consciously or unconsciously. Gut edema in end-stage cardiac failure, chronic obstructive lung disease, infection with *Helicobacter pylori*, and the impact of medications are possible factors contributing to loss of appetite and resulting weight loss.

Social and environmental factors may play significant roles in influencing eating behaviors. Elderly in institutional settings may find their preferred ethnic foods are missing from the meals and/or the foods are unappealing, or they may simply need more help with feeding than the caregivers provide. Strategies to encourage eating include: improving appearance and taste of pureed foods, increasing the flavor intensity of foods, planning meals that appeal to all of the senses, gentle treatment by caregivers, enhanced environment by such devices as soft music, supplemental use of liquid supplements, companionship when eating meals, and increased activity. Recognition of a person's right to self-determine eating behavior is discussed in this article.

aided nutritionally when those who work with them see the total picture in which they live.

Of course, adequate diet is not simply a matter of planning menus. The food must be purchased, prepared, and then served in an attractive manner in pleasant surroundings if older people are to eat and truly enjoy it. For the fortunate elderly with excellent income, a comfortable place to live, good health, and companionship, good nutritional status is a relatively simple matter. Only minor modifications from the previous dietary pattern are required.

However, for a large number of the elderly, one or more factors greatly impede an individual's efforts to be well fed. A tightly limited budget may require more marketing skill than has been acquired by previous experience if the money is to cover even the bare necessities. It may be that transportation for shopping is not readily available, so that they either must impose on someone else for grocery shopping or make numerous trips to the market if there is one within a reasonable walking distance. Economical shopping is not enhanced under transportation handicaps.

Still other older people have poor facilities for preparing food. It is difficult for anyone to become very inspired about cooking when refrigerator facilities are absent and hot foods can only be prepared on a hot plate in the same room where one eats and sleeps. Older men, who may not have had to do food preparation earlier in life, may get totally discouraged when they suddenly become responsible for all their cooking. The prospect that they will prepare tempting and nutritionally adequate meals for themselves is remote. Even older women, who usually have had considerable experience in food preparation, may fail to eat well when they have only themselves to cook for.

Problems are magnified when the individual living alone is not in good health. To the preceding picture, one certainly must add that a rather substantial amount of advertising regarding so-called "health foods" is directed toward older people. When the elderly have very limited undertstanding of the sciences of medicine and nutrition and a painful familiarity with the various physical problems they have acquired as they aged, there is little reason to be surprised that they are courted into parting with some of their limited dollars to buy products that are touted to cure existing problems or to prevent the development of others yet unknown.

Although not all of these problems confront any one person, the general picture for the elderly is that care must be given to planning and eating an adequate diet. With some attention, many older people can handle this phase of their lives very adequately for a number of years. For numerous others, some form of assistance is needed if good nutrition is to be achieved.

One interesting approach to the problems of the elderly is the Congregate Feeding Programs, which provide a highly nourishing, hot lunch served in a congenial setting to all interested senior citizens who live in the service area. Leftover foods that do not require refrigeration are given to participants who wish to take them home, thus adding to the nutritional benefit of the programs. To date, the programs have been very well received by the numerous elderly who participate regularly in this sociable and nourishing event. Obviously, such a service can alleviate loneliness, provide at least some good food each week, and teach a little about shopping and preparation of nourishing food the remainder of the week. This program is a very useful aid for the aged, but unfortunately cannot provide a guarantee that its participants will be well fed all week. Community support, in the form of money, facilities, and volunteer labor, is needed for this type of program.

Meals-on-Wheels programs have been available as an assistance to the elderly who are living in their own homes, but who may have difficulty in preparing adequate meals for themselves. The mechanics of the programs vary from city to city, but the underlying goal of Meals-on-Wheels is to provide a low-cost hot meal in the home each weekday. The meals usually are prepared in a central kitchen, then delivered by truck to the participants in the program. The success of this approach to good nutrition for the elderly is largely dependent upon the local situation. When supervision, planning, and administration are good, the food is of high quality and reasonable in price. In short, the program is highly successful. Where quality control and other facets of administration have been weak, the program has failed. Certainly, the basic concepts of this type of program are sound. Meals-on-Wheels has the potential to enable many elderly people to maintain their independence longer than they could if they did not have this nutritional assistance available to them.

STRATEGIES FOR OPTIMIZING NUTRITION

MEAL PLANNING

People who are living independently at home assume the responsibility of meal planning, shopping, and preparation themselves or of arranging for some other means of obtaining the food they need. If they are handling the responsibilities themselves, seniors need to be sure to provide the necessary amount and variety of food required to maintain their health optimally. The Food Guide Pyramid is a suitable basis for this planning.

Particular attention needs to be paid to adequate milk and dairy, a variety of protein foods (emphasizing eggs, fish, and poultry, but also red meats), and a wide and plentiful variety of fruits and vegetables. Nonfat dairy choices are wise for most seniors. Ideally, milk (preferably low fat or fat free) will be consumed regularly as the beverage at most meals and/or as snacks. Where possible, milk also should be used in cooking.

Eggs may be a source of protein that needs some endorsement because many seniors are convinced that the cholesterol level in eggs is extremely harmful to them. In fact, many seniors are not faced with a definite need for sharply restricting their cholesterol intakes. However, many of them are finding that budgetary problems make it hard for them to eat healthily, and protein sources are expensive. Eggs provide excellent quality protein at a reasonable price and can be included in the diet at least once or twice a week.

Just as was true in the middle years, seniors need to include such protein sources as fish and poultry. The relatively short safe storage period for these foods, particularly fish, means that they need to be prepared and eaten after a storage period of no more than three days. If shopping is a problem, the plan should be to use the fish first, followed by the poultry that was purchased. Frozen fish and poultry can be purchased or frozen as soon as they are brought home if it is going to be necessary to serve them later in the week. Red meats are recommended occasionally to help provide adequate iron. The comparative ease of utilizing iron from red meats is of particular merit, but the amount and type of fat in red meats may be detrimental. These contradictory qualities explain why limited amounts of red meat are suggested.

Ample amounts of a wide variety of fruits and vegetables need to be a big part of the diet for seniors. Not only are they valuable sources of essential nutrients, but they also are high in fiber. The need for fiber to promote intestinal motility is particularly important for older people to help counteract the constipation that tends to accompany the aging process. Fresh fruits and vegetables are recommended, but some seniors may find that preparing them is too much trouble or that they have trouble eating them before they start to spoil. For such situations, use of frozen and canned products may be wise, at least to augment fresh produce that may be used.

Breads and cereals should be prominent in seniors' diets, for they provide an abundance of the key B vitamins (including added folate) and also fiber if whole grain products are selected. Cereals may also be a way to encourage greater milk consumption. Seniors generally find that breads and/or cereals are pleasing to eat, convenient to prepare, and easy to shop for and store. The comparatively light loaves of bread and boxes of cereals are easy to carry from the market into the house. Furthermore, bread can be frozen without harm to its eating quality, which makes it possible to buy a loaf of bread and eat it while it is still pleasing to eat even when people are living alone. Choices among whole-grain products are numerous, and all of these are wise choices. Some of them may be quite expensive, but usually some whole wheat or other whole grain bread can be found at a reasonable price. A particularly good choice from the perspective of nutrition is oatmeal, whether it is in the form of a hot cereal or in bread.

Only limited intake of fats and oils is recommended. Butter may be a good choice for a spread because it does not have the trans fatty acids that are found in hydrogenated margarines and shortenings. The importance of avoiding consumption of trans fatty acids is not totally clear at this point. Probably a wise choice in the meantime is to use only a little butter and/or margarine. The total intake of fat is the really critical nutritional point. Inclusion of some olive oil and soybean or canola oil will provide the necessary essential fatty acids.

Although it is posible to obtain all of the nutrients needed for good health simply by eating the right foods in appropriate amounts, seniors often do not eat enough food to provide all essential nutrients in adequate amounts. A vitamin pill providing 100% of the recommended levels specified in Tables 12.1 and

12.2 can be taken daily to insure that the necessary vitamins are available to the body.

Even when a healthy diet has been planned and the groceries have been purchased, there is still a possibility that the meals may not become a reality. Sometimes lack of sufficient energy to prepare, serve, and clean up after a meal may cause seniors to prepare only a part of the meal or even to skip the meal completely. This is more likely to be a problem among seniors who live alone. The incentive to cook for just oneself may simply be lacking at times. Poor health (including difficulty in seeing, arthritic pain, poor balance, or other limitations) can make food preparation much more of a physical challenge than a joy. Snacking on whatever food is easily available may begin to be the general eating pattern. Unfortunately, these problems that interfere with preparing good meals interfere with the chance of consuming a nutritionally adequate diet. This may hasten physical deterioration, and the situation perpetuates itself in a negative manner.

INDEPENDENT LIVING

People who live alone or as couples and who want to maintain their independence as long as possible need to strategize so that they achieve adequate nutrition all of the time. This approach to living helps to optimize health and places at least part of the responsibility with the individual. The key to being successful with preparing and consuming an adequate diet is to develop patterns that are pleasing and make meals a pleasure rather than a burden. This is easy to say, but individuals have to find their own solutions to making good nutrition happen when they become seniors. For people who enjoy cooking, the practice of trying new recipes frequently may be the answer. Boredom can be avoided and motivation can be gained by inviting others over for meals. This provides important sociability for the person preparing the food and also for the friends who attend. Food always seems to taste better when it is shared with others.

For people who prefer to stay out of the kitchen as much as possible, frozen meals and carry-out from restaurants or delicatessens may be the best way to assure a good diet. This approach generally may be a bit more expensive than cooking foods from their basic ingredients, but it makes food very accesible with a minimum of effort. Another approach is to dine out fairly often. Skill in ordering is needed to assure that a good diet is obtained when restaurant dining is a significant part of the total eating experience. Fast food and short order restaurants tend to result in meals that are relatively high in fat and low in milk, fruits, and vegetables. Many restaurants have excellent meal choices available. The portions often are far more than a senior needs for a meal, but it is an accepted practice these days to take leftovers home. This way another good meal also is available for almost no effort. The common availability of microwave ovens makes reheating leftovers a very simple matter. Perhaps the biggest drawback to eating frequently at restaurants is the high cost that may be the result of healthful dining at good restaurants. This may not be an issue for some older people, but dining at restaurants may not be an option for most seniors who are on limited incomes.

People who are doing their own food preparation may need to find ways of eating well without doing quite as much work. One approach to reducing work is to make full recipes of items that will freeze well or that will be able to be enjoyed again at a meal within a day or two. If leftovers are frozen in serving portions, they can be stored for use later when time or energy may make this a welcome cornstone of a meal. It is sometimes convenient to prepare an extra serving of a fresh vegetable and refrigerate it for use later. This saves the time of having to prepare the vegetable from its raw state. Reheating in the microwave oven is quick and simple and results in a pleasing product. These are just some of the ways that seniors can make meal preparation a bit easier.

Assisted Living

Eventually, many seniors opt to move into a retirement home or community rather than continuing to live totally independently. The actual situation varies. Some retirement homes provide all meals in a large dining room; some may include one meal a day in the dining room, but provide kitchenettes so that people may prepare their other meals in their rooms or apartments. This latter arrangement is popular because the major burden of meal preparation is eliminated, but the opportunity is readily available to prepare personal favorites and to tailor some meals to suit individual preferences. The cost of living in retirement homes or communities is highly variable and so is the quality. Whether this lifestyle approach is a good choice depends upon the persons involved and on economic feasibility.

NURSING HOMES

Of growing importance in the feeding of the elderly have been nursing and convalescent homes. As the number of older citizens has been increasing, institutional care for the elderly has grown significantly. The quality of the meals in these various institutions is highly variable, again reflecting the general competence and skills of the person supervising this aspect of the unit. Theoretically, trained personnel can provide optimum nutrition and very broad acceptance of food in these institutions for the elderly. Meals need not be eaten alone, meal preparation and planning are done by persons skilled in the art and science of feeding people, and the total physical environment is centered around the needs and interests of this age group. In practice, this idealized circumstance is achieved in some nursing and convalescent homes, but undoubtedly some owners and managers are motivated more by profits and practical concerns than they are by the desire to care for the elderly to the best of their ability. Nursing homes can brighten the lives of their patients if the staff recognizes the role of good food as a link with the past. Mealtime may be the only pleasurable activity for some patients. Good food is a real morale builder.

SUMMARY

The elderly are a very rapidly increasing segment of the population, which is raising considerable concern regarding the economic and social burden this is placing on the general population and on families now and in the future. One important way of approaching this circumstance is to optimize the nutrition of seniors to help promote their quality of life and reduce their health care requirements for as long as possible.

Aging involves many physiological changes, some of which occur quite gradually. The actual physical condition of individual seniors is determined by many factors, including genetics, dietary patterns over a lifetime, and lifestyle choices over the years. Adjustments in dietary patterns and lifestyles (especially activity and exercise) can be made during this period to promote health. Diet choices based on the Food Guide Pyramid and in appropriate quantities to achieve and maintain an appropriate weight are desirable, whether people are living alone or with someone else independently, in a retirement home or community, or in a health care facility.

BIBLIOGRAPHY

BLUMBERG, J.   Nutritional needs of seniors. *J. Am. College Nutr. 16(6):* 517. 1997.

CAMPBELL, W.W., ET AL   Increased protein requirements in the elderly: new data and retrospective assessments. *Am. J. Clin. Nutr. 60:* 501. 1994.

CAMPBELL, W.W.   Dietary protein requirements of older people: is the RDA adequate? *Nutr. Today 31(5):* 192. 1996.

CLARK, R., ET AL   Hyperhomocysteinemia: risk factor for extracranial carotid artery atherosclerosis. *Ir. J. Med. Sci. 161:* 61. 1992.

COULSTON, A.M., ET AL   Meals-on-Wheels applicants are a population at risk for poor nutritional status. *J. Am. Diet. Assoc. 96(8):* 570. 1996.

FLEGAL, K.M., ET AL   Overweight and obesity in the United States 1960–1994. *Int. J. Obes. 22:* 39. 1998.

FOGT, E.J., ET AL   Nutrition assessment of the elderly. In *Geriatric Nutrition.* 2nd ed. Raven Press. New York. 1995.

GILBRIDE, J.A., ET AL   Nutrition and health status assessment of community-residing elderly in New York City: pilot study. *J. Am. Diet. Assoc. 98(5):* 554. 1998.

GLOTH, M., ET AL   Nutrient intakes in a frail homebound elderly population in the community vs. a nursing home population. *J. Am. Diet. Assoc. 96(6):* 605. 1996.

IBBOML, J.B., ET AL   Vitamin B_{12}, Vitamin B_6, and folate nutritional status in men with hyperhomocysteinemia. *Am. J. Clin. Nutr. 57:* 47. 1993.

JENSEN, G.L. AND J. ROGERS   Obesity in older persons. *J. Am. Diet. Assoc. 98(11):* 1306. 1998.

KOEHLER, K.M., ET AL   Folate nutrition and older adults: challenges and opportunities. *J. Am. Diet. Assoc. 97(2):* 167. 1997.

KRUMHOLZ, H.M., ET AL   Lack of association between cholesterol and coronary heart disease mortality and morbidity and all-cause mortality in perons older than 70. *J. Am. Med. Assoc. 272:* 1335. 1996.

MARCUS, E.L. AND E.M. BERRY   Refusal to eat in the elderly. *Nutr. Rev. 56:* 163. 1998.

MELNIK, T.A., ET AL   Screening elderly in the community. Relationship between dietary adequacy and nutritional risk. *J. Am. Diet. Assoc. 94(12):* 1425. 1994.

PACKARD, P.T. AND R.P. HEANEY   Medical nutrition therapy for patients with osteoporosis. *J. Am. Diet. Assoc. 97(4):* 414. 1997.

PERRY, I.J., ET AL   Prospective study of serum total homocysteine concentration and risk of stroke in middle-aged British men. *Lancet 346:* 1395. 1995.

ROSE, C.S., ET AL   Age differences in vitamin B_6 status of 617 men. *Am. J. Clin. Nutr. 29:* 847. 1976.

RUSSELL, R.M.   New views on the RDAs for older adults. *J. Am. Diet. Assoc. 97(5):* 515. 1997.

STAMPFER, M.J., ET AL   Prospective study of plasma homocysteine and risk of mycardial infarction in U.S. physicians. *J. Am. Med. Assoc. 268:* 877. 1992.

VAILAS, L.I., ET AL   Risk indicators for malnutrition are associated inversely with quality of life for participants in meal programs for older adults. *J. Am. Diet. Assoc. 98(5):* 548. 1998.

WELLMAN, N.S., ET AL   Elder insecurities: poverty, hunger, and malnutrition. *J. Am. Diet. Assoc. 97:* S20. 1997.

YAMAGUCHI, L.Y., ET AL   Improvement in nutrient intake by elderly Meals-on Whjeels participants receiving a liquid nutrition supplement. *Nutr. Today 33(1):* 37. 1998.

ZYLSTRA, R.C.E., ET AL   Who's at risk in Washington State? Demographic characteristics affect nutritional risk behaviors in elderly meal particpants. *J. Am. Diet. Assoc. 95(3):* 358. 1995.

SECTION FIVE

Appendices

Height-Weight Tables

APPENDIX A

Table A.1   Weight and Length of Boys from Birth to 2 Years

Age	Measurement		Percentile						
			3	10	25	50	75	90	97
Birth	Weight	pounds	5.8	6.3	6.9	7.5	8.3	9.1	10.1
		kilograms	2.63	2.86	3.13	3.4	3.76	4.13	4.58
	Length	inches	18.2	18.9	19.4	19.9	20.5	21.0	21.5
		centimeters	46.3	48.1	49.3	50.6	52.0	53.3	54.6
3 months	Weight	pounds	10.6	11.1	11.8	12.6	13.6	14.5	16.4
		kilograms	4.81	5.03	5.35	5.72	6.17	6.58	7.44
	Length	inches	22.4	22.8	23.3	23.8	24.3	24.7	25.1
		centimeters	56.8	57.8	59.3	60.4	61.8	62.8	63.7
6 months	Weight	pounds	14.0	14.8	15.6	16.7	18.0	19.2	20.8
		kilograms	6.35	6.71	7.08	7.58	8.16	8.71	9.43
	Length	inches	24.8	25.2	25.7	26.1	26.7	27.3	27.7
		centimeters	63.0	63.9	65.2	66.4	67.8	69.3	70.4
9 months	Weight	pounds	16.6	17.8	18.7	20.0	21.5	22.9	24.4
		kilograms	7.53	8.07	8.48	9.07	9.75	10.39	11.07
	Length	inches	26.6	27.0	27.5	28.0	28.7	29.2	29.9
		centimeters	67.7	68.6	69.8	71.2	72.9	74.2	75.9
12 months	Weight	pounds	18.5	19.6	20.9	22.2	23.8	25.4	27.3
		kilograms	8.39	8.89	9.48	10.07	10.8	11.52	12.38
	Length	inches	28.1	28.5	29.0	29.6	30.3	30.7	31.6
		centimeters	71.3	72.4	73.7	75.2	76.9	78.1	80.3
15 months	Weight	pounds	19.8	21.0	22.4	23.7	25.4	27.2	29.4
		kilograms	8.98	9.53	10.16	10.75	11.52	12.34	13.33
	Length	inches	29.3	29.8	30.3	30.9	31.6	32.1	33.1
		centimeters	74.4	75.6	77.0	78.5	80.3	81.5	84.2
18 months	Weight	pounds	21.1	22.3	23.8	25.2	26.9	29.0	31.5
		kilograms	9.57	10.12	10.8	11.43	12.2	13.15	14.29
	Length	inches	30.5	31.0	31.6	32.2	32.9	33.5	34.7
		centimeters	77.5	78.8	80.3	81.8	83.7	85.0	88.2
2 years	Weight	pounds	23.3	24.7	26.3	27.7	29.7	31.9	34.9
		kilograms	10.57	11.2	11.93	12.56	13.47	14.47	15.83
	Length	inches	32.6	33.1	33.8	34.4	35.2	35.9	37.2
		centimeters	82.7	84.2	85.8	87.5	89.4	91.1	94.6

Source: H. C. Stuart, in Nelson, *Textbook of Pediatrics*, 8th ed., Saunders, Philadelphia, 1964.

Table A.2   Weight and Height of Boys from 2 to 5 Years

Age	Measurement		3	10	25	50	75	90	97
			Percentile						
2 years	Weight	pounds	23.3	24.7	26.3	27.7	29.7	31.9	34.9
		kilograms	10.57	11.2	11.93	12.56	13.47	14.47	15.83
	Height	inches	32.6	33.1	33.8	34.4	35.2	35.9	37.2
		centimeters	82.7	84.2	85.8	87.5	89.4	91.1	94.6
2½ years	Weight	pounds	25.2	26.6	28.4	30.0	32.2	34.5	37.0
		kilograms	11.43	12.07	12.88	13.61	14.61	15.65	16.78
	Height	inches	34.2	34.8	35.5	36.3	37.0	37.9	39.2
		centimeters	86.9	88.5	90.2	92.1	94.1	96.2	99.5
3 years	Weight	pounds	27.0	28.7	30.3	32.2	34.5	36.8	39.2
		kilograms	12.25	13.02	13.74	14.61	15.65	16.69	17.78
	Height	inches	35.7	36.3	37.0	37.9	38.8	39.6	40.5
		centimeters	90.6	92.3	93.9	96.2	98.5	100.5	102.8
3½ years	Weight	pounds	28.5	30.4	32.3	34.3	36.7	39.1	41.5
		kilograms	12.93	13.79	14.65	15.56	16.65	17.74	18.82
	Height	inches	37.1	37.8	38.4	39.3	40.3	41.1	41.9
		centimeters	94.3	96.0	97.5	99.8	102.5	104.5	106.5
4 years	Weight	pounds	30.1	32.1	34.0	36.4	39.0	41.4	44.3
		kilograms	13.65	14.56	15.42	16.51	17.69	18.78	20.09
	Height	inches	38.4	39.1	39.7	40.7	41.9	42.7	43.5
		centimeters	97.5	99.3	100.8	103.4	106.5	108.5	110.4
4½ years	Weight	pounds	31.6	33.8	35.7	38.4	41.4	43.9	47.4
		kilograms	14.33	15.33	16.19	17.42	18.78	19.91	21.5
	Height	inches	39.6	40.3	40.9	42.0	43.3	44.2	45.0
		centimeters	100.6	102.4	104.0	106.7	109.9	112.3	114.3
5 years	Weight	pounds	33.6	35.5	37.5	40.5	44.1	46.7	50.4
		kilograms	15.24	16.1	17.01	18.37	20.0	21.18	22.86
	Height	inches	40.2	40.8	41.7	42.8	44.2	45.2	46.1
		centimeters	102.0	103.7	105.9	108.7	112.3	114.7	117.1

Source: H. C. Stuart, in Nelson, *Textbook of Pediatrics*, 8th ed., Saunders, Philadelphia, 1964.

Table A.3   Weight and Height of Boys from 5 to 18 Years

Age	Measurement		3	10	25	50	75	90	97
						Percentile			
5 years[a]	Weight	pounds	34.5	36.6	39.6	42.8	46.5	49.7	53.2
		kilograms	15.65	16.6	17.96	19.41	21.09	22.54	24.13
	Height	inches	40.2	41.5	42.6	43.8	45.0	45.9	47.0
		centimeters	102.1	105.3	108.3	111.3	114.2	116.7	119.5
6 years	Weight	pounds	38.5	40.9	44.4	48.3	52.1	56.4	61.1
		kilograms	17.46	18.55	20.14	21.91	23.63	25.58	27.71
	Height	inches	42.7	43.8	44.9	46.3	47.6	48.6	49.7
		centimeters	108.5	111.2	114.1	117.5	120.8	123.5	126.2
7 years	Weight	pounds	43.0	45.8	49.7	54.1	58.7	64.4	69.9
		kilograms	19.5	20.77	22.54	24.54	26.63	29.21	31.71
	Height	inches	44.9	46.0	47.4	48.9	50.2	51.4	52.5
		centimeters	114.0	116.9	120.3	124.1	127.6	130.5	133.4
8 years	Weight	pounds	48.0	51.2	55.5	60.1	65.5	73.0	79.4
		kilograms	21.77	23.22	25.17	27.26	29.71	33.11	36.02
	Height	inches	47.1	48.5	49.8	51.2	52.8	54.0	55.2
		centimeters	119.6	123.1	126.6	130.0	134.2	137.3	140.2
9 years	Weight	pounds	52.5	56.3	61.1	66.0	72.3	81.0	89.8
		kilograms	23.81	25.54	27.71	29.94	32.8	36.74	40.73
	Height	inches	48.9	50.5	51.8	53.3	55.0	56.1	57.2
		centimeters	124.2	128.3	131.6	135.5	139.8	142.6	145.3
10 years	Weight	pounds	56.8	61.1	66.3	71.9	79.6	89.9	100.0
		kilograms	25.76	27.71	30.07	32.61	36.11	40.78	45.36
	Height	inches	50.7	52.3	53.7	55.2	56.8	58.1	59.2
		centimeters	128.7	132.8	136.3	140.3	144.4	147.5	150.3
11 years	Weight	pounds	61.8	66.3	71.6	77.6	87.2	99.3	111.7
		kilograms	28.03	30.07	32.48	35.2	39.55	45.04	50.67
	Height	inches	52.5	54.0	55.3	56.8	58.7	59.8	60.8
		centimeters	133.4	137.3	140.5	144.2	149.2	151.8	154.4
12 years	Weight	pounds	67.2	72.0	77.5	84.4	96.0	109.6	124.2
		kilograms	30.48	32.66	35.15	38.28	43.55	49.71	56.34
	Height	inches	54.4	56.1	57.2	58.9	60.4	62.2	63.7
		centimeters	138.1	142.4	145.2	149.6	153.5	157.9	161.9

Age	Measurement		3	10	25	50	75	90	97
			\multicolumn{7}{c}{Percentile}
13 years	Weight	pounds	72.0	77.1	83.7	93.0	107.9	123.2	138.0
		kilograms	32.66	34.97	37.97	42.18	48.94	55.88	62.6
	Height	inches	56.0	57.7	58.9	61.0	63.3	65.1	66.7
		centimeters	142.2	146.6	149.7	155.0	160.8	165.3	169.5
14 years	Weight	pounds	79.8	87.2	95.5	107.6	123.1	136.9	150.6
		kilograms	36.2	39.55	43.32	48.81	55.84	62.1	68.31
	Height	inches	57.6	59.9	61.6	64.0	66.3	67.9	69.7
		centimeters	146.4	152.1	156.5	162.7	168.4	172.4	177.1
15 years	Weight	pounds	91.3	99.4	108.2	120.1	135.0	147.8	161.6
		kilograms	41.41	45.09	49.08	54.48	61.23	67.04	73.3
	Height	inches	59.7	62.1	63.9	66.1	68.1	69.6	71.6
		centimeters	151.7	157.8	162.3	167.8	173.0	176.7	181.8
16 years	Weight	pounds	103.4	111.0	118.7	129.7	144.4	157.3	170.5
		kilograms	46.9	50.35	53.84	58.83	65.5	71.35	77.34
	Height	inches	61.6	64.1	65.8	67.8	69.5	70.7	73.1
		centimeters	156.5	162.8	167.1	171.6	176.6	179.7	185.6
17 years	Weight	pounds	110.5	117.5	124.5	136.2	151.4	164.6	175.6
		kilograms	50.12	53.3	56.47	61.78	68.67	74.66	79.65
	Height	inches	62.6	65.2	66.8	68.4	70.1	71.5	73.5
		centimeters	159.0	165.5	169.7	173.7	178.1	181.6	186.6
18 years	Weight	pounds	113.0	120.0	127.1	139.0	155.7	169.0	179.0
		kilograms	51.26	54.43	57.65	63.05	70.62	76.66	81.19
	Height	inches	62.8	65.5	67.0	68.7	70.4	71.8	73.9
		centimeters	159.6	166.3	170.5	174.5	178.9	182.4	187.6

[a]Several measurements at 5 years differ slightly from their counterparts in Table A.2 because they were obtained from a different population of children.

Source: The data in this table are from studies by and are reproduced by courtesy of Howard V. Meredith, Ph.D., Professor of Child Somatology, Institute of Child Behavior and Development, University of Iowa.

Table A.4   Weight and Length of Girls from Birth to 2 Years

Age	Measurement		Percentile						
			3	10	25	50	75	90	97
Birth	Weight	pounds	5.8	6.2	6.9	7.4	8.1	8.6	9.4
		kilograms	2.63	2.81	3.13	3.36	3.67	3.9	4.26
	Length	inches	18.5	18.8	19.3	19.8	20.1	20.4	21.1
		centimeters	47.1	47.8	49.0	50.2	51.0	51.9	53.6
3 months	Weight	pounds	9.8	10.7	11.4	12.4	13.2	14.0	14.9
		kilograms	4.45	4.85	5.17	5.62	5.99	6.35	6.76
	Length	inches	22.0	22.4	22.8	23.4	23.9	24.3	24.8
		centimeters	55.8	56.9	57.9	59.5	60.7	61.7	63.1
6 months	Weight	pounds	12.7	14.1	15.0	16.0	17.5	18.6	20.0
		kilograms	5.76	6.4	6.8	7.26	7.94	8.44	9.07
	Length	inches	24.0	24.6	25.1	25.7	26.2	26.7	27.1
		centimeters	61.1	62.5	63.7	65.2	66.6	67.8	68.8
9 months	Weight	pounds	15.1	16.6	17.8	19.2	20.8	22.4	24.2
		kilograms	6.85	7.53	8.03	8.71	9.43	10.16	10.98
	Length	inches	25.7	26.4	26.9	27.6	28.2	28.7	29.2
		centimeters	65.4	67.0	68.4	70.1	71.7	72.9	74.1
12 months	Weight	pounds	16.8	18.4	19.8	21.5	23.0	24.8	27.1
		kilograms	7.62	8.35	8.98	9.75	10.43	11.25	12.29
	Length	inches	27.1	27.8	28.5	29.2	29.9	30.3	31.0
		centimeters	68.9	70.6	72.3	74.2	75.9	77.1	78.8
15 months	Weight	pounds	18.1	19.8	21.3	23.0	24.6	26.6	29.0
		kilograms	8.21	8.98	9.66	10.43	11.16	12.07	13.15
	Length	inches	28.3	29.0	29.8	30.5	31.3	31.8	32.6
		centimeters	71.9	73.7	75.6	77.6	79.4	80.8	82.8
18 months	Weight	pounds	19.4	21.2	22.7	24.5	26.2	28.3	30.9
		kilograms	8.8	9.62	10.3	11.11	11.88	12.84	14.02
	Length	inches	29.5	30.2	31.1	31.8	32.6	33.3	34.1
		centimeters	74.9	76.8	79.0	80.9	82.9	84.5	86.7
2 years	Weight	pounds	21.6	23.5	25.3	27.1	29.2	31.7	34.4
		kilograms	9.8	10.66	11.48	12.29	13.25	14.38	15.6
	Length	inches	31.5	32.3	33.3	34.1	35.0	35.8	36.7
		centimeters	80.1	82.0	84.7	86.6	88.9	91.0	93.3

Source: H. C. Stuart, in Nelson, *Textbook of Pediatrics*, 8th ed., Saunders, Philadelphia, 1964.

Table A.5   Weight and Height of Girls from 2 to 5 Years

Age	Measurement		Percentile						
			3	10	25	50	75	90	97
2 years	Weight	pounds	21.6	23.5	25.3	27.1	29.2	31.7	34.4
		kilograms	9.8	10.66	11.48	12.29	13.25	14.38	15.6
	Height	inches	31.5	32.3	33.3	34.1	35.0	35.8	36.7
		centimeters	80.1	82.0	84.7	86.6	88.9	91.0	93.3
2½ years	Weight	pounds	23.6	25.5	27.4	29.6	31.9	34.6	38.2
		kilograms	10.7	11.57	12.43	13.43	14.47	15.69	17.33
	Height	inches	33.3	34.0	35.2	36.0	36.9	37.9	38.9
		centimeters	84.5	86.3	89.3	91.4	93.8	96.4	98.7
3 years	Weight	pounds	25.6	27.6	29.6	31.8	34.6	37.4	41.8
		kilograms	11.61	12.52	13.43	14.42	15.69	16.96	18.96
	Height	inches	34.8	35.6	36.8	37.7	38.6	39.8	40.7
		centimeters	88.4	90.5	93.4	95.7	98.1	101.1	103.5
3½ years	Weight	pounds	27.5	29.5	31.5	33.9	37.0	40.4	45.3
		kilograms	12.47	13.38	14.29	15.38	16.78	18.33	20.55
	Height	inches	36.2	37.1	38.1	39.2	40.2	41.5	42.5
		centimeters	92.0	94.2	96.9	99.5	102.0	105.4	108.0
4 years	Weight	pounds	29.2	31.2	33.5	36.2	39.6	43.5	48.2
		kilograms	13.25	14.15	15.2	16.42	17.96	19.73	21.86
	Height	inches	37.5	38.4	39.5	40.6	41.6	43.1	44.2
		centimeters	95.2	97.6	100.3	103.2	105.8	109.6	112.3
4½ years	Weight	pounds	30.7	32.9	35.3	38.5	42.1	46.7	50.9
		kilograms	13.93	14.92	16.01	17.46	19.1	21.18	23.09
	Height	inches	38.6	39.7	40.8	42.0	43.0	44.7	45.7
		centimeters	98.1	100.9	103.6	106.8	109.3	113.5	116.2
5 years	Weight	pounds	32.1	34.8	37.4	40.5	44.8	49.2	52.8
		kilograms	14.56	15.79	16.96	18.37	20.32	22.32	23.95
	Height	inches	39.4	40.5	41.6	42.9	44.0	45.4	46.8
		centimeters	100.0	103.0	105.7	109.1	111.7	115.4	118.8

Source: H. C. Stuart, in Nelson, *Textbook of Pediatrics*, 8th ed., Saunders, Philadelphia, 1964.

Table A.6   Weight and Height of Girls from 5 to 18 Years

Age	Measurement		3	10	25	50	75	90	97
			colspan Percentile						

Age	Measurement		Percentile						
			3	10	25	50	75	90	97
5 years[a]	Weight	pounds	33.7	36.1	38.6	41.4	44.2	48.2	51.8
		kilograms	15.29	16.37	17.51	18.78	20.05	21.86	23.5
	Height	inches	40.4	41.3	42.2	43.2	44.4	45.4	46.5
		centimeters	102.6	105.0	107.2	109.7	112.9	115.4	118.0
6 years	Weight	pounds	37.2	39.6	42.9	46.5	50.2	54.2	58.7
		kilograms	16.87	17.96	19.46	21.09	22.77	24.58	26.63
	Height	inches	42.5	43.5	44.6	45.6	47.0	48.1	49.4
		centimeters	108.0	110.6	113.2	115.9	119.3	122.3	125.4
7 years	Weight	pounds	41.3	44.5	48.1	52.2	56.3	61.2	67.3
		kilograms	18.73	20.19	21.82	23.68	25.54	27.76	30.53
	Height	inches	44.9	46.0	46.9	48.1	49.6	50.7	51.9
		centimeters	114.0	116.8	119.2	122.3	125.9	128.9	131.7
8 years	Weight	pounds	45.3	48.6	53.1	58.1	63.3	69.9	78.9
		kilograms	20.55	22.04	24.09	26.35	28.71	31.71	35.79
	Height	inches	46.9	48.1	49.1	50.4	51.8	53.0	54.1
		centimeters	119.1	122.1	124.8	128.0	131.6	134.6	137.4
9 years	Weight	pounds	49.1	52.6	57.9	63.8	70.5	79.1	89.9
		kilograms	22.27	23.86	26.26	28.94	31.98	35.88	40.78
	Height	inches	48.7	50.0	51.1	52.3	54.0	55.3	56.5
		centimeters	123.6	127.0	129.7	132.9	137.1	140.4	143.4
10 years	Weight	pounds	53.2	57.1	62.8	70.3	79.1	89.7	101.9
		kilograms	24.13	25.9	28.49	31.89	35.88	40.69	46.22
	Height	inches	50.3	51.8	53.0	54.6	56.1	57.5	58.8
		centimeters	127.7	131.7	134.6	138.6	142.6	146.0	149.3
11 years	Weight	pounds	57.9	62.6	69.9	78.8	89.1	100.4	112.9
		kilograms	26.26	28.4	31.71	35.74	40.42	45.54	51.21
	Height	inches	52.1	53.9	55.2	57.0	58.7	60.4	62.0
		centimeters	132.3	137.0	140.3	144.7	149.2	153.4	157.4
12 years	Weight	pounds	63.6	69.5	78.0	87.6	98.8	111.5	127.7
		kilograms	28.85	31.52	35.38	39.74	44.82	50.58	57.92
	Height	inches	54.3	56.1	57.4	59.8	61.6	63.2	64.8
		centimeters	137.8	142.6	145.9	151.9	156.6	160.6	164.6

Age	Measurement		Percentile						
			3	10	25	50	75	90	97
13 years	Weight	pounds	72.2	79.9	89.4	99.1	111.0	124.5	142.3
		kilograms	32.75	36.24	40.55	44.95	50.35	56.47	64.55
	Height	inches	56.6	58.7	60.1	61.8	63.6	64.9	66.3
		centimeters	143.7	149.1	152.6	157.1	161.5	164.8	168.4
14 years	Weight	pounds	83.1	91.0	99.8	108.4	119.7	133.3	150.8
		kilograms	37.69	41.28	45.27	49.17	54.29	60.46	68.4
	Height	inches	58.3	60.2	61.5	62.8	64.4	65.7	67.2
		centimeters	148.2	153.0	156.1	159.6	163.7	167.0	170.7
15 years	Weight	pounds	89.0	97.4	105.1	113.5	123.9	138.1	155.2
		kilograms	40.37	44.18	47.67	51.48	56.2	62.64	70.4
	Height	inches	59.1	61.1	62.1	63.4	64.9	66.2	67.6
		centimeters	150.2	155.2	157.7	161.1	164.9	168.1	171.6
16 years	Weight	pounds	91.8	100.9	108.4	117.0	127.2	141.1	157.7
		kilograms	41.64	45.77	49.17	53.07	57.7	64.0	71.53
	Height	inches	59.4	61.5	62.4	63.9	65.2	66.5	67.7
		centimeters	150.8	156.1	158.6	162.2	165.7	169.0	172.0
17 years	Weight	pounds	93.9	102.8	110.4	119.1	129.6	143.3	159.5
		kilograms	42.59	46.63	50.08	54.02	58.79	65.0	72.35
	Height	inches	59.4	61.5	62.6	64.0	65.4	66.7	67.8
		centimeters	151.0	156.3	159.0	162.5	166.1	169.4	172.2
18 years	Weight	pounds	94.5	103.5	111.2	119.9	130.8	144.5	160.7
		kilograms	42.87	46.95	50.44	54.39	59.33	65.54	72.89
	Height	inches	59.4	61.5	62.6	64.0	65.4	66.7	67.8
		centimeters	151.0	156.3	159.0	162.5	166.1	169.4	172.2

^aSeveral measurements at 5 years differ slightly from their counterparts in Table A.5 because they were obtained from a different population of children.
Source: The data in this table are from studies by and are reproduced by courtesy of Howard V. Meredith, Ph.D., Professor of Child Somatology, Institute of Child Behavior and Development, University of Iowa.

The source of these data is Nutritive Value of Foods, Home and Garden Bulletin 72, revised, U.S. Department of Agriculture, Washington, D.C. Data for some cooked and prepared foods are taken from Church and Church, Food Values of Portions Commonly Used — Bowes and Church, Ninth Edition, Lippincott, Philadelphia.

The abbreviation for trace (tr) is used to indicate fatty acid and vitamin values that would round to zero with the number of deicmal places carried in these tables. For other components that would round to zero, a zero is used.

Dashes show that no basis could be found for imputing a value although there was some reason to believe that a measurable amount of the constituent might be present.

Other abbreviations used are:

av	average
c	cup
diam	diameter
hp	heaping
jc	juice
lb	pound
lg	large
lv	leaves
oz	ounce
%	percent
pc	piece
qt	quart
sc	section
serv	serving
sl	slice
sm	small
sq	square
tbsp	tablespoon

APPENDIX B

Nutritive Values of the Edible Part of Foods

Table B.1   Composition of Zwieback, Rice Cereal, and Strained Orange Pudding

Nutrients and Units	BAKED PRODUCTS Zwieback — Amount in Edible Portion of Common Measures of Food — Approximate Measure and Weight		CEREALS Rice, dry — Amount in Edible Portion of Common Measures of Food — Approximate Measure and Weight		DESSERTS Orange pudding, strained — Amount in Edible Portion of Common Measures of Food — Approximate Measure and Weight	
	1 piece = 7 g	1 oz = 28.35g	½ oz = 14.2 g	1 tbsp = 2.4 g	1 jar = 135 g	1 oz = 28.35 g
Proximate						
Water, g	0.3	1.3	1.0	0.2	107.7	22.6
Food energy, kcal	30	121	56	9	108	23
kj	125	506	232	39	451	95
Protein (N × 5.70), g	0.7	2.9	1.0	0.2	1.5	0.3
Total lipid (fat), g	0.7	2.8	0.7	0.1	1.2	0.03
Carbohydrate, total, g	5.2	21.0	11.0	1.9	23.8	5.0
Fiber, g	0.0	0.1	0.1	0.0	0.5	0.1
Ash, g	0.1	0.4	0.5	0.1	0.8	0.2
Minerals						
Calcium, mg	1	6	121	20	43	9
Iron, mg	0.04	0.17	10.19	1.77	0.14	0.03
Magnesium, mg	1	4	29	5	7	2
Phosphorus, mg	4	16	84	14	38	8
Potassium, mg	21	86	55	9	117	24
Sodium, mg	16	66	5	1		
Zinc, mg	0.038	0.153	0.282	0.048	0.230	0.048
Copper, mg			0.047	0.008		
Vitamins						
Ascorbic acid, mg	0.4	1.5	0.3	0.1	12.3	2.6
Thiamin, mg	0.015	0.059	0.376	0.063	0.054	0.011
Riboflavin, mg	0.017	0.068	0.315	0.053	0.077	0.016
Niacin, mg	0.092	0.374	4.437	0.750	0.161	0.034
Pantothenic acid, mg						
Vitamin B$_6$, mg	0.006	0.023	0.068	0.011	0.036	0.008
Folacin, mcg			3.5	0.6	10.6	2.2
Vitamin B$_{12}$, mcg						
Vitamin A, RE	0	2			16	3
IU	4	16	—	—	155	33

Table B.2   Composition of a Strained Dinner, High Meat or Cheese Dinner, and Fruit

Nutrients and Units	DINNERS Beef and egg noodles, strained		DINNERS, HIGH MEAT OR CHEESE Cottage cheese with pineapple, strained		FRUITS Peaches, strained	
	Amount in Edible Portion of Common Measures of Food		Amount in Edible Portion of Common Measures of Food		Amount in Edible Portion of Common Measures of Food	
	Approximate Measure and Weight		Approximate Measure and Weight		Approximate Measure and Weight	
	1 jar = 123 g	1 oz = 28.35 g	1 jar = 135 g	1 oz = 28.35 g	1 jar = 135 g	1 oz = 28.35 g
Proximate						
Water, g	113.4	25.1	97.2	20.4	108.1	22.7
Food energy, kcal	66	15	157	33	96	20
kj	286	63	655	138	402	84
Protein (N × 5.98), g	2.9	0.6	8.5	1.8	0.7	0.7
Total lipid (fat), g	2.2	0.5	3.0	0.6	0.0	0.0
Carbohydrate, total, g	9.0	2.0	25.4	5.3	25.5	5.4
Fiber, g	0.4	0.1	1.2	0.3	1.0	0.2
Ash, g	0.5	0.1	0.9	0.2	0.5	0.1
Minerals						
Calcium, mg	12	3	88	18	8	2
Iron, mg	0.53	0.12	1.14	0.03	0.32	0.07
Magnesium, mg	9	2	9	2	2	2
Phosphorus, mg	37	8	98	21	16	3
Potassium, mg	61	13	128	27	46	46
Sodium, mg	37	8	201	42	8	2
Zinc, mg	0.480	0.106	0.385	0.081	0.115	0.024
Copper, mg	0.038	0.009			0.072	0.015
Vitamins						
Ascorbic acid, mg	1.5	0.3	1.9	0.4	42.4	8.9
Thiamin, mg	0.045	0.010	0.051	0.011	0.015	0.003
Riboflavin, mg	0.054	0.012	0.192	0.040	0.045	0.009
Niacin, mg	0.925	0.205	0.144	0.030	0.822	0.173
Pantothenic acid, mg	0.274	0.061			0.176	0.037
Vitamin B_6, mg	0.061	0.014	0.063	0.013	0.020	0.004
Folacin, mcg	6.5	1.4			5.2	1.1
Vitamin B_{12}, mcg	0.115	0.026	0.304	0.064		
Vitamin A, RE	141	31	10	2	22	5
IU	1053	233	104	22	217	46

Table B.3   *Composition of Strained Egg Yolks and a Vegetable*

Nutrients and Units	MEATS AND EGG YOLKS Egg yolks, strained		VEGETABLES Squash, strained	
	Amount in Edible Portion of Common Measures of Food		Amount in Edible Portion of Common Measures of Food	
	Approximate Measure and Weight		Approximate Measure and Weight	
	1 jar = 94 g	1 oz = 28.35 g	1 jar = 128 g	1 oz = 28.35 g
Proximate				
Water, g	66.3	20.0	118.7	26.3
Food energy, kcal	191	58	30	7
kj	799	241	127	28
Protein (N × 6.25), g	9.4	2.8	1.1	0.2
Total lipid (fat), g	16.3	4.9	0.2	0.1
Carbohydrate, total, g	0.9	0.3	7.2	1.6
Fiber, g			0.9	0.2
Ash, g	1.1	0.3	0.8	0.2
Minerals				
Calcium, mg	72	22	30	7
Iron, mg	2.60	0.78	0.38	0.08
Magnesium, mg	6	2	16	3
Phosphorus, mg	270	81	20	4
Potassium, mg	73	22	229	51
Sodium, mg	37	11	3	1
Zinc, mg	1.800	0.543	0.180	0.040
Copper, mg	0.066	0.020	0.069	0.015
Vitamins				
Ascorbic acid, mg	1.3	0.4	9.8	2.2
Thiamin, mg	0.068	0.020	0.014	0.003
Riboflavin, mg	0.250	0.075	0.072	0.016
Niacin, mg	0.024	0.007	0.453	0.100
Pantothenic acid, mg	2.012	0.607	0.282	0.062
Vitamin B_6, mg	0.150	0.045	0.081	0.018
Folacin, mcg	86.6	26.1	19.7	4.4
Vitamin B_{12}, mcg	1.448	0.437		
Vitamin A, RE	353	107	259	57
IU	1176	355	2590	574

Table B.4 INFANT FORMULA (Meat Base) Average Nutrient Values per 100 Grams and of Amounts Commonly Purchased or Used. (Tables B.4–B.21 reproduced by permission of Gerber Products Co.)

PRODUCT	MEASURE*	WEIGHT g	WEIGHT oz	CALORIES	PROTEIN g	FAT g	CARBOHYDRATE g	ASH g	TOTAL SOLIDS g	CALCIUM mg	PHOSPHORUS mg	IRON mg	COPPER mg	SODIUM mg	POTASSIUM mg	CHLORIDE mg	MAGNESIUM mg
MBF™ (Meat Base Formula) AS PURCHASED, CONCENTRATED	3.2 fl oz / 1 fl oz or 2 tbsp.	100	3.5	126	5.4	6.3	12.0	0.80	24.2	189	126	2.65	0.08	35.0	73.0	40.0	7.6
	15 fl oz or 1 can	32	1.2	40	1.7	2.0	3.8	0.25	7.7	60	40	0.84	0.02	11.0	23.0	13.0	2.4
		475	16.7	600	25.8	30.0	57.0	3.80	115.2	900	600	12.60	0.36	164.0	346.0	190.0	36.0
1:1 DILUTION	3.3 fl oz / 1 fl oz or 2 tbsp.	100	3.5	65	2.8	3.3	6.2	0.40	12.5	98	65	1.37	0.04	18.0	38.0	21.0	4.0
	30 fl oz	31	1.1	20	0.9	1.0	1.9	0.13	3.8	30	20	0.48	0.01	5.4	11.5	6.3	1.2
		918	32.4	600	25.8	30.0	57.0	3.80	115.2	900	600	12.60	0.36	164.0	346.0	190.0	36.0

PRODUCT continued	MEASURE*	WEIGHT g	WEIGHT oz	IODINE µg	SULFUR mg	VITAMIN A IU	THIAMIN mg	RIBOFLAVIN mg	NIACIN mg	VITAMIN B6 mg	VITAMIN B12 µg	FOLACIN µg	PANTOTHENIC ACID mg	ASCORBIC ACID mg	VITAMIN D IU	VITAMIN E IU
MBF™ (Meat Base Formula) AS PURCHASED, CONCENTRATED	3.2 fl oz / 1 fl oz or 1 tbsp.	100	3.5	40	6.3	337	0.11	0.19	1.39	0.16	1.60	5.1	0.38	11.4	88	1.1
	15 fl oz or 1 can	32	1.2	13	2.0	107	0.04	0.06	0.44	0.05	0.52	1.6	0.12	3.6	28	0.4
		475	16.7	190	30.0	1600	0.54	0.90	6.60	0.78	7.80	24.0	1.80	54.0	420	5.4
1:1 DILUTION	3.3 fl oz / 1 fl oz or 1 tbsp.	100	3.5	21	3.0	174	0.06	0.10	0.72	0.08	0.80	2.6	0.20	5.9	46	0.6
	30 fl oz	31	1.1	6	1.0	53	0.02	0.03	0.22	0.03	0.26	0.8	0.10	1.8	14	0.2
		918	32.4	190	30.0	1600	0.54	0.90	6.60	0.78	7.80	24.0	1.80	54.0	420	5.4

AMINO ACID CONTENT PER 100 GRAMS AND PER **30 FLUID OUNCES AS FED

PRODUCT	MEASURE*	WEIGHT g	WEIGHT oz	TRYPTOPHAN mg	THREONINE mg	ISOLEUCINE mg	LEUCINE mg	LYSINE mg	METHIONINE mg	CYSTINE mg	PHENYLALANINE mg	TYROSINE mg
MBF™ (Meat Base Formula)	3.3 fl oz	100	3.5	29.8	112.6	126.1	235.7	218.3	101.6	26.8	133.8	104.2
1:1 DILUTION	30 fl oz	918	32.4	274.0	1034.0	1158.0	2164.0	2004.0	933.0	246.0	1229.0	957.0

PRODUCT continued	MEASURE*	WEIGHT g	WEIGHT oz	VALINE mg	ARGININE mg	HISTIDINE mg	ALANINE mg	ASPARTIC ACID mg	GLUTAMIC ACID mg	GLYCINE mg	PROLINE mg	SERINE mg
MBF™ (Meat Base Formula)	3.3 fl oz	100	3.5	138.9	205.3	81.5	159.6	255.2	409.5	137.8	161.9	93.5
1:1 DILUTION	30 fl oz	918	32.4	1275.0	1884.0	748.0	1465.0	2343.0	3759.0	1265.0	1487.0	858.0

ELECTROLYTE CONTENT PER 100 GRAMS AND PER **30 FLUID OUNCES AS FED

PRODUCT	MEASURE*	WEIGHT g	WEIGHT oz	SODIUM mEq	POTASSIUM mEq	CALCIUM mEq	PHOSPHORUS mEq	CHLORIDE mEq	MAGNESIUM mEq	SULFUR mEq	TOTAL mEq
MBF™ (Meat Base Formula)	3.3 fl oz	100	3.5	0.8	1.0	4.9	6.3	0.6	0.3	1.3	15.2
1:1 DILUTION	30 fl oz	918	32.4	7.1	8.8	44.9	58.1	5.3	3.0	11.8	139.2

*All measures level   tsp. = tablespoon   oz = ounce   g = gram   mEq = milliequivalent   µg = microgram   mg = milligram   IU = International Unit

**30 fl oz is the quantity which will result with 1:1 dilution of one can of MBF

Table B.5 READY-TO-SERVE DRY CEREALS
Nutrition Information per Serving (Serving Size—½ oz (14.2g) 6 Tbsp)

PRODUCT	SERVING SIZE DRY-½ oz (14.2 g) WITH MILK 2.4 fl oz (70 ml)	AVERAGE NUTRIENT CONTENT PER SERVING				PERCENT OF U.S. RECOMMENDED DAILY ALLOWANCES FOR INFANTS									
		CALORIES	PROTEIN g	CARBO-HYDRATE g	FAT g	PROTEIN	VITAMIN A	VITAMIN C	THIAMIN (VIT. B₁)	RIBO-FLAVIN (VIT. B₂)	NIACIN	CALCIUM	IRON	VITAMIN B₆	PHOS-PHORUS
BARLEY	Dry	60	2	11	1	6	*	*	45	45	25	15	45	15	15
	With milk	100	4	14	3	15	6	2	50	70	25	30	45	20	25
HIGH PROTEIN	Dry	50	5	6	1	20	*	*	45	45	25	15	45	15	15
	With milk	110	8	10	4	35	6	2	45	70	25	25	45	25	30
HIGH PROTEIN CEREAL WITH APPLE & ORANGE	Dry	60	4	8	1	15	*	*	45	45	25	15	45	15	15
	With milk	90	6	11	3	25	6	2	50	70	25	30	45	25	30
MIXED	Dry	60	2	10	1	8	*	*	45	45	25	15	45	8	15
	With milk	100	5	13	3	20	6	2	50	70	25	30	45	15	25
MIXED CEREAL WITH BANANA	Dry	60	1	11	1	6	*	*	45	45	25	15	45	15	10
	With milk	100	4	14	3	15	6	2	50	70	25	30	45	25	20
OATMEAL	Dry	60	2	10	1	8	*	*	45	45	25	15	45	6	20
	With milk	100	5	13	4	20	6	2	50	70	25	30	45	15	30
OATMEAL WITH BANANA	Dry	60	2	10	1	8	*	*	45	45	25	15	45	15	10
	With milk	110	4	14	4	20	6	2	50	70	25	30	45	25	20
RICE	Dry	60	1	11	1	4	*	*	45	45	25	15	45	20	15
	With milk	100	4	14	3	15	6	2	50	70	25	30	45	30	30
RICE CEREAL WITH BANANA	Dry	60	1	11	1	4	*	*	45	45	25	15	45	20	10
	With milk	100	4	14	3	15	6	2	50	70	25	30	45	30	20

Legend: g = gram   fl oz = fluid ounce   ml = milliliter   * = Contains less than 2% of the U.S. RDA for these nutrients

SERVINGS PER PACKAGE: 1 oz = 2
8 oz = 16
16 oz = 32

Table B.6 BAKED GOODS
Nutrition Information per Serving (Serving Size Listed Below)

PRODUCT	AVERAGE NUTRIENT CONTENT PER SERVING						PERCENT OF U.S. RECOMMENDED DAILY ALLOWANCES FOR INFANTS AND CHILDREN 1-4 YEARS OF AGE								
	WEIGHT g	WEIGHT oz	CALORIES	PROTEIN g	CARBO-HYDRATE g	FAT g	PROTEIN	VITAMIN A	VITAMIN C	THIAMIN (VIT. B₁)	RIBO-FLAVIN (VIT. B₂)	NIACIN	CALCIUM	IRON	VITAMIN B₆
ARROWROOT COOKIES	11	0.4	50	1	8	2	(c) 4	*	*	8	4	4	*	2	*
COOKIES ANIMAL SHAPED	13	0.4	60	2	9	2	(c) 6	*	2	20	35	15	2	4	45
PRETZELS	12	0.4	45	1	10	0	(c) 4	*	*	10	6	8	*	6	*
TEETHING BISCUITS	11	0.4	45	1	8	1	(1) 4	*	*	6	10	6	2	2	2
ZWIEBACK TOAST	14	0.5	60	1	10	2	(c) 4	*	2	4	4	2	*	*	2

Legend: g = gram   oz = ounce   * = Contains less than 2% of the U.S. RDA for these nutrients

SERVING SIZE:
ARROWROOT COOKIES—2 Cookies (11g)
COOKIES (ANIMAL SHAPED)—2 Cookies (13g)
PRETZELS—2 Pretzels (12g)
TEETHING BISCUITS—1 Biscuit (11g)
ZWIEBACK TOAST—2 Toasts (14g)

Table B.7   STRAINED JUICES
Nutrition Information per Serving (Serving Size—1 Container • Servings per Container—1)

PRODUCT	WEIGHT ml	oz	CALORIES	PROTEIN g	CARBO-HYDRATE g	FAT g	PROTEIN	VITAMIN A	VITAMIN C	THIAMIN (VT. B₁)	RIBO-FLAVIN (VT. B₂)	NIACIN	CALCIUM	IRON	VITAMIN B₆
				AVERAGE NUTRIENT VALUES PER CONTAINER					**PERCENT OF U.S. RECOMMENDED DAILY ALLOWANCES FOR INFANTS**						
APPLE	124	4.2	60	0	16	0	*	*	120	*	2	*	*	4	10
APPLE-CHERRY	124	4.2	70	0	16	1	*	*	120	2	4	*	*	4	10
APPLE-GRAPE	124	4.2	60	0	16	0	*	*	120	2	4	2	*	4	10
APPLE-PEACH	124	4.2	60	0	15	0	*	4	120	*	2	4	*	2	8
APPLE-PLUM	124	4.2	60	0	16	0	*	2	120	2	6	2	*	2	8
MIXED FRUIT	124	4.2	70	0	18	0	*	2	120	8	4	2	*	*	15
ORANGE	124	4.2	70	1	14	1	2	4	120	15	6	4	*	2	15
ORANGE-APPLE	124	4.2	80	1	16	1	2	6	120	8	4	2	*	2	15
ORANGE-APPLE BANANA	124	4.2	80	1	16	1	2	4	120	8	6	2	*	2	20
ORANGE-APRICOT	124	4.2	70	1	16	0	4	20	120	15	6	4	*	2	20
ORANGE-PINEAPPLE	124	4.2	80	1	18	0	2	4	120	15	6	4	2	2	25
PRUNE-ORANGE	124	4.2	90	1	21	0	4	8	120	10	30	6	*	2	20

Legend: ml = milliliter   fl oz = fluid ounce   g = gram   * = Contains less than 2% of the U.S.RDA for these nutrients

Table B.8 STRAINED MEATS AND EGG YOLKS
Nutrition Information per Serving (Serving Size—1 Jar • Servings per Jar—1)

PRODUCT	AVERAGE NUTRIENT VALUES PER JAR						PERCENT OF U.S. RECOMMENDED DAILY ALLOWANCES FOR INFANTS								
	WEIGHT g	oz	CALORIES	PROTEIN g	CARBO-HYDRATE g	FAT g	PROTEIN	VITAMIN A	VITAMIN C	THIAMIN (VIT. B_1)	RIBO-FLAVIN (VIT. B_2)	NIACIN	CALCIUM	IRON	VITAMIN B_6
BEEF	99	3.5	90	13	0	4	70	6	6	2	20	40	*	8	30
BEEF WITH BEEF HEART	99	3.5	90	13	1	4	70	8	6	2	60	45	*	15	30
BEEF LIVER	99	3.5	90	14	2	3	80	1690	50	6	260	100	*	30	70
CHICKEN	99	3.5	140	14	0	9	80	4	4	2	25	40	10	6	35
EGG YOLKS	94	3.33	180	9	1	16	50	25	6	10	35	*	10	20	35
HAM	99	3.5	110	13	1	6	70	2	6	20	25	30	*	6	50
LAMB	99	3.5	100	14	1	4	80	2	2	2	35	30	*	10	35
PORK	99	3.5	110	13	1	6	70	2	6	20	30	25	*	6	45
TURKEY	99	3.5	120	14	1	7	80	10	8	2	35	40	4	6	40
VEAL	99	3.5	90	13	1	4	70	4	6	2	25	45	*	6	35

Legend: g = gram   oz = ounce   * = Contains less than 2% of the U.S.RDA for these nutrients

Table B.9 STRAINED VEGETABLES
Nutrition Information per Serving (Serving Size—1 Jar • Servings per Jar—1)

PRODUCT	AVERAGE NUTRIENT VALUES PER JAR						PERCENT OF U.S. RECOMMENDED DAILY ALLOWANCES FOR INFANTS								
	WEIGHT g	WEIGHT oz	CALORIES	PROTEIN g	CARBO-HYDRATE g	FAT g	PROTEIN	VITAMIN A	VITAMIN C	THIAMIN (VIT. B₁)	RIBO-FLAVIN (VIT. B₂)	NIACIN	CALCIUM	IRON	VITAMIN B₆
BEETS	128	4.5	40	1	10	0	6	2	6	2	8	2	2	2	8
CARROTS	128	4.5	40	1	8	0	4	120	25	6	8	6	4	2	25
CREAMED CORN	128	4.5	90	2	18	1	10	*	8	2	10	10	4	*	15
CREAMED SPINACH	128	4.5	70	4	9	2	15	120	15	6	20	4	20	8	15
GARDEN VEGETABLES	128	4.5	50	3	7	1	10	200	25	15	15	10	6	6	25
GREEN BEANS	128	4.5	40	2	7	0	6	25	15	8	15	6	6	4	8
MIXED VEGETABLES	128	4.5	60	2	10	1	6	120	8	6	4	6	2	2	15
PEAS	128	4.5	60	4	10	1	15	30	25	20	10	15	2	8	20
SQUASH	128	4.5	40	1	8	0	4	90	30	4	8	6	4	2	15
SWEET POTATOES	135	4.75	80	1	19	0	6	120	40	6	6	6	2	2	30

Legend: g = gram   oz = ounce   * = Contains less than 2% of the U.S. RDA for these nutrients

NUTRITION FOR THE GROWING YEARS

Table B.10   STRAINED HIGH MEAT DINNERS
Nutrition Information per Serving (Serving Size—1 Jar • Servings per Jar—1)

PRODUCT	AVERAGE NUTRIENT VALUES PER JAR						PERCENT OF U.S. RECOMMENDED DAILY ALLOWANCES FOR INFANTS								
	WEIGHT g	WEIGHT oz	CALORIES	PROTEIN g	CARBO-HYDRATE g	FAT g	PROTEIN	VITAMIN A	VITAMIN C	THIAMIN (VIT. B₁)	RIBO-FLAVIN (VIT. B₂)	NIACIN	CALCIUM	IRON	VITAMIN B₆
BEEF WITH VEGETABLES	128	4.5	110	7	9	5	40	30	2	6	10	25	*	6	25
CHICKEN WITH VEGETABLES	128	4.5	130	8	8	7	45	60	6	2	10	15	10	8	15
COTTAGE CHEESE WITH PINEAPPLE	135	4.75	150	8	26	2	45	*	4	10	15	2	15	*	15
HAM WITH VEGETABLES	128	4.5	110	8	10	4	45	25	8	25	15	25	*	4	35
TURKEY WITH VEGETABLES	128	4.5	120	8	9	6	45	35	6	4	15	10	10	6	15
VEAL WITH VEGETABLES	128	4.5	90	8	9	3	45	4	4	4	10	25	*	6	25

Legend g = gram   oz = ounce   * = Contains less than 2% of the U.S.RDA for these nutrients

APPENDIX B: NUTRITIVE VALUES OF THE EDIBLE PART OF FOODS   485

Table B.11   STRAINED FRUIT—NO SUGAR ADDED
(Serving Size—1 Jar • Servings per Jar—1)

| | AVERAGE NUTRIENT VALUES PER JAR | | | | | PERCENT OF U.S. RECOMMENDED DAILY ALLOWANCE FOR INFANTS | | | | | | | | |
	WEIGHT g / oz.	CALORIES	PROTEIN (g)	CARBO-HYDRATE (g)	FAT (g)	PROTEIN	VITAMIN A	VITAMIN C	THIAMIN	RIBO-FLAVIN	NIACIN	CALCIUM	IRON	VITAMIN B6
Apple Blueberry	128 4.5	70	0	16	1	*	*	45	4	8	2	*	*	10
Applesauce	128 4.5	70	0	16	1	*	2	45	2	8	*	*	*	8
Applesauce & Apricots	128 4.5	80	0	18	1	*	15	45	2	6	2	*	*	10
Applesauce w/ Pineapple	128 4.5	60	0	16	0	*	*	45	4	6	*	*	*	10
Apricots w/ Tapioca	128 4.5	70	1	14	1	2	70	45	4	2	4	*	*	15
Bananas w/ Tapioca	128 4.5	80	1	16	1	2	2	45	4	6	4	*	*	35
Bananas w/Pine. & Tapioca	128 4.5	70	0	16	1	*	2	45	2	4	2	*	*	30
Peaches	128 4.5	70	1	14	1	2	15	45	2	6	10	*	*	*
Pears	128 4.5	70	1	15	1	2	2	45	4	6	4	*	*	2
Pears & Pineapple	128 4.5	80	1	16	1	2	2	45	6	6	2	2	*	6
Plums w/Tapioca	128 4.5	90	1	19	1	2	10	2	4	6	4	*	*	8
Prunes w/Tapioca	135 4.75	110	1	25	1	4	20	20	4	20	8	2	2	25

These are preliminary values representing products with recent formulation changes.

LEGEND: g = grams   oz. = ounces   *Contains less than 2% of the U.S.RDA for these nutrients.

Table B.12   STRAINED CEREALS WITH FRUIT—NO SUGAR ADDED
(Serving Size—1 Jar • Servings per Jar—1)

			AVERAGE NUTRIENT VALUES PER JAR				PERCENT OF U.S. RECOMMENDED DAILY ALLOWANCE FOR INFANTS									
	WEIGHT		CALORIES	PROTEIN (g)	CARBO-HYDRATE (g)	FAT (g)	PROTEIN	VITAMIN A	VITAMIN C	THIAMIN	RIBO-FLAVIN	NIACIN	CALCIUM	IRON	VITAMIN B6
	g	oz.													
Mixed Cereal w/ Applesauce & Bananas	128	4.5	90	2	18	1	8	*	45	45	45	45	*	45	45
Oatmeal Cereal w/ Applesauce & Bananas	128	4.5	80	2	15	1	8	*	45	45	45	45	*	45	45
Rice Cereal w/ Applesauce & Bananas	135	4.75	100	2	20	1	6	*	45	45	45	45	2	45	45

Table B.13 STRAINED VEGETABLES AND MEATS
Nutrition Information per Serving (Serving Size—1 Jar • Servings per Jar—1)

PRODUCT	AVERAGE NUTRIENT VALUES PER JAR					PERCENT OF U.S. RECOMMENDED DAILY ALLOWANCES FOR INFANTS								
	WEIGHT g / oz	CALORIES	PROTEIN g	CARBO-HYDRATE g	FAT g	PROTEIN	VITAMIN A	VITAMIN C	THIAMIN (VT. B₁)	RIBO-FLAVIN (VT. B₂)	NIACIN	CALCIUM	IRON	VITAMIN B₆
BEEF & EGG NOODLES WITH VEGETABLES	128 / 4.5	80	4	12	2	15	35	4	10	10	10	*	4	15
CEREAL & EGG YOLK	128 / 4.5	70	2	10	2	10	6	2	4	10	2	6	2	8
CHICKEN & NOODLES	128 / 4.5	70	3	11	2	10	35	4	8	10	10	4	2	10
CREAM OF CHICKEN SOUP	128 / 4.5	80	3	10	3	10	30	4	4	10	6	8	2	10
MACARONI & CHEESE	128 / 4.5	90	4	12	3	15	2	2	10	15	8	10	2	8
MACARONI-TOMATO WITH BEEF	128 / 4.5	80	3	12	2	10	40	4	10	8	10	2	2	15
TURKEY & RICE WITH VEGETABLES	128 / 4.5	70	3	10	2	10	40	6	2	6	10	4	2	15
VEGETABLES & BACON	128 / 4.5	100	2	11	5	10	100	4	10	6	10	2	2	25
VEGETABLES & BEEF	128 / 4.5	80	3	11	3	10	70	4	4	6	10	*	2	15
VEGETABLES & CHICKEN	128 / 4.5	60	3	8	2	10	80	4	4	6	2	2	2	6
VEGETABLES & HAM	128 / 4.5	70	2	10	2	8	45	4	10	4	6	*	*	15
VEGETABLES & LAMB	128 / 4.5	90	3	11	4	10	100	4	6	6	8	*	2	15
VEGETABLES & LIVER	128 / 4.5	70	3	12	1	10	120	8	10	70	20	*	20	25
VEGETABLES & TURKEY	128 / 4.5	70	2	10	2	10	40	4	2	4	6	4	2	10

Legend: g = gram   oz = ounce   * = Contains less than 2% of the U.S. RDA for these nutrients

Table B.14   STRAINED DESSERTS
Nutrition Information per Serving (Serving Size—1 Jar • Servings per Jar—1)

PRODUCT	WEIGHT g	WEIGHT oz	CALORIES	PROTEIN g	CARBO-HYDRATE g	FAT g	PROTEIN	VITAMIN A	VITAMIN C	THIAMIN (VIT. B₁)	RIBO-FLAVIN (VIT. B₂)	NIACIN	CALCIUM	IRON	VITAMIN B₆
	AVERAGE NUTRIENT VALUES PER JAR						PERCENT OF U.S. RECOMMENDED DAILY ALLOWANCES FOR INFANTS								
CHERRY VANILLA PUDDING	135	4.75	100	0	24	1	*	15	4	*	2	*	*	2	4
CHOCOLATE CUSTARD PUDDING	128	4.5	120	3	23	2	15	4	4	4	20	*	10	4	4
COTTAGE CHEESE WITH PINEAPPLE	135	4.75	120	4	24	1	25	2	45	4	10	*	6	*	4
DUTCH APPLE DESSERT	135	4.75	110	0	22	2	*	4	25	2	2	*	*	*	4
FRUIT DESSERT	135	4.75	100	0	23	1	*	20	10	6	2	2	2	2	10
HAWAIIAN DELIGHT	128	4.5	120	2	27	1	8	2	45	10	10	2	6	*	10
ORANGE PUDDING	135	4.75	120	1	24	2	6	10	20	10	10	2	6	2	8
PEACH COBBLER	135	4.75	110	1	24	1	2	6	35	2	2	4	*	*	2
RASPBERRY DESSERT WITH YOGURT	128	4.5	100	1	21	1	6	*	*	4	10	*	6	*	4
VANILLA CUSTARD PUDDING	128	4.5	120	2	21	3	10	6	2	2	15	*	10	2	6

Legend: g = gram   oz = ounce   * = Contains less than 2% of the U.S. RDA for these nutrients

Table B.15 *JUNIOR MEATS*
Nutrition Information per Serving (Serving Size—1 Jar • Servings per Jar—1)

PRODUCT		WEIGHT g	WEIGHT oz	CALORIES	PROTEIN g	CARBO-HYDRATE g	FAT g	AGE	PROTEIN	VITAMIN A	VITAMIN C	THIAMIN (VIT. B₁)	RIBO-FLAVIN (VIT. B₂)	NIACIN	CALCIUM	IRON	VITAMIN B₆
BEEF	INFANT	99	3.5	100	14	1	4	INFANT	80	4	6	*	20	45	*	10	30
	CHILD							CHILD	70	2	4	*	15	40	*	15	15
CHICKEN	INFANT	99	3.5	140	14	0	9	INFANT	80	2	4	2	25	45	6	8	40
	CHILD							CHILD	70	2	4	*	20	45	6	10	25
CHICKEN STICKS	INFANT	71	2.5	130	10	1	10	INFANT	50	*	2	2	15	15	6	8	15
	CHILD							CHILD	50	*	2	*	15	15	6	10	10
HAM	INFANT	99	3.5	120	15	1	6	INFANT	80	2	6	20	25	35	*	6	50
	CHILD							CHILD	70	*	6	15	20	30	*	10	25
LAMB	INFANT	99	3.5	100	15	1	4	INFANT	80	*	2	2	25	40	*	10	40
	CHILD							CHILD	70	*	2	*	20	35	*	15	20
MEAT STICKS	INFANT	71	2.5	130	10	1	6	INFANT	60	2	2	6	15	15	4	8	10
	CHILD							CHILD	50	*	*	4	10	15	2	10	6
TURKEY	INFANT	99	3.5	130	15	0	8	INFANT	80	2	8	2	30	45	4	6	40
	CHILD							CHILD	80	*	6	2	25	40	2	10	25
TURKEY STICKS	INFANT	71	2.5	140	10	1	11	INFANT	60	*	2	*	15	15	10	6	15
	CHILD							CHILD	50	*	2	*	15	15	8	10	8
VEAL	INFANT	99	3.5	100	15	0	4	INFANT	80	2	6	*	25	50	*	6	35
	CHILD							CHILD	70	*	6	*	20	45	*	10	20

AVERAGE NUTRIENT VALUES PER JAR

PERCENT OF U.S. RECOMMENDED DAILY ALLOWANCES FOR INFANTS AND CHILDREN 1–4 YEARS OF AGE

Legend: g = gram   oz = ounce   * = Contains less than 2% of the U.S.RDA for these nutrients

Table B.16   JUNIOR VEGETABLES
Nutrition Information per Serving (Serving Size—1 Jar • Servings per Jar—1)

PRODUCT	CALORIES	PROTEIN g	CARBO-HYDRATE g	FAT g	CRUDE FIBER g	TOTAL SOLIDS g	CALCIUM mg	PHOS-PHORUS mg	IRON mg	SODIUM mg	POTAS-SIUM mg	VITAMIN A I U	THIAMIN mg	RIBO-FLAVIN mg	NIACIN mg	VITAMIN B₁ mg	VITAMIN C mg
CARROTS	27	0.9	5.6	0.2	0.7	8.1	18	20	0.2	52	172	15000	0.02	0.04	0.41	0.08	7.0
CREAMED CORN	69	2.0	14.0	0.5	0.2	17.1	20	35	0.1	11	64	11	0.01	0.05	0.77	0.07	3.8
CREAMED GREEN BEANS	43	1.6	8.6	0.2	0.3	11.0	36	23	0.4	12	73	97	0.02	0.06	0.21	0.03	2.6
CREAMED SPINACH	49	3.0	6.0	1.4	0.4	11.7	91	49	1.0	55	222	2270	0.02	0.14	0.26	0.07	14.5
MIXED VEGETABLES	40	1.5	7.9	0.3	0.5	10.7	11	28	0.3	36	131	5860	0.03	0.03	0.62	0.05	2.9
SQUASH	27	0.8	5.4	0.2	0.8	7.5	20	17	0.2	1	179	1740	0.02	0.05	0.45	0.06	7.7
SWEET POTATOES	60	1.2	13.5	0.1	0.6	16.3	13	24	0.2	23	262	6040	0.03	0.03	0.35	0.12	14.1

Legend: g = gram   mg = milligram   I U = International Unit

Table B.17   *JUNIOR HIGH MEAT DINNERS*
Nutrition Information per Serving (Serving Size—1 Jar • Servings per Jar—1)

| | AVERAGE NUTRIENT VALUES PER JAR | | | | | | PERCENT OF U.S. RECOMMENDED DAILY ALLOWANCES FOR INFANTS AND CHILDREN 1–4 YEARS OF AGE | | | | | | | | | |
PRODUCT	WEIGHT g	oz	CALORIES	PROTEIN g	CARBO-HYDRATE g	FAT g	AGE	PROTEIN	VITAMIN A	VITAMIN C	THIAMIN (VIT. B₁)	RIBO-FLAVIN (VIT. B₂)	NIACIN	CALCIUM	IRON	VITAMIN B₆
BEEF WITH VEGETABLES	128	4.5	120	8	11	5	INFANT CHILD	45 40	60 35	4 4	4 4	15 10	25 20	2 *	6 10	30 15
CHICKEN WITH VEGETABLES	128	4.5	140	8	9	8	INFANT CHILD	45 40	100 60	4 4	4 2	15 10	15 10	10 8	6 8	15 8
HAM WITH VEGETABLES	128	4.5	120	8	10	5	INFANT CHILD	45 40	10 8	6 4	30 20	15 10	20 15	* *	6 8	30 20
TURKEY WITH VEGETABLES	128	4.5	130	8	10	6	INFANT CHILD	45 40	45 30	8 6	4 4	15 10	10 10	15 10	6 8	10 6
VEAL WITH VEGETABLES	128	4.5	100	8	11	3	INFANT CHILD	45 40	45 25	8 6	6 4	15 10	25 20	* *	4 6	25 15

Legend: g = gram   oz = ounce   * = Contains less than 2% of the U.S.RDA for these nutrients

Table B.18 JUNIOR FRUITS—NO SUGAR ADDED
(Serving Size—1 Jar • Servings per Jar—1)

	WEIGHT g	oz.	CALORIES	PROTEIN (g)	CARBO-HYDRATE (g)	FAT (g)	AGE	PROTEIN	VITAMIN A	VITAMIN C	THIAMIN	RIBO-FLAVIN	NIACIN	CALCIUM	IRON	VITAMIN B6
Apple Blueberry	213	7.5	120	1	27	1	INFANT	2	4	45	6	15	2	*	2	15
							CHILD	2	2	40	4	10	2	*	2	8
Applesauce	213	7.5	100	0	24	1	INFANT	*	4	45	6	10	2	*	*	15
							CHILD	*	2	40	4	8	2	*	2	8
Applesauce & Apricots	213	7.5	120	1	26	1	INFANT	2	35	45	6	10	4	2	2	20
							CHILD	2	20	40	4	8	4	*	4	10
Applesauce w/ Pineapple	213	7.5	100	0	23	1	INFANT	*	4	45	10	8	2	*	2	20
							CHILD	*	2	40	8	6	2	*	2	10
Apricot w/ Tapioca	213	7.5	110	1	24	1	INFANT	4	100	45	6	4	6	2	2	20
							CHILD	2	60	40	4	2	6	2	4	10
Bananas w/ Tapioca	213	7.5	120	1	27	1	INFANT	4	6	45	6	10	6	2	2	70
							CHILD	4	4	40	4	10	6	*	4	45
Bananas w/Pine. & Tapioca	213	7.5	120	1	26	1	INFANT	2	4	45	6	6	4	2	*	50
							CHILD	2	2	40	4	4	2	*	2	30
Peaches	213	7.5	100	1	23	1	INFANT	6	25	45	4	10	15	*	*	8
							CHILD	4	15	40	2	8	15	*	2	6
Pears	213	7.5	120	1	26	1	INFANT	4	4	45	6	8	4	2	2	4
							CHILD	4	2	40	4	6	4	2	2	2
Pears & Pineapple	213	7.5	120	1	26	1	INFANT	4	4	45	10	8	4	2	2	8
							CHILD	2	2	40	8	6	4	2	4	4
Plums w/Tapioca	213	7.5	140	1	33	1	INFANT	2	15	2	2	10	6	2	2	15
							CHILD	2	8	2	2	8	4	2	4	8
Prunes w/Tapioca	220	7.75	180	1	43	1	INFANT	6	35	30	6	25	15	4	4	40
							CHILD	4	20	25	4	20	10	4	6	25

AVERAGE NUTRIENT VALUES PER JAR / *PERCENT OF U.S. RECOMMENDED DAILY ALLOWANCE FOR INFANTS AND CHILDREN 1 – 4 YEARS OF AGE*

These are preliminary values representing products with recent formulation changes.

LEGEND: g = grams oz. = ounces *Contains less than 2% of the U.S. RDA for these nutrients.

Table B.19 JUNIOR VEGETABLES AND MEATS
Nutrition Information per Serving (Serving Size—1 Jar • Servings per Jar—1)

PRODUCT	WEIGHT g	WEIGHT oz	CALORIES	PROTEIN g	CARBO-HYDRATE g	FAT g	AGE	PROTEIN	VITAMIN A	VITAMIN C	THIAMIN (VIT. B_1)	RIBO-FLAVIN (VIT. B_2)	NIACIN	CALCIUM	IRON	VITAMIN B_6
BEEF & EGG NOODLES WITH VEGETABLES	213	7.5	130	6	20	3	INFANT	25	100	4	15	15	15	2	6	20
							CHILD	20	70	4	10	10	15	*	8	15
CEREAL & EGG YOLK	213	7.5	120	4	16	4	INFANT	15	10	4	6	15	4	8	4	10
							CHILD	15	8	4	4	10	4	6	6	6
CHICKEN & NOODLES	213	7.5	110	5	16	3	INFANT	20	70	8	10	8	15	6	6	10
							CHILD	15	40	6	6	6	10	4	8	6
MACARONI & CHEESE	213	7.5	140	6	19	4	INFANT	25	2	4	15	20	15	15	2	10
							CHILD	20	*	4	10	15	15	15	4	6
MACARONI-TOMATO WITH BEEF	213	7.5	120	5	20	2	INFANT	20	100	6	15	15	15	4	6	20
							CHILD	20	60	6	10	10	15	4	8	10
SPAGHETTI-TOMATO SAUCE & BEEF	213	7.5	150	6	24	3	INFANT	25	80	10	25	20	25	6	6	35
							CHILD	20	50	8	20	15	25	4	10	20
SPLIT PEAS WITH HAM	213	7.5	150	7	24	3	INFANT	30	120	10	20	15	15	6	6	30
							CHILD	25	70	8	15	10	15	4	8	15
TURKEY & RICE WITH VEGETABLES	213	7.5	130	5	19	4	INFANT	20	130	10	6	15	15	6	4	25
							CHILD	15	80	8	4	10	10	4	6	15
VEGETABLES & BACON	213	7.5	190	5	20	10	INFANT	20	150	6	20	10	15	2	6	25
							CHILD	15	90	4	15	8	10	2	8	15
VEGETABLES & BEEF	213	7.5	130	6	21	3	INFANT	25	90	6	15	15	15	2	6	30
							CHILD	20	50	6	10	10	15	2	8	20
VEGETABLES & CHICKEN	213	7.5	120	4	19	3	INFANT	15	100	10	6	6	10	4	4	20
							CHILD	15	60	8	4	4	10	4	6	10
VEGETABLES & HAM	213	7.5	120	5	16	4	INFANT	20	50	8	10	8	8	*	2	15
							CHILD	15	30	8	8	6	8	*	4	8
VEGETABLES & LAMB	213	7.5	140	4	18	6	INFANT	15	130	8	10	10	10	2	4	20
							CHILD	15	80	8	6	8	10	*	6	10
VEGETABLES & LIVER	213	7.5	110	4	18	2	INFANT	15	200	10	10	80	35	2	20	35
							CHILD	15	120	8	6	60	30	2	25	20
VEGETABLES & TURKEY	213	7.5	110	4	18	3	INFANT	15	100	6	6	6	10	6	4	15
							CHILD	15	60	6	4	4	8	4	6	10

AVERAGE NUTRIENT VALUES PER JAR

PERCENT OF U.S. RECOMMENDED DAILY ALLOWANCES FOR INFANTS AND CHILDREN 1-4 YEARS OF AGE

Legend: g = gram   oz = ounce   * = Contains less than 2% of the U.S.RDA for these nutrients

Table B.20   *JUNIOR DESSERTS*
Nutrition Information per Serving (Serving Size—1 Jar • Servings per Jar—1)

PRODUCT	WEIGHT g	WEIGHT oz	CALORIES	PROTEIN g	CARBO- HYDRATE g	FAT g	AGE	PROTEIN	VITAMIN A	VITAMIN C	THIAMIN (VIT. B₁)	RIBO- FLAVIN (VIT. B₂)	NIACIN	CALCIUM	IRON	VITAMIN B₆
CHERRY VANILLA PUDDING	220	7.75	170	1	40	1	INFANT	2	30	6	4	4	*	2	2	6
							CHILD	2	15	4	2	4	*	2	4	4
COTTAGE CHEESE WITH PINEAPPLE	220	7.75	210	7	41	2	INFANT	40	2	45	8	20	*	6	*	6
							CHILD	35	*	40	6	15	*	4	2	4
DUTCH APPLE DESSERT	220	7.75	180	0	40	2	INFANT	*	8	45	2	6	*	2	*	6
							CHILD	*	4	40	2	4	*	*	2	4
FRUIT DESSERT	220	7.75	160	1	38	1	INFANT	2	20	20	6	4	4	2	2	20
							CHILD	2	10	15	4	2	4	2	4	10
HAWAIIAN DELIGHT	220	7.75	200	3	44	1	INFANT	10	6	45	15	15	4	15	2	20
							CHILD	10	4	40	10	15	2	10	4	10
PEACH COBBLER	220	7.75	170	1	40	1	INFANT	4	10	45	4	4	8	*	2	4
							CHILD	2	6	40	2	4	6	*	2	2
RASPBERRY DESSERT WITH YOGURT	213	7.5	160	2	35	1	INFANT	8	*	2	6	20	2	10	*	8
							CHILD	8	*	2	4	15	*	8	*	4
VANILLA CUSTARD PUDDING	220	7.75	210	4	37	5	INFANT	20	6	6	4	25	*	15	4	8
							CHILD	20	4	4	4	20	*	10	6	4

Legend: g = gram   oz = ounce   * = Contains less than 2% of the U.S. RDA for these nutrients

Table B.21 TODDLER MEALS
Nutrition Information per Serving (Serving Size— 1 Jar • Servings per Jar—1)

PRODUCT	AVERAGE NUTRIENT VALUES PER JAR						PERCENT OF U.S. RECOMMENDED DAILY ALLOWANCES FOR CHILDREN 1-4 YEARS OF AGE								
	WEIGHT g	WEIGHT oz	CALORIES	PROTEIN g	CARBO-HYDRATE g	FAT g	PROTEIN	VITAMIN A	VITAMIN C	THIAMIN (VIT. B₁)	RIBO-FLAVIN (VIT. B₂)	NIACIN	CALCIUM	IRON	VITAMIN B₆
BEEF LASAGNA	177	6.25	110	7	17	2	25	50	10	10	15	15	4	15	15
BEEF & RICE WITH TOMATO SAUCE	177	6.25	140	8	17	4	25	15	15	6	10	20	2	10	20
BEEF STEW	177	6.25	120	10	13	3	35	90	15	4	15	25	2	10	20
CHICKEN STEW	170	6	140	8	12	7	30	70	10	6	15	20	8	10	10
GREEN BEANS POTATOES & HAM CASSEROLE	177	6.25	130	7	14	5	25	15	20	10	10	15	4	10	20
SPAGHETTI & MEAT BALLS	177	6.25	130	9	19	2	30	15	20	10	20	30	4	15	20
VEGETABLES & TURKEY CASSEROLE	177	6.25	150	9	15	6	30	100	15	6	20	15	10	10	15

Legend: g = gram   oz = ounce

The source of these data is *Nutritive Value of Foods*, Home and Garden Bulletin 72, revised, U.S. Department of Agriculture, Washington, D.C. Data for some cooked and prepared foods are taken from Church and Church, *Food Values of Portions Commonly Used—Bowes and Church*, Ninth Edition, Lippincott, Philadelphia.

The abbreviation for trace (tr) is used to indicate fatty acid and vitamin values that would round to zero with the number of decimal places carried in these tables. For other components that would round to zero, a zero is used.

Dashes show that no basis could be found for imputing a value although there was some reason to believe that a measurable amount of the constituent might be present.

Other abbreviations used are:

av-average	oz-ounce
c-cup	%-percent
diam-diameter	pc-piece
hp-heaping	qt-quart
jc-juice	sc-section
lb-pound	serv-serving
lg-large	sl-slice
lv-leaves	sm-small
med-medium	sq-square
tbsp-tablespoon	

Table C.1   Nutritive Values of the Edible Part of Foods

Food	Weight, gm	Approximate Measure	Food Energy, Cal.	Pro-tein, gm	Fat (total lipid), gm
Almonds, shelled	142	1 c	850	26	77
Apple, raw	150	1 med	70	tr	tr
Apple brown betty	230	1 c	345	4	8
Apple butter	20	1 tbsp	37	tr	tr
Apple juice, bottled or canned	249	1 c	120	tr	tr
Applesauce, sweetened	254	1 c	230	1	tr
Apricots:					
raw	114	3 apricots	55	1	tr
sirup pack	259	1 c	220	2	tr
dried, uncooked	150	1 c	390	8	1
dried, cooked	285	1 c	240	5	1
Asparagus:					
fresh, cooked	175	1 c	35	4	tr
canned, green	96	6 spears	20	2	tr
Bacon:					
broiled or fried	16	2 sl	100	5	8
Canadian, cooked	21	1 sl	65	6	4
Banana, raw	150	1 med	85	1	tr
Beans:					
baked, with tomato sauce, with pork	261	1 c	320	16	7
baked, with tomato sauce, without pork	261	1 c	310	16	1
green snap, fresh cooked	125	1 c	30	2	tr
green snap, canned	239	1 c	45	2	tr
Lima, fresh, cooked	160	1 c	180	12	1
red kidney, canned	256	1 c	230	15	1
wax, canned	125	1 c	27	2	tr
Beef, cooked:					
cuts, braised, simmered, pot-roasted	72	2.5 oz, lean	140	22	5
cuts, braised, simmered, pot-roasted	85	3 oz, lean and fat	245	23	16
hamburger, ground lean	85	3 oz	185	23	10
hamburger, regular	85	3 oz	245	21	17
rib roast	51	1.8 oz, lean	125	14	7
rib roast	85	3 oz, lean and fat	375	17	34
round	78	2.7 oz, lean	125	24	3
round	85	3 oz, lean and fat	165	25	7
steak, sirloin	56	2 oz, lean	115	18	4
steak, sirloin	85	3 oz, lean and fat	330	20	27
Beef, canned:					
corned beef	85	3 oz	185	22	10
corned beef hash	85	3 oz	155	7	10

Table C.1   (Continued)

| Fatty Acids | | | | | | | | | | |
| Satur-ated (total), gm | Unsaturated | | Carbo-hydrate, gm | Cal-cium, mg | Iron, mg | Vitamin A Value, IU | Thia-min mg | Ribo-flavin, mg | Niacin, mg | Ascorbic Acid, mg |
	Oleic, gm	Lino-leic, gm								
6	52	15	28	332	6.7	0	0.34	1.31	5.0	tr
—	—	—	18	8	0.4	50	0.04	0.02	0.1	3
4	3	tr	68	41	1.4	230	0.13	0.10	0.9	3
—	—	—	9	3	0.1	0	tr	tr	tr	tr
—	—	—	30	15	1.5	—	0.01	0.04	0.2	2
—	—	—	60	10	1.3	100	0.05	0.03	0.1	3
—	—	—	14	18	0.5	2890	0.03	0.04	0.7	10
—	—	—	57	28	0.8	4510	0.05	0.06	0.9	10
—	—	—	100	100	8.2	16350	0.02	0.23	4.9	19
—	—	—	62	63	5.1	8550	0.01	0.13	2.8	8
—	—	—	6	37	1.0	1580	0.27	0.32	2.4	46
—	—	—	3	18	1.8	770	0.06	0.10	0.8	14
3	4	1	1	2	0.5	0	0.08	0.05	0.8	—
—	—	—	3	4	—	0	0.18	0.03	1.1	0
—	—	—	23	8	0.7	190	0.05	0.06	0.7	10
3	3	1	50	141	4.7	340	0.20	0.08	1.5	5
—	—	—	60	177	5.2	160	0.18	0.09	1.5	5
—	—	—	7	62	0.8	680	0.08	0.11	0.6	16
—	—	—	10	81	2.9	690	0.08	0.10	0.7	9
—	—	—	32	75	4.0	450	0.29	0.16	2.0	28
—	—	—	42	74	4.6	tr	0.13	0.10	1.5	—
—	—	—	6	45	2.1	150	0.05	0.06	0.5	6
2	2	tr	0	10	2.7	10	0.04	0.16	3.3	—
8	7	tr	0	10	2.9	30	0.04	0.18	3.5	—
5	4	tr	0	10	3.0	20	0.08	0.20	5.1	—
8	8	tr	0	9	2.7	30	0.07	0.18	4.6	—
3	3	tr	0	6	1.8	10	0.04	0.11	2.6	—
16	15	1	0	8	2.2	70	0.05	0.13	3.1	—
1	1	tr	0	10	3.0	tr	0.06	0.18	4.3	—
3	3	tr	0	11	3.2	10	0.06	0.19	4.5	—
2	2	tr	0	7	2.2	10	0.05	0.14	3.6	—
13	12	1	0	9	2.5	50	0.05	0.16	4.0	—
5	4	tr	0	17	3.7	20	0.01	0.20	2.9	—
5	4	tr	9	11	1.7	—	0.01	0.08	1.8	—

APPENDIX C

Glossary

Acid-base balance   Relationship of alkaline and acidic compounds in the body.

Acidosis   The basic building blocks of protein; contain an organic acid radical and an amino radical.

Amylase   Enzyme that breaks down starch into smaller molecules.

Amylose   The fraction of starch that is in a straight chain.

Anabolism   Synthesis of new compounds in the body.

Anemia   A condition in which the red blood cells are abnormal either in number, shape, or size. Iron deficiency anemia is characterized by a low hemoglobin count; large red blood cells (immature) may be the result of folacin or vitamin B_{12} deficiency.

Anorexia   Loss of appetite.

Antioxidant   Compound that takes up oxygen very readily. Used to protect other substances that would be affected detrimentally by the uptake of oxygen.

Apatite   Crystalline masses that form the structure of bones and teeth, and contain a variety of chemical substances such as calciuim, phosphate, fluoride, and hydroxyl ions.

Arteriosclerosis   Disease in which the walls of the arteries become hardened and thickened.

Ascorbic acid   A synonym for vitamin C.

Atherosclerosis   Type of arteriosclerosis; fatty substances such as cholesterol form mushy depsoits in the arteries and partially obstruct blood flow.

Basal metabolic rate   Rate at which energy is used in the body to maintain vital body functions; measured in a resting postabsorptive state.

Beriberi   Condition characterized by disturbances of nerve function; caused by a deficiency of thiamin.

Biotin   A water-soluble vitamin in the B complex.

Blastocyst   Embryonic cell of a mammal.

Blastogenesis   Transmission of inherited characteristics via germ plasm; trophoblastic (external) cells and internal cells are formed and separated by fluid.

Blood serum   Fluid, colorless plasma remaining when the cells, clotting factor, and fibrin have been removed from the blood.

Calciferol   Synonym for vitamin D.

calorie   Heat required to raise the temperature of a gram of water at an atmosphere of pressure a degree Celsius.

Calorie   Heat required to raise the temperature of a kilogram of water at an atmosphere of pressure a degree Celsius. This unit is synonymous with kilocalorie and is a thousand times larger than a calorie.

Carbohydrates   Organic compounds containing carbon, hydrogen, and oxygen, with the ratio of hydrogen to oxygen being two to one. Starch and sugar are examples.

Carotenes   Yellow pigments that can be converted into vitamin A in the body; sometimes called provitamin A.

Catabolism   Process of breaking down complex compounds in the body.

Catalyst   Compound capable of altering the speed of a chemical reaction without being changed during the reaction.

Cellulose   Complex carbohydrate (polysaccharide) found in plants and important as roughage in a person's diet.

Cheilosis   Lesions on the lips and cracks at corners of mouth; condition caused by riboflavin deficiency.

Cholesterol   Steroid alcohol found in some foods and also manufactured in the body; occurs in mushy deposits in arteries in cases of atherosclerosis.

Chorionic villi   Villi (small convolutions) in the outer membrane of the placenta; contain capillaries that transport the nutrients absorbed through these villi to the fetus.

Chylomicron   Miniscule globules of fat; form in which fat is transported in the blood.

Cobalamin   Synonym for vitamin B_{12}; indicates the cobalt atom found in the vitamin molecule.

Coenzyme A   Compound containing panthothenic acid; required for metabolism of fats.

Collagen   Type of connective tissue in the body.

Colostrum   Thin, somewhat yellow fluid secreted during the first few days of lactation prior to the development of mature human milk.

Congenital   Condition present at or dating from birth.

Cytochrome system   Iron-containing enzymes functioning in the release of energy in the body.

Cytoplasm   Protoplasm of cell outside the nucleus of the cell.

Deamination   Removal of the amino (nitrogen-containing) group from an amino acid.

Decalcification   Loss of calcium from bones and/or teeth.

Denaturation   Change in physical properties of protein (usually by heat).

Dermatitis   Inflammation of the skin.

Dextrins   Polysaccharides somewhat smaller than starch and often formed from starch.

Digestion   Breakdown process whereby the protein, lipid, and carbohydrate components of foods are converted into simpler substances that can be transported (absorbed) through the membranes (primarily the small intestine wall) into the body.

Diglyceride   Fat molecule containing two fatty acids.

Disaccharide   Sugars that are composed of two monosaccharides united into a single molecule by the loss of a molecule of water. Lactose is a disaccharide found in milk.

DNA   Deoxyribonucleic acid.

Eclampsia   Severe toxemia in pregnancy; convulsions are symptomatic.

Ectoderm   Outer germinal layer formed during the embryonic period; brain, nervous system, outer skin, hair, and nails develop from this layer.

Edema .   Accumulation of fluid in the tissues.

Embryo   The developing being, from implantation to the end of the second month of pregnancy (in humans).

Emulsify   To form an emulsion.

Emulsion   Colloidal dispersion of two immiscible liquids; suspension of small droplets of a liquid (such as an oil) in another liquid (such as water).

Endemic   Occurring with some constancy in a geographic region.

Endocrine gland   Any of the glands comprising the endocrine system; a gland that secretes hormones in the body.

Endoderm   Inner germinal layer formed during the embryonic period; inner linings of the digestive and respiratory tracts and the glands (including liver and pancreas) develop from this layer.

Enzymes   Proteins that catalyze reactions in the body.

Epiphysis   The bony formation that gradually replaces cartilage at the ends of bones.

Epithelium   Outer layer of skin and mucous membranes.

Essential fatty acid   Linoleic acid; fatty acid needed by the body and that must be supplied by the diet because the body cannot synthesize this specific unsaturated fatty acid.

FAD   Flavin-adenine dinucleotide.

Fatty acid   Organic acid that can combine with glycerol to form a fat.

Fetus   Developing, unborn being; fetal period for humans if from third month to birth.

Flavin-adenine dinucleotide   Coenzyme required for normal cellular respiration; contains riboflavin. Synonym is FAD.

Flavoprotein   Protein containing riboflavin; functions in release of energy in the body.

Fluorapatite   Protein containing riboflavin; functions in release of energy in the body.

Fluoridation   Process of regulating fluoride level in water at a desirable level, normally at one part fluoride per million parts of water.

Fluorosis   Condition characterized by a mottled appearance of teeth caused by a very high intake of fluoride over an extended period of time.

Folacin   Also termed folic acid; one of the water-soluble B vitamins.

Fructose   A simple sugar or monosaccharide; a specific carbohydrate.

Galactose   A simple sugar resulting from the breakdown of lactose in milk; a specific carbohydrate.

Gastric lipase   Enzyme in the stomach that initiates the digestion of emulsified fats.

Gastrulation   Formation of the three germinal layers during the embryonic period.

Gestation   Pregnancy.

Glucagon   Pancreatic hormone that releases glucose from storage in the liver.

Glucose   A simple sugar or monosaccharide; a specific carbohydrate. The type of sugar found in the blood; the most common of the monosaccharides.

Glyceride   Fatty compound formed when glycerol and fatty acids are combined.

Glycogen   Polysaccharide; form in which carbohydrate is stored in man and animals. Starch is the counterpart in plants.

Goiter   Enlargement of the thyroid gland in the throat; caused by lack of iodine.

Hemoglobin   Iron-containing protein in red blood cells.

Hemosiderosis   Condition caused by toxic levels of iron in the diet.

Hormone   Compound secreted by an endocrine gland that influences the functioning of an organ in another part of the body.

Hydrogenation   Addition of hydrogen to an unsaturated fatty acid; process raises the melting point and increases the firmness of the fatty acid.

Hydrolysis   Chemical splitting of a compound by the addition of a water molecule.

Hydroxyapatite   Structural splitting of a compound by the addition of a water molecule.

Hydroxyapatit   Structural compound of bones and teeth; can be replaced by fluorapatite, a harder compound, when fluoride is available.

Hypercalcemia   Exessive calcium in the blood.

Hypervitaminosis   Condition caused by an excessive intake of a vitamin; vitamin A and vitamin D excesses have been found to lead to this condition.

Hypothyroidism   Inadequate levels of thyroxine, resulting in a low basal metabolic rate.

INCAP   Institute of Nutrition for Central America and Panama.

Incaparina   Food formulation that, when reconstituted, makes a beverage similar to a Central American beverage called "atole." Designed to provide needed nutritional supplementation at a relatively low cost.

Intestinal lipase   Enzyme in the intestine that digests emulsified fats to fatty acids and glycerol.

Keratin   Insoluble structural protein in epidermis, hair, and nails.

Ketone bodies   Compounds (acetone, acetoacetic acid, and beta-hydroxybutyric acid) that cause ketosis when they accumulate in the body; can lead to coma and even death.

Ketosis   Condition caused by the accumulation of ketone bodies; occurs when insufficient carbohydrate derivatives are available for normal metabolism of fats in the body.

Kilocalorie   Amount of heat required to raise a kilogram of water at an atmosphere of pressure a degree Celsius; synonymous with Calorie.

Kwashiorkor   Condition in children caused by inadequate intake of protein.

Lactase   Enzyme required for digestion of lactose, the sugar in milk.

Lactation   Production of milk by the mammry glands.

Lactose   The carbohydrate in milk; also called milk sugar. Upon digestion, this sugar yields equal amounts of glucose and galactose.

Lacunae   Intervillous spaces in the placenta containing the maternal blood supply to the placenta.

Linoleic acid   Esential fatty acid; contains 18 carbons and 3 double bonds.

Lipase   Enzyme that digests fats.

Lipids   Organic compounds composed of carbon, hydrogen, and oxygen; fat or fat-like substances.

Lipoprotein   Compound containing a lipid and a protein.

Macrocytic anemia   Condition in which the red blood cells fail to mature; hence the cells remain large.

Maltase   Enzyme that digests maltose to glucose.

Maltose   Disaccharide made up of two glucose units linked together.

Marasmus   Condition caused by a severely restricted caloric (and usually protein) intake; starvation.

Megaloblastic anemia   Blood condition in which the red blood cells do not mature.

Melanin   Dark pigments in skin and hair.

Mesoderm   Middle germinal layer formed during the embryonic period; voluntary muscles, execretory system, the covering of internal organs, inner skin layer, circulatory system (including heart), and bones and cartilage develop from this layer.

Metabolism   Chemical changes involved in utilizing nutrients for the functioning of the body; general term covering both anabolism and catabolism.

Microvilli   Extremely tiny structures on the villi of the intestine that greatly increase the surface area available for absorption of nutrients.

Mitochondria   Rod-shaped organelles in cells where energy-releasing reactions take place.

Monoglyceride   Compound composed of a fatty acid attached to glycerol.

Monosaccharide   Carbohydrate in its simplest form; common examples are galactose, fructose, and glucose.

Myelin   Protective, sheath-like, coating around nerves.

NAD   Nicotinamide adenine dinucleotide.

Niacin   One of the water-soluble B vitamins.

Nicotinamide adenine dinucleotide   Coenzyme containing niacin that is needed in the release of energy; also called NAD.

Night blindness   Limited ability to adapt to changes in light intensity; occurs in a deficiency of vitamin A.

Obesity   Condition of being 20 percent or more above desirable weight.

Osmotic pressure   The force that enables a solvent to pass through a semipermeable membrane when the concentrations of solutes on both sides of the membrane are different.

Ossification   Formation of bone.

Ovum   Egg.

Pancreatic amylase   Starch-digesting enzyme formed in the pancreas and acting in the small intestine.

Pancreatic lipase   Enzyme that is produced in the pancreas, but that acts in the small intestine to digest lipids.

Pantothenic acid   A water-soluble B vitamin; component of coenzyme A.

Pectin   Carbohydrate composed of methylated galacturonic acid units.

Pellagra   Deficiency condition due to insufficient niacin.

Pernicious anemia   Condition in which nerve function and red blood cell development are modified; caused by inadequate vitamin B_{12} in the body.

Phenyketonuria   Condition caused by an inborn metabolic error that causes phenylalanine to accumulate in the blood, resulting in premanent brain damage; also called PKU.

Phenyalanine   An essential amino acid.

Phospholipid   Fat in which phosphate and a nitrogenous substance have replaced one of the fatty acids.

Pinosytosis   Process by which a cell can take up fluid by invagination and pinching off the cell membrane.

Placenta   The organ of reproduction responsible for the nourishment and excretory functions of the developing being.

Polysaccharide   Carbohydrate of very large molecular size; examples include starch, cellulose, glycogen, and pectin.

Polyunsaturated fatty acid   Fatty acid with more than one double bond; commonly of two or three double bonds.

Protease   Enzyme that digests protein.

Protein   Organic compound composed of amino acids; contains carbon, hydrogen, oxygen, and nitrogen.

Protein-calorie malnutrition   Condition caused by inadequate intake of protein and calories; also called PCM.

Ptyalin   Enzyme in the mouth that initiates digestion of starch; also called salivary amylase.

Pyridoxine   A water-soluble B vitamin.

RDA   Recommended dietary allowances; nutrient levels recommended by the Food and Nutrition Board, National Academy of Sciences — National Research Council. Revised at approximately 5-year intervals.

Renal solute load   Level of ions in the kidney.

Reticulum   Network in the placenta.

Rhodopsin   Compound formed int he rods of the retina of the eye and required for vision in dim light; also called visual purple. Vitamin A is needed for formation of rhodopsin.

Riboflavin   A water-soluble B vitamin.

Ribonucleic acid   Compound playing a prominent role in protein synthesis in the cell; also called RNA.

Ribosome   Organelle in which protein is synthesized in the cell.

Rickets   Deficiency condition in which insufficient vitamin D is available to promote adequate absorption of calcium.

Salivary amylase   Starch splitting enyzme in mouth; also called ptyalin.

Saturated fatty acid   Fatty acid containing as much hydrogen as it is capable of holding.

Scurvy   Deficiency condition caused by inadequate intake of ascorbic acid.

Starch   Carbohydrate composed of many glucose units linked together into very large molesucles.

Sterile field sterilization   Method of formula preparation in which the bottles and other equipment are sterilized separately before sterilized formula is poured into the bottles.

Terminal sterilization   Preparation of formula by sterilizing the formula already poured into the bottles.

Thiamin   A water-soluble B vitamin; occasionally called vitamin B.

Thiamin pyrophosphate   Thiamin-containing coenzyem utilized in releasing energy in the body; also called TPP.

Thyroxine   Hormone containing iodine and secreted by the thyroid gland to regulate basal metabolic rate.

Tocopherol   Compound with vitamin E activity.

Transamination   Transfer of an amino group from an amino acid to another compound to form a new, nonessential amino acid in the body.

Trophoblastic cells   Cells formed during blastogenesis and that form the external cover of the embryo.

U.S. RDA   Levels of nutrients used as the basis for nutritional labeling. Levels are established for: infants, children under 4 years of age, adults and children 4 or more years of age, and pregnant or lactating women.

Vitamin A   Fat-soluble vitamin.

Vitamin B$_6$ Water-soluble B vitamin; also called pyridoxine.

Vitamin B$_{12}$ Water-soluble vitamin; also called cobalamin.

Vitamin C   Water-soluble vitamin: also called ascorbic acid.

Vitamin D   Fat-soluble vitamin.

Vitamin E   Fat-soluble vitamin.

Xerophthalmia   Disease of the eye that can result in blindness; caused by a vitamin A deficiency.

Photo Credit List

INDEX

Fructose, 3
Fruitarian, 350
Fruit,
　baby foods, 226-227
　group, 53-54
　preparation, 262
Functional foods, 423-425
Gastric lipase, 11
Gavage feeding, 197
Geophagia, 146
Glucose solution, 197
Glycerol, 8
Glycogen, 7
Goiter, 32
Growth, 74-79
Gums, 3
HDL, 419
Head circumference, 83-84
Height, 74-79
　boys 0-3, 75
　boys 4-18, 77
　girls 0-3, 75
　girls 4-18, 77
Hemochromatosis, 30
Hemodilution, 134
Hemoglobin, 25, 29
Hemosiderosis, 30
High-density lipoprotein, 9
HIV-1, 184
Homogenization, 164
Honey, 167
Human milk, 160-162, 208
Hydrogenation, 9
Hyperbilirubinemia, 135
Hyperhomocysteinemia, 449
Hyperparathyroidism, 21
Hyperplasia, 67, 80
Hypertension, 144, 418
Hypertrophy, 80, 82
Hypervitaminosis A, 35
Hypervitaminosis D, 36
Hypothermia, 385
Hypothyroidism, 21
IgG, 72, 172
Immunoglobulin, 72

A, 172
E, 172
Inborn errors of metabolism, 20
INCAP, 17
Incomplete protein, 15-16
Incremental lines, 88
Infancy, 202-242
　beikost, 217-218
　feeding schedules, 213-215, 229-230
　menus, 228-229
　milk for, 156-200
　nutrition in, 205-211, 219-220
　prevention of obesity, 376-379
　RDA, 205-208
　serving size, 228
　supplements, 209-213
　weight concerns, 220, 233-234,
　　378-379
Inner cell mass, 65
Institute of Nutrition,
　Central America and Panama, 17
Insulin, 25
Intellectual growth, 104-108
Intestinal lipase, 11
Iodine, 26, 31-32
Iodized salt, 32
Iron, 25, 26, 29-30
　deficiency anemia, 29
Ischemia, 418
Ketone bodies, 12
Ketosis, 14
Kilocalories, 4, 20
Kreb's cycle, 7-8
Kwashiorkor, 108-109
Lactase, 6
Lactation, 148-150, 181-188
Lactiferous ducts, 182
Lactiferous sinuses, 182
Lactobacillus bifidus, 167
Lacto-ovo-vegetarian, 349-350, 352
Lactose, 3-4, 55
　intolerance, 55, 427
La Leche League, 180
Latency, 294-326
LDL, 419